SCHEUER'S
Liver Biopsy
Interpretation

Commissioning Editor: *Michael Houston*
Development Editor: *Joanne Scott*
Editorial Assistant: *Kirsten Lowson*
Project Manager: *Priya Dauntess*
Design: *Stewart Larking*
Illustration Manager: *Bruce Hogarth*
Illustrator: *Deborah Maizels*
Marketing Manager(s) (UK/USA): *Richard Jones/Radha Mawrie*

SCHEUER'S
Liver Biopsy Interpretation

EIGHTH EDITION

Jay H. Lefkowitch

Professor of Clinical Pathology
College of Physicians and Surgeons of Columbia University
New York

For additional online content visit
www.expertconsult.com

Expert | CONSULT

SAUNDERS
ELSEVIER

SAUNDERS an imprint of Elsevier Limited

© 2010, Elsevier Limited. All rights reserved.

First edition 1968
Second edition 1973
Third edition 1980
Fourth edition 1988
Fifth edition 1994
Sixth edition 2000
Seventh edition 2005
Eighth edition 2010

Notices

Knowledge and best practice in this field are constantly changing. As new research and experience broaden our understanding, changes in research methods, professional practices, or medical treatment may become necessary. Practitioners and researchers must always rely on their own experience and knowledge in evaluating and using any information, methods, compounds, or experiments described herein. In using such information or methods they should be mindful of their own safety and the safety of others, including parties for whom they have a professional responsibility.

With respect to any drug or pharmaceutical products identified, readers are advised to check the most current information provided (i) on procedures featured or (ii) by the manufacturer of each product to be administered, to verify the recommended dose or formula, the method and duration of administration, and contraindications. It is the responsibility of practitioners, relying on their own experience and knowledge of their patients, to make diagnoses, to determine dosages and the best treatment for each individual patient, and to take all appropriate safety precautions.

To the fullest extent of the law, neither the Publisher nor the authors, contributors, or editors, assume any liability for any injury and/or damage to persons or property as a matter of products liability, negligence or otherwise, or from any use or operation of any methods, products, instructions, or ideas contained in the material herein.

ISBN: 978-0-7020-3410-7

British Library Cataloguing in Publication Data
A catalogue record for this book is available from the British Library

Library of Congress Cataloging in Publication Data
A catalog record for this book is available from the Library of Congress

Printed in China
Last digit is the print number: 9 8 7 6 5 4 3 2 1

Contents

Peter J. Scheuer, MD. 1928–2006.
(Photograph by Charles Manley, Columbia University).

Preface

The present edition of this book is the first without the direct imprimature of its founding and longtime author Professor Peter J. Scheuer, who very sadly died in 2006. The younger reader may not know that *Liver Biopsy Interpretation* was the first book of its kind, a fairly slender volume written by Peter when he was Senior Lecturer in Morbid Anatomy at the Royal Free Hospital Medical School, London, and published just over 40 years ago in 1968. At the time the percutaneous needle liver biopsy technique of Menghini had been in regular use only for a decade, so Peter's concept of a book 'intended as a practical aid to liver biopsy diagnosis' (as he wrote in the Preface to the first edition) was both timely and prescient. Preparation of the subsequent editions was a source of great satisfaction to him, particularly the integration of advances in the fields of hepatology and hepatic pathology. Peter's unique ability to distill the essence of a diagnostic problem to its crystalline core, both conceptually and in writing, was a quality much in evidence in his lectures and publications. Many friends, trainees and colleagues benefited from his generously given advice and counsel, myself included. Peter's optimistic view of the world and the pursuit of academe were informed by his gentle good humour and love of music (a prodigiously talented cellist and chamber music enthusiast), the Italian language and the arts. He is greatly missed. The book's new title, *Scheuer's Liver Biopsy Interpretation*, honours Peter Scheuer and his many contributions to the way we think about pathology of the liver.

For this edition there are both new illustrations and references which address recently described entities as well as current diagnostic problems in practice including chronic hepatitis and fatty liver disease. The principle of a concise 'bench' book for use by the microscope has been kept to the fore and the reader is encouraged to take advantage of larger textbooks and Internet sources for new information. It is to be hoped that the material in this book will serve not only as a foundation for interpreting liver biopsies, but also to stimulate encorporation of the many advances in genomic and molecular diagnostics that are now available.

Jay H. Lefkowitch
2010

Acknowledgements

The preparation of this edition has been greatly helped by the many challenging questions regarding liver biopsies posed by clinicians and pathologists at my home institution and in consultation from other centres, and much gratitude is due them. My expert colleagues in the Department of Pathology and other departments at Columbia have brought their breadth of knowledge to bear on many difficult diagnostic issues, for which I am indebted. Thanks are also due to Drs Elizabeth Brunt and Milton Finegold, whose thoughtful discussions have provided insights on liver pathology in general and in their specific areas of expertise. On the home front, it has been most gratifying in recent years to work with pathology residents and Fellows who have taken up an interest in liver pathology as an avenue for their future careers. The administrative tasks involved in producing this book have been in the amiable and capable hands of Ms Casey Schadie.

Oversight of the exceptionally fine histopathology and immunohistochemistry laboratories in pathology at Columbia is provided by Sunilda Valladares-Silva and Suzy Alexander, respectively, and thanks are also due to them and their responsive and congenial staff. It has been a longtime pleasure to know and work with Jackie Lewin in Electron Microscopy at the Royal Free Hospital, London, who continues to find new ways of looking at liver ultrastructure. Paul Bates, Francis Moll and John Difford, also of the Department of Histopathology at the Royal Free, have immeasurably contributed to the genesis of this book throughout the years.

Warm thanks are owed to Michael Houston, our Commissioning Editor at Elsevier, who has provided an ideal environment for preparing this book and its previous editions. His knowledge of publishing pathology textbooks and sensitivity to the authors' needs are *non pareil*. It has likewise been a pleasure to work with Joanne Scott, our Development Editor in Elsevier's London office and with Priya Dauntess who managed book production.

Special thanks and much gratitude go to Louise Scheuer, anatomist and forensic anthropologist and wife of the late Professor Scheuer, for her unfailing support and advice through the years on matters both academic and quotidien. She and Michael Houston lent critical enthusiasm to the idea of bringing out this new edition re-named 'Scheuer's Liver Biopsy Interpretation'. Finally, it goes without saying that the influence of the giants of the 'golden age' of hepatology and hepatic pathology remains felt in very many aspects of this book, among whom Hans Popper, Dame Sheila Sherlock, Kamal Ishak and Peter Scheuer most notably should be highlighted.

General Principles of Biopsy Assessment

Introduction

Liver biopsy is one of many diagnostic tools used in the evaluation and management of patients with liver disease. It continues to play an important role because the concepts and classifications of liver disease are rooted in morphology. Moreover, looking at a liver biopsy specimen through the microscope is a very direct way of visualising the morphological changes that affect the liver in disease. The pathologist's *interpretation* (rather than mere enumeration) of these changes is used to answer important clinical questions such as disease causation and activity, and is important in therapeutic decision-making.[1] A thorough and informed interpretation of liver biopsy findings therefore stands to have substantial impact on patient care. It bears emphasising that the evidence base[2] for much of liver biopsy interpretation rests on the large body of important observations reported in the pathology literature during the past five decades, since Menghini in 1958 first introduced the technique of percutaneous needle biopsy.[3] Questions of a more basic pathobiological nature can also be addressed by applying contemporary techniques of molecular and genomic medicine to liver biopsy material.

There are many reasons for liver biopsy (**Table 1.1**), as will be apparent from the contents of this book. Establishing a tissue diagnosis of neoplastic disease, evaluation of jaundice of uncertain cause and assessment of pyrexia of unknown aetiology continue to be common diagnostic problems. Pathologists are well familiar with the need for formal grading and staging of chronic hepatitis (covered in **Ch. 9**). The ubiquitous 'elevated liver function tests' inscribed on biopsy requisitions are now very often explained by steatosis, steatohepatitis or related conditions (**Ch. 7**) stemming from the wide prevalence of obesity, diabetes, hyperlipidaemia and metabolic syndrome. Indeed, in evaluating abnormal liver function tests in patients with negative serological studies, liver biopsy is rarely normal.[4] The work-up of liver dysfunction following liver, kidney or haematopoietic cell transplantation is also reliant on information from liver biopsies, which must be reported promptly and

Table 1.1 Reasons for liver biopsy

Evaluation of abnormal liver function tests
Investigation of pyrexia of unknown aetiology
Diagnosis of neoplasms
Evaluation of ascites and portal hypertension
Grading and staging of chronic hepatitis
Documentation of steatosis and its possible complications
Evaluation of liver dysfunction after liver, kidney and bone marrow transplantation
Investigation of jaundice of unclear aetiology
Determination of the effects of therapy

©2010 Elsevier Ltd
DOI: 10.1016/B978-0-7020-3410-7.00007-1

with due consideration that the pathological changes in these patients may reflect more than one aetiological factor.

Type and adequacy of liver biopsy specimen

Several liver biopsy techniques and routes are now available for use (**Table 1.2**), each with inherent diagnostic advantages and disadvantages.[1] Liver biopsy is an invasive technique which requires a skilled operator and all possible safeguards to minimise the risk of complications. Precise guidelines vary from one centre to another.[5] Following the biopsy procedure the needle track may be plugged with gelatin sponge (**Fig. 1.1**) or other materials[6] (**Fig. 1.2**) to prevent bleeding.[7] The standard percutaneous suction needle biopsy popularised by Menghini[3] continues to be in active use, while biopsy samples obtained with thin needles under computed tomography guidance and by the transjugular route are now seen more often. Whatever method is chosen, the operator should carefully consider whether the specimen obtained is likely to be adequate for the intended purpose. For example, a small needle specimen obtained with a small-bore needle guided by ultrasound imaging may be adequate for the diagnosis of hepatocellular carcinoma, but not necessarily suitable for the diagnosis and histological evaluation of chronic hepatitis.[8] With needles of the Menghini type the biopsy core is aspirated and may fragment if the liver is cirrhotic. This is discussed further in **Chapter 10**. Cutting needles have been reported to produce better specimens,[9] but in patients with focal lesions aspiration needles often sample both the lesion itself and the adjacent liver; this is helpful in planning treatment.

Table 1.2 Liver biopsy techniques and routes
Percutaneous
Suction (e.g. Menghini, Klatskin, Jamshidi needles)
Cutting (e.g. Vim–Silverman, Tru-cut needles)
Spring-loaded
Transjugular
Thin-needle with ultrasound/CT guidance
Laparoscopic
Operative wedge
Fine-needle aspiration

Figure 1.1 Foreign material.
This is absorbable gelatin which was used to plug a needle track. A small amount of liver tissue is seen at the point of the arrow. (Needle biopsy, H&E.)

Figure 1.2 Foreign material.
Material used to plug a needle track has here escaped and produced a peritoneal foreign-body giant-cell reaction.[6] (H&E.)

Biopsy pathology differs from autopsy pathology in that there are pitfalls peculiar to small samples. A needle biopsy specimen of liver represents perhaps one fifty-thousandth of the whole organ and there is thus an obvious possibility of sampling error. Some diseases of the liver are diffuse and involve every acinus, so that sampling error is unlikely; these can be diagnosed with confidence even in small specimens. A diagnosis of acute viral hepatitis can be established in a needle specimen only a few millimetres long, whereas a specimen of similar size may not be adequate for the accurate diagnosis and evaluation of chronic liver disease, for assessment of bile duct numbers, for assessing the full extent of steatosis[10] or for the detection of focal lesions such as tumour deposits or granulomas. Focal or unevenly distributed lesions cannot be entirely excluded on the basis of their absence from an unguided needle biopsy specimen. When focal lesions are suspected, multiple biopsies may help to reduce sampling error.

Chronic hepatitis and cirrhosis present particular sampling problems. In some patients with hepatitis there is a zone of extensive necrosis immediately adjacent to the capsule, whereas the deeper parenchyma is less severely affected. A small specimen consisting of tissue from the subcapsular zone of the liver would then give a misleadingly pessimistic impression (**Fig. 1.3**). In cirrhosis the structure of a nodule is sometimes very similar to that of normal liver, so that a sample consisting almost entirely of the parenchyma from within a nodule may present serious diagnostic difficulties (**Fig. 1.4**). These are accentuated by the resistance of dense fibrous tissue; in a patient with cirrhosis an aspiration biopsy needle may glance off fibrous septa and selectively sample the softer nodular parenchyma. For this reason, some clinicians prefer to use cutting needles in patients with suspected cirrhosis.[11]

Abnormalities in a liver biopsy may represent changes remote from a pathological lesion rather than the lesion itself. In large bile-duct obstruction, for example, the results of the obstruction are clearly seen in the biopsy sample, whereas the cause of the obstruction is usually not visible. The biopsy may be taken from the vicinity of a focal liver lesion such as metastatic carcinoma, and present one or more of a range of pathological features, often puzzling to the interpreter (**Fig. 1.5**). Similarly, disease elsewhere in the body may

Figure 1.3 Subcapsular necrosis.
There is a zone of multiacinar necrosis immediately deep to the liver capsule (right) in this patient with chronic hepatitis. The changes are less severe in the deeper tissue to the left. A small superficial sample would have presented problems of interpretation. (Needle biopsy, H&E.)

Figure 1.4 Cirrhosis.
Appearances are nearly normal because the sample is from the centre of a nodule and does not include septa. A portal tract (at right, below centre) is small and poorly formed. (Needle biopsy, H&E.)

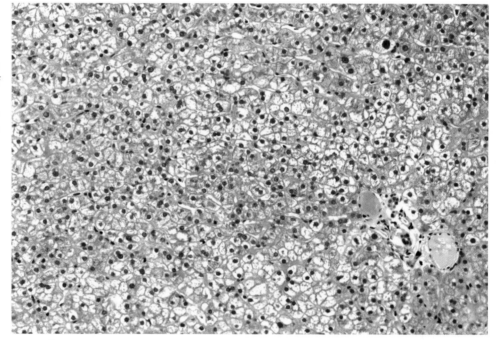

give rise to reactive changes in the liver; biopsy appearances are not normal, but at the same time do not indicate primary liver disease.

Biopsies reveal lesions or diseases rarely seen at autopsy because of their relatively benign course, such as sarcoidosis. In other conditions the evolution of a disease to an end stage means that the earlier and more characteristic pathological features are rarely seen at autopsy or even at liver transplantation. In such cases liver biopsies provide valuable insights into the pathology of the disease.

**Figure 1.5
Changes near
metastatic tumour.**
Portal changes like
those of biliary
obstruction are seen
(left, and top right),
and there is
sinusoidal dilatation
in the perivenular
area (bottom right).
(Needle biopsy,
H&E.)

Liver biopsy does not always provide a final or complete diagnosis. Sometimes it even fails to give helpful information. In most cases, however, an adequate and properly processed biopsy is an important item among the diagnostic tests to which the patient is subjected. The relatively limited range of morphological reactions of the liver to injury determines a need for full clinical, biochemical, immunological and imaging data to complement the biopsy findings. Pathologists need this information in order to avoid writing clinically unhelpful, or even misleading, reports, though they may prefer to read the slides before the clinical data to avoid bias.[12] Conversely, it is important that pathologists should produce clear and full reports on the biopsy findings for their clinical colleagues. Every report should attempt to answer one or more clinical questions, whether or not these are explicitly stated on the request form. The use of a standardised checklist has been advocated as a means of ensuring that no potentially useful information is omitted.[13] However, most pathologists currently write unstructured reports. These can be supplemented by a summary giving the essential message which the pathologist wants to convey.

The specimen at the bedside and in the laboratory

Before a liver biopsy is undertaken, the clinician may wish to discuss with the pathologist the need for any special treatment of the specimen, such as freezing part of the specimen or taking tissue for electron microscopy.[12] Accurate assessment of the often subtle changes in a liver biopsy requires sections of high quality. The pathologist is usually aware of possible artefacts in liver biopsy material, as in any histological specimen. Artefacts should obviously be avoided whenever possible, and recognised as such when they do occur. A biopsy of adequate size may be made undiagnosable by rough handling (**Fig. 1.6**), poor fixation, overheating, poor microtome technique and bad staining, all of which can obscure the criteria on which histological diagnoses are based. Poor fixation sometimes leads to potentially confusing liver-cell swelling, recognisable as artefact by its location away from the edges of the specimen (**Fig. 1.7**). False-positive staining for iron is unrelated to particular cells or structures, or is in a different focal plane from the tissue.

5

Figure 1.6 Traumatic artefact.
The triangular spaces, which slightly resemble blood vessels, are artefacts caused by rough packing of the specimen between pieces of foam sponge. (H&E.)

Figure 1.7 Fixation artefact.
Hepatocytes in the central part of the specimen are swollen and pale-staining because of poor fixation. (Needle biopsy, H&E.)

This book is mainly about changes seen in conventionally stained paraffin sections and cytological preparations. There are many other ways of looking at or investigating a tissue sample, some of them helpful in routine diagnosis. Immunohistochemistry is frequently an essential aspect of liver biopsy evaluation. Its value in individual diseases is covered in the subsequent chapters. A small cross-section of the issues that can be addressed is illustrated in **Fig. 1.8**. For example, the functional heterogeneity and 'zonation' of the

Figure 1.8 Immunohistochemistry in liver biopsy interpretation.
A: Glutamine synthetase immunostain shows positivity localised to a rim of perivenular hepatocytes, while the mid-zone and periportal regions are negative. P, portal tract.
B: A vigorous ductular reaction has developed in this case of primary sclerosing cholangitis as demonstrated with cytokeratin 7 immunostain. The native bile duct (bd) can be identified with this method.

Figure 1.8, cont'd
C: In this case of Alagille's syndrome (syndromatic paucity of intrahepatic bile ducts) an unpaired artery (a) is seen, without an accompanying bile duct. This cytokeratin 7 immunostain shows a line of hepatocyte-like 'intermediate hepatobiliary cells' on either side of the tract, quite unlike the well-developed ductular reaction seen in panel B.
D: Immunostain for CD10 demonstrates only partial display on bile canaliculi in the left-hand portion of the field, but is missing from a substantial part of the parenchyma in this case of Alagille's syndrome. Note the absence of a native bile duct in the portal tract (PT).

normal liver lobule or acinus is based upon oxygenation[14] and Wnt/β-catenin signalling,[15] and can be demonstrated using immunohistochemical stains for enzymes localised to particular acinar zones. A striking example is glutamine synthetase (GS), which is involved in ammonia metabolism and is only present in the several layers of hepatocytes surrounding efferent venules (**Fig. 1.8A**). Demonstration of the ductular reaction using antibody to cytokeratin 7 (or 19) (**Fig. 1.8B**) is important in several chronic biliary tract diseases, in fibrosing cholestatic hepatitis after liver transplantation, and in the progression of fibrosis in steatohepatitis. Conversely, defining the absence of a well-defined ductular reaction can be a key point for differentiating among several paediatric cholestatic disorders. Alagille's syndrome is such an instance[16] (**Fig. 1.8C**) and should be distinguished from the vigorous bile ductular proliferation seen in biliary atresia. Similarly, clusters of differentiation marker CD10 (neutral endopeptidase) are normally identified by immunohistochemistry on bile canaliculi, but are absent before the age of 24 months and also in Alagille's syndrome[17] (**Fig. 1.8D**). Immunostains are useful in demonstration of viral hepatitis antigens (**see Ch. 9**) and are the most accurate way of diagnosing α_1-antitrypsin deficiency morphologically. Immunohistochemistry is used extensively in the evaluation of primary and secondary tumours of the liver (**see Ch. 11**). Electron microscopy has a well-defined place in liver pathology and is dealt with in the last chapter.

In situ hybridisation has been applied to liver tissue for the identification or assessment of replication of hepatitis viruses and cytomegalovirus. The polymerase chain reaction (PCR) can be applied to liver tissue, and provides more direct evidence of virus infection in the liver than serum PCR. DNA extracted from biopsy tissue can be used in analysis of viral infections and several inherited metabolic diseases.

Part of the biopsy specimen can be analysed for copper, iron or abnormally stored substances, and enzyme activities can be assayed by micromethods. In the case of copper and iron, these measurements can if necessary be made after paraffin embedding, as discussed in **Chapter 14**. Elution of Sirius red from sections provides an accurate method for the measurement of tissue collagen,[18] and this stain is also used for image analysis of collagen.[19] *In situ* demonstration of enzymes can be achieved by immunocytochemical methods or by means of enzyme histochemistry as has been described in the functional zonation of human liver.[20,21]

Well-established techniques of morphometry and image analysis have been applied to tissue sections to obtain data on relative volumes of tissue components in normal human liver[22,23] and in disease. Three-dimensional reconstruction using a computer has helped in the understanding of disease processes and of the relationship between anatomical structures.[24–26]

References

1 Rockey DC, Caldwell SH, Goodman ZD, et al. Liver biopsy. *Hepatology* 2009; **49**: 1017–1044.

2 Crawford JM. Evidence-based interpretation of liver biopsies. *Lab Invest* 2006; **86**: 326–334.

3 Menghini G. One-second needle biopsy of the liver. *Gastroenterology* 1958; **35**: 190–199.

4 Skelly MM, James PD, Ryder SD. Findings on liver biopsy to investigate abnormal liver function tests in the absence of diagnostic serology. *J Hepatol* 2001; **35**: 195–199.

5 Sue M, Caldwell SH, Dickson RC, et al. Variation between centers in technique and guidelines for liver biopsy. *Liver* 1996; **16**: 267–270.

6 Thompson NP, Scheuer PJ, Dick R, et al. Intraperitoneal Ivalon mimicking peritoneal malignancy after plugged percutaneous liver biopsy. *Gut* 1993; **34**: 16–35.

7 Sawyer AM, McCormick PA, Tennyson GS, et al. A comparison of transjugular and plugged-percutaneous liver biopsy in patients with impaired coagulation. *J Hepatol* 1993; **17**: 81–85.

8 Petz D, Klauck S, Röhl FW, et al. Feasibility of histological grading and staging of chronic viral hepatitis using specimens obtained by thin-needle biopsy. *Virchows Arch* 2003; **442**: 238–244.

9 Sada PN, Ramakrishna B, Thomas CP, et al. Transjugular liver biopsy: a comparison of aspiration and Trucut techniques. *Liver* 1997; **17**: 257–259.

10   Ratziu V, Charlotte F, Heurtier A, et al. Sampling variability of liver biopsy in nonalcoholic fatty liver disease. *Gastroenterology* 2005; **128**: 1898–1906.

11   Gerber MA, Thung SN, Bodenheimer HC Jr., et al. Characteristic histologic triad in liver adjacent to metastatic neoplasm. *Liver* 1986; **6**: 85–88.

12   Desmet VJ. What more can we ask from the pathologist? *J Hepatol* 1996; **25** (Suppl 1): 25–29.

13   Foschini M, Sarti F, Dina RE, et al. Standardized reporting of histological diagnoses for non-neoplastic liver conditions in needle biopsies. *Virchows Arch* 1995; **426**: 593–596.

14   Jungermann K, Kietzmann T. Oxygen: modulator of metabolic zonation and disease of the liver. *Hepatology* 2000; **31**: 255–260.

15   Burke ZD, Reed KR, Phesse TJ, et al. Liver zonation occurs through a β-catenin-dependent, c-Myc-independent mechanism. *Gastroenterology* 2009; **136**: 2316–2324.

16   Fabris L, Cadamuro M, Guido M, et al. Analysis of liver repair mechanisms in Alagille syndrome and biliary atresia reveals a role for Notch signaling. *Am J Pathol* 2007; **171**: 641–653.

17   Byrne JA, Meara NJ, Rayner AC, et al. Lack of hepatocellular CD10 along bile canaliculi is physiologic in early childhood and persistent in Alagille syndrome. *Lab Invest* 2007; **87**: 1138–1148.

18   Jimenez W, Pares A, Caballeria J, et al. Measurement of fibrosis in needle liver biopsies: evaluation of a colorimetric method. *Hepatology* 1985; **5**: 815–818.

19   Pape L, Olsson K, Petersen C, von Wasilewski R, Melter M. Prognostic value of computerized quantification of liver fibrosis in children with biliary atresia. *Liver Transplant* 2009; **15**: 876–882.

20   Lamers WH, Hilberts A, Furt E, et al. Hepatic enzymic zonation: a reevaluation of the concept of the liver acinus. *Hepatology* 1989; **10**: 72–76.

21   Sokal EM, Trivedi P, Cheeseman P, et al. The application of quantitative cytochemistry to study the acinar distribution of enzymatic activities in human liver biopsy sections. *J Hepatol* 1989; **9**: 42–48.

22   Ranek L, Keiding N, Jensen ST. A morphometric study of normal human liver cell nuclei. *Acta Pathol Microbiol Scand A* 1978; **83**: 467–476.

23   Rohr HP, Luthy J, Gudat F, et al. Stereology: a new supplement to the study of human liver biopsy specimens. In: Progress in Liver Diseases, **Vol. V**, 1st edn. Popper H, Schaffner F, eds. New York, NY: Grune & Stratton, 1976: 24.

24   Yamada S, Howe S, Scheuer PJ. Three-dimensional reconstruction of biliary pathways in primary biliary cirrhosis: a computer-assisted study. *J Pathol* 1987; **152**: 317–323.

25   Nagore N, Howe S, Boxer L, et al. Liver cell rosettes: structural differences in cholestasis and hepatitis. *Liver* 1989; **9**: 43–51.

26   Ludwig J, Ritman EL, LaRusso NF, et al. Anatomy of the human biliary system studied by quantitative computer-aided three-dimensional imaging techniques. *Hepatology* 1998; **27**: 893–899.

Laboratory Techniques 2

Processing of the specimen

As soon as a needle biopsy specimen is obtained from the patient it should be expelled gently into fixative or onto a piece of glass, card or wood. Filter paper is less suitable because fibres tend to adhere to the tissue and may interfere with sectioning. The specimen must be treated with great care and excessive manipulation should be rigorously avoided; distortion of the specimen by rough handling at this stage may seriously interfere with accurate diagnosis, because diagnosis often depends on subtle criteria. At this stage, minute pieces can be put into an appropriate fixative for electron microscopy (**Ch. 17**), preferably by an operator experienced in this technique, and samples taken for chemical analysis or freezing. Frozen sections may be needed for demonstration of lipids. If porphyria is suspected, a very small amount of the unfixed tissue can be examined under ultraviolet light or with a suitable quartz halogen source, either whole or smeared onto a glass slide.

Tissue for paraffin embedding should be transferred to a fixative as soon as possible. When transit to the laboratory is likely to involve much movement, it is helpful to fill the container to the brim with fixative. Buffered formalin and formol saline are both suitable for routine fixation, which is accomplished after 3 h at room temperature or less at higher temperatures (**Table 2.1**). Operative wedge biopsies and larger specimens need longer fixation. Fixatives other than formalin are successfully used in some centres; handbooks of laboratory technique should be consulted for optimum times and conditions for each fixative.

Minute fragments can be hand-processed more quickly than larger pieces and this also avoids undue shrinkage and hardening. Automated vacuum embedding allows the time of processing of needle specimens to be drastically reduced, as shown in **Table 2.1**; the ultra-rapid method by which a good section can be produced in about 2 h has become important because of the need for rapid decisions on treatment in patients who have undergone liver transplantation. Frozen sections, occasionally needed for a decision at surgery, can be cut by a standard method using a cryostat. They are sometimes adequate for diagnosis of obvious lesions such as neoplasms, but are unsuitable for recognition of subtle changes, and can even be dangerously misleading.

The exact number of sections routinely cut from a block varies widely from one laboratory to another. In Scheuer's former laboratory at the Royal Free Hospital in London, ten or more consecutive sections 3–5 μm thick are cut from each block and alternate sections used for the staining procedures outlined in the next paragraphs. The remaining sections are stored. Step sections are used when discrete lesions such as granulomas or tumour

©2010 Elsevier Ltd
DOI: 10.1016/B978-0-7020-3410-7.00008-3

Table 2.1 Sample tissue schedules for liver biopsies

Agent	Manual overnight automatic (vacuum)[a]	Routine overnight automatic	Routine automatic (vacuum)[a]	Ultra-rapid
Buffered formalin	3 h	3 h	2 h	30 min
Formalin–ethanol–water (1:8:1)	Overnight	–	–	–
70% ethanol	–	3 h	1 h	3 min
90% ethanol	–	3 h	1 h	2 min
100% ethanol	2 × 1 h	2 × 2 h	3 × 1 h	3 × 2 min
Xylene	3 × 1 h	3 × 1 h	4 × 1 h	4 × 5 min
Wax (60°C)	2 × 1 h	2 × 1 h	3 × 1 h	3 × 5 min
Total time	24 h	18 h	14 h	1 h 16 min

[a]All at 50°C except for wax step.

deposits are suspected or for identification of bile ducts when duct paucity is suspected. Serial or near-serial sections are helpful when utilising multiple immunohistochemical stains.

Choice of stains

The stains routinely applied to liver biopsies vary according to local custom. The minimum advised is haematoxylin and eosin (H&E) and a reliable method for connective tissue. The author prefers a silver preparation for reticulin as the principal method for showing connective tissue for reasons discussed below, but trichrome stains also have important applications and can reveal changes not easily seen in a reticulin, such as the pericellular fibrosis of steatohepatitis. Routine staining for iron enables the biopsy to be used to screen for iron storage disease and the periodic acid–Schiff stain after diastase digestion (DPAS or PASD) provides a relatively crude, but practicable screening procedure for α_1-antitrypsin deficiency as well as showing activated macrophages and bile-duct basement membranes. Stains for copper-associated protein, elastic fibres and hepatitis B surface antigen are useful and arguably essential additions to the routine list. Some pathologists like to see two H&E-stained sections, one from the beginning and the other from the end of a series of consecutive sections. Other methods are used as required for particular purposes. The extent to which 'special' stains form part of the routine set must be decided by each pathologist.

A **reticulin** preparation is important for accurate assessment of structural changes. Without it, thin layers of connective tissue and hence cirrhosis may be missed, as may foci of well-differentiated hepatocellular carcinoma in which the reticulin structure is often highly abnormal (**see Fig. 11.12**). Counterstaining is sometimes used, but is apt to distract rather than help, bearing in mind that the chief function of the reticulin preparation is to provide a sensitive low-power indicator of structural changes.

Stains for **collagen** such as chromotrope–aniline blue (CAB) are important for the detection of new collagen formation, especially in alcoholic steatohepatitis and its imitators (**see Ch. 7**). Collagen staining is therefore advised for any biopsy showing substantial steatosis. It also helps to show blocked veins within scars; these are easily missed on H&E staining. It is therefore wise to use a trichrome stain when vascular disease is suspected.

A stain for **elastic fibres** such as the orcein stain, Victoria blue or elastic–Van Gieson is also useful to identify blocked vessels. The stains often enable the pathologist to distinguish between recent collapse and old fibrosis, since only the latter is positive (**see Ch. 6**). Again, this distinction may be very difficult to make on H&E and even with the help of stains for collagen and reticulin. The orcein and Victoria blue also show copper-associated protein and hepatitis B surface material.

Staining for **iron** by Perls' or other similar method enables not only iron but also bile, lipofuscin and other pigments to be evaluated, as discussed in **Chapter 3**. Counterstaining should be light to avoid obscuring small amounts of pigment.

Staining of **glycogen** by means of the PAS method or Best's carmine demonstrates the extent of any liver-cell loss, and shows focal areas devoid of hepatocytes such as granulomas. **Glycoproteins** may be demonstrated by the PAS method after digestion with diastase to remove glycogen. This stain serves to accentuate hypertrophied macrophages, such as Kupffer cells filled with ceroid pigment after an acute hepatitis or episode of cholestasis. Alpha$_1$-antitrypsin bodies stain strongly, but the stain is not sufficiently sensitive to enable all examples of α_1-antitrypsin deficiency to be detected.

Staining for **copper** is mainly used in suspected Wilson's disease, although, as explained in **Chapter 14**, it is not always helpful and may even be negative. The rhodanine method is preferred because it is easy to distinguish the orange-red colour of copper from bile, a distinction which is occasionally difficult with rubeanic acid. In Wilson's disease, there is variable correlation between the presence of stainable copper and staining for **copper-associated protein**. In chronic cholestasis, however, the two usually correspond.

Other non-immunological methods useful on occasion include the Ziehl–Neelsen stain for mycobacteria and for the ova of *Schistosoma mansoni*. Specific staining for bilirubin is rarely necessary, but conjugated bilirubin stains a bright green colour by the Van Gieson method (**Fig. 4.3**). **Amyloid** is stained by the usual techniques.

For **immunohistochemical staining**, standard techniques are applied. Among antibodies that are helpful in everyday practice are those against components of the hepatitis B virus, the delta agent, cytomegalovirus and α_1-antitrypsin. Neoplasms of doubtful histogenesis or differentiation are investigated by appropriate panels of antibodies, as in any other organ. In hepatocellular carcinoma, bile canaliculi between tumour cells may stain with a polyclonal anti-CEA (carcinoembryonic antigen) antibody, cross-reacting with a canalicular antigen. Assessment of bile-duct loss may require staining of cytokeratins 7 and 19, characteristic of bile-duct rather than liver-cell cytoplasm and of the ductular reaction (**see Ch. 4**). The application of immunohistochemistry as well as of other modern techniques is discussed in more detail in **Chapter 17**.

Most of the staining methods mentioned above are used routinely in many laboratories, and can be found in the books listed under General reading at the end of this chapter. A selection of methods is given below (see **Box 2.1**).

Box 2.1 Staining methods

Silver impregnation for reticulin fibres (Gordon & Sweets)

1. Bring section to distilled water.
2. Treat with acidified potassium permanganate for 10 min; wash in distilled water.
3. Leave section in 1% oxalic acid until pale (about 1 min). Wash well in several changes of distilled water.
4. Mordant in 2.5% iron alum for 10 min. Wash in several changes of distilled water.
5. Treat with silver solution until section is transparent (about 10–15 s). Wash in several changes of distilled water.

Box 2.1 Staining methods continued

6. Reduce in 10% formalin (4% aqueous solution of formaldehyde) for 30 s. Wash in tap water followed by distilled water.
7. Tone if desired in 0.2% gold chloride for 1 min. Rinse in distilled water.
8. Fix in 2.5% sodium thiosulphate for 5 min. Wash several times in tap water.
9. Transfer section to ethanol, clear and mount.

   Reticulin appears black. The colour of the collagen varies according to whether step 7 is used; in untoned preparations it is yellow-brown.

Silver solution

To 5 ml of 10% aqueous silver nitrate, add strong ammonia (sp. gr. 0.88) drop by drop until the precipitate which forms is just dissolved. Add 5 ml of 3% sodium hydroxide. Add strong ammonia drop by drop until the resulting precipitate dissolves. The solution does not clear completely. Make up to 50 ml with distilled water. Scrupulously clean glassware should be used throughout.

Acidified potassium permanganate

To 95 ml of 0.5% potassium permanganate, add 5 ml of 3% sulphuric acid.

Chromotrope–aniline blue (CAB) method for collagen and Mallory bodies

(As used at Mount Sinai Hospital, New York; modified from Roque[1] and Churg & Prado[2])

1. Bring section to water.
2. Stain nuclei by the celestine blue–Lillie Mayer sequence or other method. Rinse in distilled water.
3. Immerse in 1% phosphomolybdic acid for 1–3 min. Rinse well in distilled water.
4. Stain with CAB solution for 8 min. Rinse well in distilled water. Blot.
5. Dehydrate quickly, clear and mount.

   Collagen is stained blue. Mallory bodies stain blue or sometimes red. Giant mitochondria stain red.

CAB solution

1.5 g aniline blue is dissolved in 2.5 ml HCl and 200 ml distilled water with gentle heat; 6 g chromotrope 2R is added. The pH should be 1.0.

Orcein stain for copper-associated protein, elastic fibres and hepatitis B surface material[3]

1. Bring section to water.
2. Treat with acidified potassium permanganate for 15 min.
3. Rinse in water and de-colorise in 2% oxalic acid.
4. Rinse in distilled water, then wash in tap water for 3 min.
5. Stain in commercial orcein solution for 30–60 min, at room temperature.
6. Rinse in water, then differentiate if necessary in 1% HCl in 70% ethanol.
7. Dehydrate, clear and mount.

   Elastic fibres, copper-associated protein and hepatitis B surface material (HBsAg) stain brown. The method is less sensitive for HBsAg than immunohistochemical techniques. However, of the components listed, copper-associated protein is often the most difficult to stain reliably. Natural orceins seem to be more satisfactory than synthetic ones, but are difficult or impossible to obtain. In case of difficulty, doubling the concentration of orcein and the amount of HCl may help (Hans Popper, personal communication).

Box 2.1 Staining methods continued

Acidified potassium permanganate

To 95 ml of 0.5% potassium permanganate, add 5 ml of 3% sulphuric acid.

Rhodanine stain for copper[4]

1. Bring section to distilled water.
2. Incubate in rhodanine working solution for 18 h at 37°C or 3 h at 56°C.
3. Rinse in several changes of distilled water and stain with Carazzi's haematoxylin for 1 min.
4. Rinse with distilled water and then quickly in borax solution. Rinse well in distilled water.
5. Dehydrate, clear and mount.

Copper deposits stain bright red. Bile stains green. Weakly positive stains tend to fade, but fading can be reduced by staining at the higher temperature and by using certain mounting media (e.g. Ralmount (Raymond A. Lamb), DPX or Diatex). Note the two alternative times and temperatures for the rhodanine working solutions. The staining time can be shortened further.[5]

Rhodanine stock solution

p-Dimethylaminobenzylidene rhodanine	0.2 g
Ethanol	100 ml

The working solution is prepared by diluting 3 ml of the well-shaken stock solution with 47 ml distilled water.

Borax solution

Disodium tetraborate	0.5 g
Distilled water	100 ml

Victoria blue method for copper-associated protein, elastic fibres and hepatitis B surface material[6]

1. Bring section to distilled water.
2. Treat with acidified potassium permanganate (see Gordon & Sweets' reticulin, above) for 5 min.
3. Treat with 4% aqueous sodium metabisulphite for 1 min.
4. Wash in running tap water.
5. Wash well with 70% ethanol.
6. Stain in Victoria blue solution in a Coplin jar for a minimum of 4 h, and preferably overnight.
7. Wash well with 70% ethanol. This is the differentiation step; ensure that the background of the section is clear.
8. Wash in running tap water for 1 min.
9. Stain with nuclear fast red solution for 5 min.
10. Wash in running water for 2 min.
11. Dehydrate, clear and mount.

Copper-associated protein, elastic fibres and hepatitis B surface material are stained blue on a pink background.

Victoria blue solution

Distilled water	200 ml
Dextrine	0.5 g
Victoria blue	2 g
Resorcinol	4 g

Box 2.1 Staining methods continued

Slowly warm the mixture of the above until it boils. Gradually add 25 ml of boiling 29% ferric chloride solution and boil for a further 3 min. Cool and filter through fine paper. Dry the filtrate on the filter paper to complete dryness in a 56°C oven. Dissolve the filtrate in 400 ml 70% ethanol. Finally add 4 ml concentrated HCl and 6 g phenol. The solution is best left for 2 weeks before use.

Nuclear fast red

Dissolve 0.1 g nuclear fast red in 100 ml warmed 5% aluminium sulphate. Filter when cool.

References

1 Roque AL. Chromotrope aniline blue method of staining Mallory bodies of Laennec's cirrhosis. *Lab Invest* 1953; **2:** 15–21.

2 Churg J, Prado A. A rapid Mallory trichrome stain (Chromotrope–aniline blue). *Arch Pathol* 1956; **62:** 505–506.

3 Shikata T, Uzawa T, Yoshiwara N, et al. Staining methods of Australia antigen in paraffin section – detection of cytoplasmic inclusion bodies. *Jpn J Exp Med* 1974; **44:** 25–36.

4 Lindquist RR. Studies on the pathogenesis of hepatolenticular degeneration. II. Cytochemical methods for the localization of copper. *Arch Pathol* 1969; **87:** 370–379.

5 Emanuele P, Goodman ZD. A simple and rapid stain for copper in liver tissue. *Ann Diagn Pathol* 1998; **2:** 125–126.

6 Tanaka K, Mori W, Suwa K. Victoria blue-nuclear fast red stain for HBs antigen detection in paraffin section. *Acta Pathol Jpn* 1981; **31:** 93–98.

General reading

Bancroft JD, Gamble M, eds. Theory and Practice of Histological Techniques, 5th edn. London: Churchill Livingstone, 2002.

Kiernan JA. Histological and Histochemical Methods: Theory and Practice, 3rd edn. Oxford: Butterworth-Heinemann, 1999.

Lefkowitch JH. Special stains in diagnostic liver pathology. *Semin Diagn Pathol* 2006; **23:** 190–198.

Polak JM, van Noorden S. Introduction to Immunocytochemistry, 2nd edn. Microscopy Handbooks 37. Oxford: Bios Scientific Publishers, 1997.

Prophet EB, Mills B, Arrington JB, Sobin LH, eds. Laboratory Methods in Histotechnology. Washington, DC: American Registry of Pathology, 1992.

The Normal Liver

Structures and components

Functional units and nomenclature

Under the low power of the light microscope, normal liver is seen to have a regular structure based on portal tracts and efferent veins. The smallest portal tracts contain portal venules, hepatic arterioles and small interlobular bile ducts. Blood from both venules and arterioles passes through the sinusoidal system to reach efferent hepatic venules. From these, the blood drains into successively larger veins to reach the inferior vena cava. Bile flows from the smallest ducts into larger ducts, to reach the small intestine by way of the common bile duct.

The functional relationship between these various structures has been the subject of much debate. The most widely used models are the classic lobule and Rappaport's acinus.[1] The lobule has an efferent venule at its centre and portal tracts at its periphery (**Fig. 3.1**). The acinus is based on a terminal portal tract, with blood passing from this, through successively less well-oxygenated parenchymal zones 1, 2 and 3, to efferent venules. It is worth emphasising that both lobules and acini are concepts rather than fixed anatomical structures. Several other models have been proposed, as well as modifications to the original lobular model.[2-4] From a pathologist's point of view, both lobular and acinar concepts have their merits in different situations. To give examples, the sinusoidal congestion of venous outflow obstruction is often more easily understood on the basis of the lobule, with maximum intensity at its centre. Bridging hepatic necrosis, however, is difficult to understand in terms of the lobule and has been explained as death of hepatocytes in acinar zones 3, the zones in which oxygen saturation is relatively low. In everyday practice it seems best to use words compatible with either model as far as possible. In this book we have therefore used the term 'periportal' to describe the part of the parenchyma lying nearest to a small portal tract, and 'perivenular' for the parenchyma near an efferent venule.

Portal tracts

Portal tracts of different size may be seen in biopsies (**see Fig. 4.1**). The smallest represent terminal tracts from which blood enters the parenchyma. Larger portal tracts contain vessels and ducts which convey blood and bile to and from the smaller tracts. Pathological processes do not necessarily affect large and small tracts to the same extent.

©2010 Elsevier Ltd
DOI: 10.1016/B978-0-7020-3410-7.00009-5

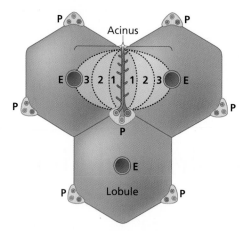

Figure 3.1 Diagrammatic representation of a simple acinus.
It is divided into zones 1, 2 and 3, with three adjacent lobules for comparison. Portal tracts (P) contain bile ducts, arterioles and venules. E, efferent vein (central vein or terminal hepatic venule).

Figure 3.2 Normal adult liver.

A small portal tract contains a portal venule (V), arteriole (A) and interlobular bile duct (B). (Needle biopsy, H&E.)

A typical small portal tract contains a bile duct, portal venule, hepatic arteriole and lymphatics, all embedded in connective tissue (**Fig. 3.2**). A few lymphocytes and mast cells may be seen even in normal subjects and nerve fibres can be demonstrated by appropriate staining. The exact contents are variable, however, depending in part on the angle of sectioning. In a study of 16 needle biopsies from normal subjects,[5] 38%, 9% and 7% of tracts did not contain a portal-vein branch, hepatic arteriole or bile duct, respectively. Most, but by no means all, hepatic artery branches are accompanied by bile ducts. These observations have obvious implications for the histological diagnosis of bile duct or blood vessel loss. A confident diagnosis requires examination of several portal tracts.

Figure 3.3 Bile ductules and canals of Hering. These are unusually prominent in this cirrhotic liver. A liver-cell plate is seen in continuity with a ductular structure (arrow). (Needle biopsy, H&E.)

Bile ducts

Near or at the margins of the small portal tracts, the bile canaliculi, formed as spaces between adjacent hepatocytes, communicate with the canals of Hering.[6–8] These are lined partly by hepatocytes and partly by biliary epithelial cells. From the canals of Hering, bile drains into bile ductules lined entirely by biliary epithelium (**see Fig. 5.1**). Neither canals of Hering nor ductules are easily seen in normal liver, but they may become apparent in disease (**Fig. 3.3**). The exact location of the junction between the canals of Hering and bile ductules varies, the ductules sometimes having an intraparenchymal portion, seen in two-dimensional sections as apparently isolated ductules among hepatocytes. The canals of Hering and bile ductules have received much attention in recent years, because they appear to be the site of a progenitor-cell compartment which becomes activated when a need for new hepatocytes and bile ducts cannot be adequately met otherwise.[8–10] Progenitor cells can be immunostained for cytokeratins CK7 and CK19, EpCAM (epithelial cell adhesion molecule) and NCAM (neural cell adhesion molecule)[11] and also stain with OV-6, an antibody used on frozen tissue to mark similar cells ('oval cells') in rodents.[11,12] The response to various types of liver injury may also involve participation of hepatoblasts derived from progenitor cells.[12]

The interlobular ducts into which the ductules drain have an internal diameter of less than 100 μm and are more or less centrally located in the small portal tracts. They are lined by cuboidal or low columnar epithelium and have a basement membrane associated with diastase periodic acid–Schiff (DPAS)-positive material. Portal venules and hepatic arterioles usually lie close to these ducts but, as already noted, not all three structures are necessarily seen in a single plane of section. Positive identification of bile ducts in pathological states can be difficult, but is made easier by cytokeratin staining; ducts contain CK7 and CK19 in addition to CK8 and CK18; the latter two are also found in hepatocytes.[13]

Bile drains from the interlobular ducts into septal bile ducts having an internal diameter of more than 100 μm. Septal ducts are lined by tall columnar epithelium, with basally located nuclei. These and larger ducts towards the hepatic hilum are sometimes associated with heterotopic exocrine pancreatic tissue.[14] Around the largest intrahepatic ducts there are peribiliary glands.[14]

Hepatic sinusoids, space of Disse and extracellular matrix

Hepatic sinusoids

The hepatic sinusoids are lined by specialised endothelial cells, which form an incomplete, porous barrier allowing easy exchange of materials between blood and hepatocytes. The endothelial cells are positive for cluster differentiation markers CD4, CD13, CD14, CD16, Cdw32, CD36 and CD54 and thus have a different phenotype from capillary endothelium, portal venules and terminal hepatic venules; these stain for CD31 and CD34 and bind *Ulex europaeus* lectin.

Within the sinusoidal lumen lie the Kupffer cells, specialised hepatic macrophages which are demonstrable with immunostain for CD68. These have irregular processes, which may straddle the sinusoidal lumen. They are more numerous near portal tracts. Activated Kupffer cells, unlike endothelial cells, are DPAS and muramidase positive. Phenotypically distinct lymphocytes are found both within the sinusoidal lumens and in the portal tracts.[15] Lymphocytes in the lumens include pit cells having natural killer (NK) activity.[16]

Space of Disse

The space of Disse, lying between the sinusoidal endothelium and the hepatocytes, is not conspicuous in paraffin-embedded biopsies, but may be artefactually prominent in autopsy material. It contains components of the extracellular matrix, nerves[17,18] and hepatic stellate cells.

Hepatic stellate cells are members of the myofibroblast family. There is international agreement that the term 'stellate cell' should be used rather than one of many synonyms in the literature[19] (see Glossary). Stellate cells are involved in fibrogenesis and in the control of sinusoidal blood flow.[20,21] They may also act as antigen-presenting cells. In childhood and adolescence, stellate cells are positive for alpha smooth muscle actin, but thereafter become negative until activated under pathological conditions.[22] Both resting and activated stellate cells are positive for synaptophysin,[23] for vinculin after microwave pretreatment of paraffin sections[24] and for cellular retinol-binding protein-1 (CRBP-1).[25] Difficult to identify in normal liver in routine sections, stellate cells can be recognised in pathological conditions by their vacuolated cytoplasm and consequently scalloped nucleus (**see Fig. 7.6**). It is likely that the hepatic stellate cell is not the only cell type in the liver concerned with collagen synthesis.[26,27]

The extracellular matrix comprises many different components. Collagen types I and III predominate. Types IV, V, VI, VIII, XIV, XVIII and XIX are also present, together with proteoglycans and glycoproteins such as fibronectin and laminin.[28] Type III collagen is the main component of reticulin fibres in the space of Disse (**Fig. 3.4**), while type I is abundant in portal tracts and in the walls of efferent veins. Elastic fibres, abundant in portal tracts, are not demonstrable in sinusoidal walls in normal liver.[29]

Hepatocytes

The hepatocytes are arranged in plates separated by the sinusoidal labyrinth (**Fig. 3.5**). The layer of hepatocytes next to a small portal tract is known as the limiting plate. In adults the hepatocyte plates are one cell thick, but in any one section a few plates will appear thicker because of tangential cutting. Widespread formation of twin-cell plates indicates hyperplasia, recent or current.

Figure 3.4 Normal adult liver.
There is a regular reticulin network between the portal tract (below right) and the efferent hepatic venule to the left. (Needle biopsy, reticulin.)

Figure 3.5 Normal adult liver.
Hepatocyte plates, for the most part one cell thick, radiate out from the terminal venule in the centre. (Wedge biopsy, H&E.)

Hepatocytes are polygonal cells with well-defined cell borders. Each cell contains one or more nuclei. Most cells contain one nucleus; a few contain two in normal subjects. Nucleoli are often visible, mitotic figures rare. Most of the nuclei are diploid,[30] but smaller numbers of tetraploid and even larger nuclei are found, especially in older subjects.[31] Polyploidy and variation in nuclear size are therefore normal characteristics of adult human liver. A few periportal nuclei may appear vacuolated because of glycogen accumulation, especially in children and adolescents.

Hepatocyte cytoplasm is normally rich in glycogen. In sections stained with haematoxylin and eosin (H&E) the cytoplasm appears granular and often pale-staining centrally, where glycogen and endoplasmic reticulum predominate. A few fat vacuoles and occasional apoptosis may be seen in the absence of obvious disease. Many different proteins can be demonstrated in or on the hepatocytes, in keeping with the liver's many metabolic functions. These include secreted proteins such as albumin and cell surface proteins such as adhesion molecules.[32] Structural proteins include cytokeratins 8 and 18. Staining with the antibody Hep Par 1 is positive,[33] but this is not exclusive to hepatocytes.

Between the hepatocytes, their walls formed by two or three cells, are the bile canaliculi, already mentioned. They are usually too small to be readily seen by light microscopy in routine paraffin sections, but are occasionally visible as minute spaces at the biliary poles of the hepatocytes. Bile is rarely seen in normal subjects. The canalicular network can be demonstrated using a polyclonal antibody to carcinoembryonic antigen (CEA), which reacts with the canalicular antigen biliary glycoprotein (**see Fig. 11.15**). Another option is antibody to CD10 (neutral endopeptidase), which is expressed on the surface microvilli of bile canaliculi (**see Fig. 1.8**) and on the apices of cholangiocytes.[34] It should be noted that physiological expression of CD10 on canaliculi develops only after 24 months of age[34] and, consequently, immunostain results will be negative in younger children and neonates.

Hepatocellular pigments (Table 3.1)

Within the hepatocytes, aggregated near the bile canaliculi and most abundant in perivenular areas, there are fine yellow-brown granules of lipofuscin pigment (**Fig. 3.6**). Lipofuscin is a normal constituent of adult liver, increasing in amount with age but also

Table 3.1 Identification of hepatocellular pigments

	Haemosiderin	Lipofuscin	Dubin–Johnson pigment	Bile	Copper-associated protein
Distribution	Periportal	Perivenular	Perivenular, often also in Kupffer cells	Often perivenular; also in canaliculi and Kupffer cells	Periportal in chronic cholestasis
Intracellular site	Pericanalicular	Pericanalicular	Pericanalicular	Pericanalicular or diffuse	Variable
Granule size (approximate)	1 μm	1 μm often	>1 μm	Variable	≤1 μm
Colour	Golden brown, refractile	Yellow-brown	Dark brown	Yellow, brown or green	Grey
Perls' stain for iron	+	–	–	–	–
Diastase–PAS stain	–	Variable	Variable	Variable	Often +
Long Ziehl–Neelsen stain	–	+	Often +	–	–
Orcein, Victoria blue stain	–	–	–	–	+

**Figure 3.6
Lipofuscin
pigment.**
In this normal liver
from an adult there
are prominent
brown lipofuscin
granules at the
biliary poles of the
hepatocytes. (Wedge
biopsy, H&E.)

sometimes found in children. The granules represent lysosomes containing materials which cannot be further degraded. The amount of the pigment varies greatly in normal liver, making assessment of an increase or decrease in disease subject to error in the absence of well-controlled morphometric data. Lipofuscin also varies in its staining properties according to its constituents and age. It is acid-fast, has reducing properties and stains variably with DPAS. Perls' stain for iron is negative.

Large amounts of lipofuscin are difficult to distinguish from Dubin–Johnson pigment by light microscopy alone, but the latter is usually coarser and darker (**see Fig. 13.19**). Intracellular bile can be distinguished from lipofuscin by its bright green staining with Van Gieson's method (**see Fig. 4.3**) and by the almost invariable presence of bile thrombi in canaliculi. An exception to this is liver following transplantation, in which diffuse intracellular bile is common in the absence of bile thrombi.

Normal liver is negative for stainable iron. All but very small amounts should be further investigated by appropriate biochemical and genetic methods. This is because it is important to identify patients with the common and treatable condition of hereditary haemochromatosis (**Ch. 14**).

Copper-associated protein is seen in high copper states as grey-brown or red intra-cytoplasmic granules (**see Fig. 15.27**), usually in a periportal location. It can be stained with orcein, Victoria blue and DPAS.

Normal appearances in childhood

Haematopoiesis is active during the fetal period (**Fig. 3.7**) and continues until a few weeks after birth. Haemopoietic cells are present in portal tracts and sinusoids (**Fig. 3.8**). Hepatocyte plates are mainly two cells thick until the age of five or six years, when the adult pattern of single cell plates is established. Hepatocytes and their nuclei vary little in size. Glycogen vacuolation of nuclei is common until adolescence. Lipofuscin pigment is absent or scanty in the first two decades of life.

Figure 3.7 Liver of fetus at 19 weeks' gestation. Many haemopoietic cells are seen in sinusoids and in the immature portal tract. A ductal plate at the margin of the tract (arrows) indicates bile-duct formation. (Post-mortem liver, H&E.)

Figure 3.8 Normal liver in a neonate. Abundant haemopoietic cells are seen in the portal tract and in the sinusoids. (Post-mortem liver, H&E.)

Ageing

The size of hepatocytes and their nuclei becomes more variable with increasing age, most notable in perivenular regions (**Fig. 3.9**). This variation is due to greater numbers of poly-ploid cells,[31] with large nuclear and cell volumes. Lipofuscin pigment in hepatocytes is often abundant, especially around terminal hepatic venules (**Fig. 3.6**). Portal connective tissue becomes denser, and arteries may be thick-walled even in normotensive subjects.

Figure 3.9 Liver in an elderly person. Hepatocyte nuclei vary considerably in size. (Needle biopsy, H&E.)

Pseudocapillarisation of the sinusoidal lining with loss of permeability may have important consequences for lipid metabolism and vascular disease.[35]

Biopsy of the normal liver

Percutaneous liver biopsies are necessarily taken though the liver capsule, which may be seen at one end of the core or as a separate piece. It sometimes contains vessels and bile ducts, but can be distinguished from a pathological septum by the density and maturity of the connective tissue. Deeper in the core, pathological septa must also be distinguished from longitudinally cut portal tracts (**Fig. 3.10**). The length and width of the liver core is often critical for diagnosis, as discussed under the heading of grading and staging in **Chapter 9**. Short pieces or slender cores taken with narrow needles may be inadequate for the diagnosis of unevenly distributed, non-neoplastic lesions.

Other organs and tissues, especially skin, pleura and intercostal muscle, are sometimes included in the specimen. Close apposition to the liver core of fibrous tissue or of tumour does not necessarily reflect hepatic fibrosis or tumour within the liver.

Transjugular biopsy is now often used and usually provides ample sized specimens, sometimes including longitudinally-cut portions of efferent vein walls.

Surgical biopsies taken from the inferior margin of the liver are in the form of wedges covered on two aspects by capsule. The structure of the immediately subcapsular zone differs somewhat from the deeper tissue (**Fig. 3.11**), but there is good correlation between the volume fraction of non-parenchymal components in subcapsular and deeper zones.[36] Appearances mimicking cirrhosis do not usually extend for more than 2 mm into the liver, and confusion is unlikely except with very small superficial samples.

In surgical biopsies taken some time after the beginning of an operation, neutrophil leucocytes accumulate under the capsule and in portal tracts, around terminal venules and focally within the parenchyma (**Fig. 3.12**). Here, there is focal loss of hepatocytes. Similar parenchymal changes have been reported after heavy sedation without full anaesthesia.[37] They are also found in patients infected with cytomegalovirus (**Ch. 15**).

Figure 3.10
Normal adult liver.
Two normal portal
tracts (P), cut
longitudinally, mimic
septa. Between
them is an efferent
hepatic venule (V).
(Needle biopsy,
reticulin.)

Figure 3.11
Normal adult liver.
The capsule is thick
and portal tracts are
prominent. (Post-
mortem liver,
trichrome.)

**Figure 3.12
Operative wedge
biopsy.**
Clumps of
neutrophils mark
sites of
hepatocellular
necrosis, resulting
from the procedure.
Part of an efferent
venule is seen (top
left). (Wedge biopsy,
H&E.)

References

1 Rappaport AM. The microcirculatory acinar concept of normal and pathological hepatic structure. *Beitr Pathol* 1976; **157**: 215–243.

2 Saxena R, Theise ND, Crawford JM, et al. Microanatomy of the human liver – exploring the hidden interfaces. Derivation of hepatocytes from bone marrow cells in mice after radiation-induced myeloablation. *Hepatology* 1999; **30**: 1339–1346.

3 Roskams T, Desmet VJ, Verslype C. Development, structure and function of the liver. In: Burt AD, Portmann BC, Ferrell LD, eds. MacSween's Pathology of the Liver, 5th edn. Edinburgh: Churchill Livingstone/Elsevier, 2007:1–74.

4 Reuben A. Now you see it, now you don't. *Hepatology* 2003; **38**: 781–784.

5 Crawford AR, Lin X-Z, Crawford JM. The normal adult human liver biopsy: a quantitative reference standard. *Hepatology* 1998; **28**: 323–331.

6 Theise ND, Saxena R, Portmann BC, et al. The canals of Hering and hepatic stem cells in humans. *Hepatology* 1999; **30**: 1425–1433.

7 Saxena R, Theise N. Canals of Hering: recent insights and current knowledge. *Semin Liver Dis* 2004; **24**: 43–48.

8 Roskams TA, Theise ND, Balabaud C, et al. Nomenclature of the finer branches of the biliary tree: canals, ductules, and ductular reactions in human livers. *Hepatology* 2004; **39**: 1739–1745.

9 Roskams TA, Libbrecht L, Desmet VJ. Progenitor cells in diseased human liver. *Semin Liver Dis* 2003; **23**: 385–396.

10 Kuwahara R, Kofman AV, Landis CS, et al. The hepatic stem cell niche: identification by label-retaining cell assay. *Hepatology* 2008; **47**: 1994–2002.

11 Roskams T, De Vos R, van Eyken P, et al. Hepatic OV-6 expression in human liver disease and rat experiments: evidence for hepatic progenitor cells in man. *J Hepatol* 1998; **29**: 455–463.

12 Zhang L, Theise N, Chua M, Reid LM. The stem cell niche of human livers: symmetry between development and regeneration. *Hepatology* 2008; **48**: 1598–1607.

13 van Eyken P, Desmet VJ. Cytokeratins and the liver. *Liver* 1993; **13**: 113–122.

14 Terada T, Nakanuma Y, Kakita A. Pathologic observations of intrahepatic peribiliary glands in 1000 consecutive autopsy livers. Heterotopic pancreas in the liver. *Gastroenterology* 1990; **98**: 1333–1337.

15 Norris S, Collins C, Doherty DG, et al. Resident human hepatic lymphocytes are phenotypically different from circulating lymphocytes. *J Hepatol* 1998; **28**: 84–90.

16 Nakatani K, Kaneda K, Seki S, Nakajima Y. Pit cells as liver-associated natural killer cells: morphology and function. *Med Electron Microsc* 2004; **37**: 29–36.

17 Tiniakos DG, Lee JA, Burt AD. Innervation of the liver: morphology and function. *Liver* 1996; **16**: 151–160.

18 Akiyoshi H, Gonda T, Terada T. A comparative histochemical and immunohistochemical study of aminergic, cholinergic and peptidergic innervation in rat, hamster, guineapig, dog and human livers. *Liver* 1998; **18**: 352–359.

19 International Consensus Group. Hepatic stellate cell nomenclature. *Hepatology* 1996; **23**: 193.

20 Pinzani M. Hepatic stellate (Ito) cells: expanding roles for a liver-specific pericyte. *J Hepatol* 1995; **22**: 700–706.

21 Rockey DC. Hepatic blood flow regulation by stellate cells in normal and injured liver. *Semin Liver Dis* 2001; **21**: 337–349.

22 Schmitt-Graff A, Kruger S, Bochard F, et al. Modulation of alpha smooth muscle actin and desmin expression in perisinusoidal cells of normal and diseased human livers. *Am J Pathol* 1991; **138**: 1233–1242.

23 Cassiman D, van Pelt J , De Vos R, et al. Synaptophysin: a novel marker for human and rat hepatic stellate cells. *Am J Pathol* 1999; **155**: 1831–1839.

24 Kawai S, Enzan H, Hayashi Y, et al. Vinculin: a novel marker for quiescent and activated hepatic stellate cells in human and rat livers. *Virchows Arch* 2003; **443**: 78–86.

25 Lepreux S, Bioulac-Sage P, Gabbiani G, et al. Cellular retinol-binding protein-1 expression in normal and fibrotic/cirrhotic human liver: different patterns of expression in hepatic stellate cells and (myo)fibroblast subpopulations. *J Hepatol* 2004; **40**: 774–780.

26 Cassiman D, Roskams T. Beauty is in the eye of the beholder: emerging concepts and pitfalls in hepatic stellate cell research. *J Hepatol* 2002; **37**: 527–535.

27 Ramadori G, Saile B. Mesenchymal cells in the liver: one cell type or two? *Liver* 2002; **22**: 283–294.

28 Schuppan D, Ruehl M, Somasundaram R, et al. Matrix as a modulator of hepatic fibrogenesis. *Semin Liver Dis* 2001; **21**: 351–372.

29 Porto LC, Chevallier M, Peyrol S, et al. Elastin in human, baboon, and mouse liver: an immunohistochemical and immunoelectron microscopic study. *Anat Rec* 1990; **228**: 392–404.

30 Deprez C, Vangansbeke D, Fastrez R, et al. Nuclear DNA content, proliferation index, and nuclear size determination in normal and cirrhotic liver, and in benign and malignant primary and metastatic hepatic tumors. *Am J Clin Pathol* 1993; **99**: 558–565.

31 Kudryatsev BN, Kudryatseva MV, Sakuta GA, et al. Human hepatocyte polyploidization kinetics in the course of life cycle. *Virchows Arch [B] Cell Pathol* 1993; **64**: 387–393.

32 Hinchliffe SA, Woods S, Gray S, et al. Cellular distribution of androgen receptors in the liver. *J Clin Pathol* 1996; **49**: 418–420.

33 Wennerberg AE, Nalesnik MA, Coleman WB. Hepatocyte paraffin 1: a monoclonal antibody that reacts with hepatocytes and can be used for differential diagnosis of hepatic tumors. *Am J Pathol* 1993; **143**: 1050–1054.

34 Byrne JA, Meara NJ, Rayner AC, Thompson RJ, Knisely AS. Lack of hepatocellular CD10 along bile canaliculi is physiologic in early childhood and persistent in Alagille syndrome. *Lab Invest* 2007; **87**: 1138–1148.

35 Le Couteur DG, Fraser R, Cogger VC, et al. Hepatic pseudocapillarisation and atherosclerosis in ageing. *Lancet* 2002; **359**: 1612–1615.

36 Ryoo JW, Buschmann RJ. Comparison of intralobular non-parenchyma, subcapsular non-parenchyma, and liver capsule thickness. *J Clin Pathol* 1989; **42**: 740–744.

37 McDonald GS, Courtney MG. Operation-associated neutrophils in a percutaneous liver biopsy: effect of prior transjugular procedure. *Histopathology* 1986; **10**: 217–222.

General reading

Crawford AR, Lin X-Z, Crawford JM. The normal adult human liver biopsy: a quantitative reference standard. *Hepatology* 1998; **28**: 323–331.

Dollé L, Best J, Mei J, et al. The quest for liver progenitor cells: a practical point of view. *J Hepatol* 2010; **52**: 117–129.

Friedman SL. Mechanisms of hepatic fibrogenesis. *Gastroenterology* 2008; **134**: 1655–1669.

Geerts A. History, heterogeneity, developmental biology, and functions of quiescent hepatic stellate cells. *Semin Liver Dis* 2001; **21**: 311–335.

Lemaigre FP. Mechanisms of liver development: concepts for understanding liver disorders and design of novel therapies. *Gastroenterology* 2009; **137**: 62–79.

Reuben A. Now you see it, now you don't. *Hepatology* 2003; **38**: 781–784.

Roskams TA, Libbrecht L, Desmet VJ. Progenitor cells in diseased human liver. *Semin Liver Dis* 2003; **23**: 385–396.

Roskams TA, Theise ND, Balabaud C, et al. Nomenclature of the finer branches of the biliary tree: canals, ductules, and ductular reactions in human livers. *Hepatology* 2004; **39**: 1739–1745.

Roskams T, Desmet VJ, Verslype C. Development, structure and function of the liver. In: Burt AD, Portmann BC, Ferrell LD, eds. MacSween's Pathology of the Liver, 5th edn. Edinburgh: Churchill Livingstone/Elsevier, 2007: 1–74.

Si-Tayeb K, Lemaigre FP, Duncan SA. Organogenesis and development of the liver. *Dev Cell* 2010; **18**: 175–189.

Zhang L, Theise N, Chua M, Reid LM. The stem cell niche of human livers: symmetry between development and regeneration. *Hepatology* 2008; **48**: 1598–1607.

Assessment and Differential Diagnosis of Pathological Features

Initial examination and reporting

Naked-eye examination and description of biopsy specimens

Although naked-eye examination and description are of limited diagnostic value, they reduce the possibility of specimen identification error. The pathologist should make sure that the whole specimen has been adequately sectioned by comparing the size of the sectioned and stained tissue with the measurement recorded on macroscopic examination. Naked-eye examination also helps in the selection of suitable areas for electron microscopy. Needle biopsy specimens from cirrhotic liver are often irregular in calibre or obviously nodular, with brown or green nodules separated by grey or white fibrous tissue. The specimen may easily break into smaller pieces on handling or processing. Specimens with metastatic tumour or primary hepatocellular carcinoma also often fragment. Normal liver, on the other hand, gives rise to cylinders of even colour and thickness, which do not fragment easily. Cholestasis imparts a green colour, whereas fatty liver is pale brown or yellow and may float in the fixative. In cholesterol ester storage disease and Wolman's disease the specimen is bright orange; this should warn the pathologist of the need to keep some tissue for frozen sectioning and electron microscopy. A black or very dark brown colour is characteristic of the Dubin–Johnson syndrome. Metastatic tumour, like fibrous tissue, is often white. Congested liver is deep red in colour. The clinician should record whether the specimen was difficult to obtain from the patient and whether the liver felt hard when the needle was inserted, as in many cases of cirrhosis, or very hard, as in congenital hepatic fibrosis.

Routine microscopy

Routine microscopy of liver biopsies should include systematic assessment of overall structure, portal tracts and their contents, terminal hepatic venules, hepatocytes and sinusoidal cells. Some pathologists use a pro forma or checklist in order to avoid omitting relevant data.[1]

The following sections are intended to help in the evaluation of pathological changes. Most of the information is also found in other parts of the book, under individual diseases.

©2010 Elsevier Ltd
DOI: 10.1016/B978-0-7020-3410-7.00010-1

There is inevitably some repetition, because many of the listed features are found in combination. The final part of the chapter contains guidance on the differential diagnosis of acute cholestasis and of individual pathological findings.

Basic patterns of injury

Structural changes, collapse and fibrosis

Minor structural changes are difficult to assess in sections stained with haematoxylin and eosin (H&E), and may indeed be missed altogether. Examination of a connective tissue preparation is therefore often important. Normal liver tissue shows a hierarchy of ramifying portal tracts of varied sizes which are present in needle and wedge biopsy samples (**Fig. 4.1**). The subdivisions of these portal tracts parallel the hierarchy of hepatic artery and portal vein branches and bile ducts as they distribute throughout the liver and can thereby be roughly subdivided into segmental, area, conducting (septal) and terminal portal tract units (**see Fig. 5.1**). For detection of the most minor abnormalities an uncounterstained silver impregnation for reticulin is generally best, although pericellular fibrosis is most easily detected in sections stained for collagen.

Using these methods, an impression may be gained that, although portal tracts and terminal venules are normally related to each other, the portal tracts are enlarged and perhaps even linked by fibrous septa. This is consistent with mild chronic viral hepatitis or with one of the conditions in which portal changes typically predominate; these include biliary tract disease, haemochromatosis, congenital hepatic fibrosis and schistosomiasis. If on the other hand the reticulin framework of the parenchyma is distorted, lesions characterised by lobular damage should be considered. These include acute and chronic hepatitis as well as forms of biliary disease in which there is also hepatocellular damage, notably

Figure 4.1 Portal tract size variations.
Biopsies contain portal tracts ranging in size from larger conducting tracts (at left) to the small terminal tracts (right top and bottom) from which blood enters the parenchyma. (Wedge biopsy, chromotrope–aniline blue.)

primary biliary cirrhosis. Venous congestion leads to regular condensation of perivenular reticulin.

Recent collapse and fibrosis are sometimes difficult to distinguish, even with the help of good collagen stains. A stain for elastic tissue can help to resolve this problem because the presence of elastic fibres outside the portal tracts is an indication of long-standing disease. Collagen stains are helpful for the recognition of blocked veins, for example in necrotic areas, alcoholic liver disease, venous outflow obstruction and epithelioid haemangioendothelioma. Collagen staining is important for the detection of pericellular fibrosis, as already indicated, and should therefore be used whenever there is substantial steatosis or a suspicion of steatohepatitis.

The histological diagnosis of cirrhosis is fully discussed in **Chapter 10**. Once cirrhosis has developed, the pattern of fibrosis is one of the features that may help to determine its cause. In primary or secondary biliary cirrhosis, for example, fibrosis expanding and linking the portal tracts is a more important early factor in pathogenesis than hepatocellular regeneration; this is reflected in the morphological picture of broad perilobular septa surrounding irregularly shaped islands of parenchyma (**see Fig. 5.11**). In hereditary haemochromatosis and chronic venous outflow obstruction the impression is also of fibrosis rather than regeneration as the principal pathogenetic factor. In these diseases with a long pre-cirrhotic phase of fibrosis, transected parenchymal peninsulas may be mistaken for true regenerative nodules. This is particularly common just deep to the liver capsule. Isolated subcapsular nodules in an otherwise not nodular biopsy should therefore be interpreted with caution.

Hepatocellular damage

Death of individual hepatocytes or small groups of these cells is loosely called **focal** necrosis, although the mechanism may in fact be apoptosis. The distinction cannot always be made easily by routine microscopy unless apoptotic bodies are seen. Focal necrosis is associated with accumulation of inflammatory cells of various types, including macrophages. **Spotty** necrosis is a term used for the same lesion in the context of acute hepatitis. Focal necrosis is a common finding which does not in itself indicate primary disease of the liver, because it is often part of a non-specific reaction to disease elsewhere in the body. While degenerating hepatocytes or cell fragments are sometimes seen within the focal inflammatory infiltrate, the inflammatory reaction is usually more obvious than the necrosis, and the latter is assumed to have taken place because of a gap in a liver-cell plate (liver-cell 'dropout').

Confluent necrosis

Confluent necrosis (**see Fig. 8.4**) refers to substantial areas of liver-cell death. The commonest cause of this type of necrosis in biopsy material is hepatitis, either viral or drug-related, in which case the necrosis is accompanied by an inflammatory reaction. Confluent necrosis with little or no inflammation is seen in hypoperfusion of the hepatic parenchyma, as in shock or left ventricular failure, and in heatstroke (**see Fig. 12.2**). Paracetamol (acetaminophen) poisoning produces a similar lesion. In all the above examples the necrosis is typically perivenular but it may, if severe and extensive, form bridges linking vascular structures (see below). Some poisons, including ferrous sulphate, typically cause periportal (zone 1) necrosis. Haphazardly distributed areas of necrosis are found in disseminated herpes virus infections (e.g. herpes simplex, varicella) (**see Fig. 15.4**) and in mycobacterial diseases. Tumour necrosis may be so extensive that no recognisable tumour tissue is present in the section; in such cases the reticulin pattern may help to establish a diagnosis.

Figure 4.2 Acute hepatitis with bridging necrosis. Collapsed reticulin here gives a false impression of chronic liver disease. A bridge or passive septum (arrowheads) links an expanded portal tract (P) with a terminal hepatic venule (V). (Needle biopsy, reticulin.)

Bridging necrosis

Bridging necrosis describes the location rather than the type of necrosis. It usually results from extensive necrosis of confluent type. The term has been used for necrosis linking any of the vascular structures, but it is now more often restricted to the linking of terminal hepatic venules (centrilobular veins) to portal tracts (**Fig. 4.2**). A possible explanation for this type of bridging is that it represents necrosis of acinar zones 3, which touch both the veins and the larger portal tracts (**as in Fig. 3.1**). Linking of portal tracts to each other is common in conditions in which portal tracts are widened, for example by chronic hepatitis or biliary tract disease; this is partly because the chance of obtaining a longitudinal section of a widened portal tract is greater than for one of normal width. Linking of perivenular areas to each other by is found in some examples of parenchymal hypoperfusion and venous outflow obstruction.

Bridging of terminal hepatic venules to portal tracts is a fairly common feature of acute hepatitis of viral type, when the bridges contain few or no elastic fibres. It is also seen in exacerbations of chronic hepatitis. Old bridges contain elastic fibres as well as collagen fibres. Such bridging fibrosis is an important component both of the more severe examples of chronic viral hepatitis and of steatohepatitis. Contraction of collagen-rich bridges may produce rapid and severe distortion of the normal hepatic microstructure, with correspondingly rapid progression to cirrhosis.

Panlobular and multilobular necrosis

Panlobular (panacinar) and multilobular (multiacinar) necrosis are terms used to describe confluent necrosis involving entire single lobules or several adjacent lobules respectively. They are further discussed in **Chapter 6**.

Interface hepatitis (piecemeal necrosis)

Interface hepatitis (piecemeal necrosis) (**see Figs 9.3, 9.4**) is a process of inflammation and erosion of the hepatic parenchyma at its junction with portal tracts or fibrous septa. The term 'interface hepatitis' was introduced because the death of hepatocytes probably involves apoptosis rather than, or as well as, necrosis,[2–5] and because it takes place at the parenchymal–connective tissue interface. It is common in chronic viral hepatitis but is also found in other conditions (**see Box 9.2**). The inflammatory infiltrate is composed mainly of lymphocytes, with or without recognisable plasma cells, and is accompanied by fibrosis of the affected areas with new formation of collagens and other extracellular matrix components.[6] The process is sometimes referred to as classical or lymphocytic piecemeal necrosis in order to distinguish it from biliary, ductular and fibrotic piecemeal necrosis, processes found in chronic biliary tract disease and described in the section on primary biliary cirrhosis in **Chapter 5**.

Cholestasis

In morphological terms, cholestasis is the presence of visible bile in tissue sections. It is also known as bilirubinostasis because the main component seen by light microscopy is bilirubin. Bile is rarely seen in normal liver, and then only in minute amounts; cholestasis should therefore be regarded as pathological. The location of the bile varies. The commonest is in dilated bile canaliculi between hepatocytes. This canalicular form of cholestasis, sometimes called acute cholestasis, may be accompanied by bile accumulation in the cytoplasm of hepatocytes and Kupffer cells. Canalicular cholestasis is typically perivenular. In contrast, in patients with chronic biliary tract disease, bile may accumulate in periportal hepatocytes. This is also known as cholate stasis because abnormal bile salts are thought to contribute to its pathogenesis.

In large bile-duct obstruction in adults, bile is not usually visible under the microscope within canals of Hering, bile ductules or bile ducts even though the biliary tree may be dilated. The commonest cause of ductular cholestasis is sepsis. Dense bile is also visible in ducts in different forms of ductal plate malformation and in extrahepatic biliary atresia.

Canalicular cholestasis

Canalicular cholestasis takes the form of bile plugs (bile thrombi) in dilated canaliculi (**see Fig. 5.2**). There is often brown or yellow pigment in nearby hepatocytes and Kupffer cells, but the distinction of this pigment from others such as lipofuscin and ceroid is not a serious practical problem; this is because the presence of bile in the canaliculi makes the diagnosis of cholestasis obvious. In general, cholestasis should only be diagnosed with great caution in the absence of bile plugs in canaliculi, although cytoplasmic liver-cell bilirubinostasis without canalicular bile is quite common after liver transplantation. The perivenular location of canalicular cholestasis is partly an artefact of paraffin embedding, but also reflects real functional differences between the various parts of the acinus.

The colour of bile under the microscope varies according to pigment concentration and the degree of oxidation. It may be dark brown, green or yellow, and is occasionally so pale as to make detection difficult at first glance. The Van Gieson stain, which stains bilirubin green, may then be helpful (**Fig. 4.3**). Pale counterstaining, as commonly used in Perls' and Prussian blue methods for iron, also makes bile easier to see. Specific histochemical methods for bilirubin are rarely necessary in ordinary diagnostic work.

When acute cholestasis is prolonged, the relationship of hepatocytes to each other may undergo focal change. Instead of the normal arrangement of two or three hepatocytes around a small bile canaliculus, the number of cells is increased and the lumen of the canaliculus considerably enlarged. The new structures are called cholestatic rosettes (**Fig. 4.4**). The lumens of the rosettes are part of the biliary tree, but the bile may be lost during

Figure 4.3
Cholestasis.
Bile thrombi in dilated canaliculi are stained bright green. The red material is collagen. (Needle biopsy, haematoxylin & van Gieson.)

Figure 4.4
Cholestasis.
Several liver-cell rosettes, glandular formations around prominent lumens, are marked by arrowheads. (Wedge biopsy, H&E.)

processing. Even apparently empty rosettes should therefore be regarded as an indication of cholestasis. Other hepatocellular changes in cholestasis are described in the **Chapter 5**, in the section on large bile-duct obstruction. Very occasionally prolonged canalicular cholestasis is associated with the accumulation of copper and copper-associated protein, but this is much more characteristic of the chronic periportal form of cholestasis, discussed below.

Canalicular cholestasis in perivenular areas is mainly seen in the conditions listed in **Tables 4.1 and 4.2**. Cholestasis of less regular distribution is common in chronic liver diseases with severe hepatocellular dysfunction or with associated sepsis.

Chronic cholestasis

Chronic cholestasis (cholate stasis, pseudoxanthomatous change, precholestasis; **see Fig. 5.10**) is seen in chronic liver diseases, especially those involving the biliary tree, and is the result of interference with bile flow at the level of the portal tracts. Bile (i.e. bilirubinostasis) may or may not be obvious, and the lesion is more easily recognised by hepatocellular swelling and pallor, and by the accumulation of copper and copper-associated protein in the affected cells. Mallory bodies may also be present. In some instances these are associated with an infiltrate of neutrophils, in which case the distinction from steatohepatitis must be made on the overall appearances and clinical context. The connective tissue adjacent to an area of chronic cholestasis is often oedematous. It may show a ductular reaction containing proliferated ductule-like structures which have the cytokeratin profile of bile ducts.[7] They express cytokeratins 7 and 19, which are not normally demonstrable in hepatocytes. Because the ductular reaction is often associated with disruption of the limiting plates of hepatocytes around the portal tracts, it has given rise to the concept of ductular piecemeal necrosis.[8] Chronic cholestasis, unlike acute canalicular cholestasis, is not necessarily associated with clinical jaundice or a high level of serum bilirubin, but the serum alkaline phosphatase level is characteristically raised.

Table 4.1 Common causes of canalicular cholestasis
Obstruction to major bile ducts
Acute hepatitis
Cholestatic drug jaundice
Sepsis
Cholestatic syndromes (**Table 5.2**)

Table 4.2 Main causes of bland intrahepatic cholestasis
Drugs (e.g. contraceptive steroids)
Sepsis
Benign recurrent intrahepatic cholestasis
Cholestasis of pregnancy
Post-transplant bile-flow impairment or rejection
Lymphomas

Differential diagnosis of individual findings

Acute cholestasis

Modern imaging methods have greatly reduced the need for liver biopsy in acutely jaundiced patients. Biopsy is nevertheless still helpful in some instances when the cause of a presumed intrahepatic jaundice is in doubt, when there is a need to distinguish between acute and chronic liver disease, and when other investigations give equivocal results. Liver transplantation has led to a striking increase in liver biopsies for evaluation of the cause of jaundice. The pathologist may also need to assess surgical biopsy specimens from jaundiced patients. Accurate histological diagnosis is important because correct treatment may depend upon it, and a wrong answer can lead to dangerous mismanagement. It has to be admitted, however, that the pathologist cannot always give a clear answer to the questions put by the clinician.

In essence, the pathologist faced with a liver biopsy from an acutely jaundiced patient is asked to decide between the options in **Table 4.3**. The last two items listed in the box are discussed in detail in **Chapters 7** and **9**, and it is only necessary here to note that it is sometimes difficult to distinguish between chronic hepatitis and severe acute hepatitis with bridging necrosis. This clinically important distinction is made more easily with the help of a stain for elastic fibres. The main problem lies in the differentiation of the first four possibilities: bile-duct obstruction, acute hepatitis and various other forms of intrahepatic cholestasis, including that due to sepsis. These can usually be distinguished by

Table 4.3 Decisions in the acutely jaundiced patient

- Are the patient's major bile ducts obstructed?
- Does the patient have an acute viral or drug-related hepatitis?
- Is there evidence for a diagnosis of sepsis?
- Does the patient have one of the intrahepatic conditions listed in **Table 4.2**?
- Does the patient have steatohepatitis?
- Does the patient have chronic liver disease with an acute exacerbation rather than acute liver disease?

careful and methodical examination of abnormalities in the lobules and in the portal tracts (**Fig. 4.5**).

Lobular changes

Obstruction to large bile ducts within or outside the liver leads to morphological cholestasis in perivenular areas. Bile canaliculi are dilated and contain bile thrombi (canalicular cholestasis). There is a variable degree of liver-cell swelling, inflammatory cell infiltration and Kupffer-cell hypertrophy in the cholestatic areas, but elsewhere the parenchyma appears substantially normal. The inflammatory infiltration is usually modest or even absent, and liver-cell plates remain for the most part intact. A few apoptotic bodies and liver-cell mitoses may be seen, reflecting increased liver-cell turnover. Bile infarcts sometimes develop in the elderly, in whom duct obstruction is a very important cause of acute jaundice; there is sometimes more liver-cell damage than in the young.

By contrast, in acute hepatitis there is usually disruption of cell plates and widespread swelling, shrinking and loss of hepatocytes, usually most striking in perivenular areas but often widely distributed. In some forms of viral hepatitis, especially hepatitis A, there is sometimes substantial necrosis and lymphoplasmacytic infiltration of the periportal parenchyma. Cholestasis may be seen in acute hepatitis, again commonly in hepatitis A, but canalicular dilatation is slight and hepatocellular changes are not confined to areas of cholestasis. In patients on immunosuppressive therapy, for example after liver transplantation, the inflammatory infiltrate of an acute viral hepatitis may be relatively inconspicuous.

In other forms of intrahepatic cholestasis, such as drug-induced cholestasis, benign recurrent cholestasis and cholestasis of pregnancy, the changes within the acini are much the same as in bile-duct obstruction, except that bile infarcts are unusual and, if present, small. Canaliculi are less dilated than in bile-duct obstruction, except in liver-cell rosettes, which often form in intrahepatic cholestases and are described and illustrated above. There may be striking liver-cell swelling and multinucleation. Inflammatory infiltration is variable; in most forms of intrahepatic cholestasis, inflammation and liver-cell damage are absent or slight, but in a minority of cases of idiosyncratic drug cholestasis they are sufficient to justify the label of cholestatic hepatitis.

Portal changes

Examination of portal tracts (**Fig. 4.6**) provides further discrimination, particularly between bile-duct obstruction and the other conditions. In bile-duct obstruction the portal tracts are typically expanded and oedematous, with a pale watery appearance to the connective tissue. There is an increased number of bile-duct profiles at the margins of the tracts, most of these ducts lying roughly parallel to the portal–parenchymal interface (see section on the ductular reaction, below). An associated inflammatory infiltrate includes neutrophils. Not all portal tracts are equally affected. Bile extravasates (see **Chapter 5**) may be seen. The margins of the portal tracts are usually irregular, leading to possible confusion with interface hepatitis. The latter is accompanied by a lymphocytic infiltrate rather than neutrophils, and the cholestasis, portal oedema and duct proliferation of duct obstruction are absent.

Paradoxically, the portal bile ducts are not always strikingly dilated when major ducts are obstructed, although the main duct system is seen to be dilated on cholangiography. When small ducts or canals of Hering are dilated, filled with bile and infiltrated or

Figure 4.5 Algorithmic approach to cholestasis. Once the site of cholestasis is identified pathologically, careful assessment of portal tracts and acinar changes allows the major differential diagnosis to be established. *In PBC, morphological cholestasis is usually only apparent in later, advanced disease.

surrounded by neutrophils, sepsis rather than bile-duct obstruction should be suspected as the cause of the patient's jaundice (**see Fig. 15.11**).

In acute hepatitis the portal infiltrate is mainly composed of lymphocytes, although a few other cells are commonly seen. Ductular reaction is not usually conspicuous but ducts may be damaged (**see Fig. 6.7**). In the less common examples of acute hepatitis in which the portal reaction mimics that of duct obstruction, the parenchymal changes of hepatitis make the diagnosis clear.

Figure 4.6 The ductular reaction in different diseases.
A: Ductular structures at the edge of the portal tract in bile-duct obstruction. **B:** Tangle of ductules in primary biliary cirrhosis.

The ductular reaction

The ductular structures which develop as a prominent feature in a variety of biliary and other conditions may arise from periportal progenitor cells, canals of Hering or other sources (**see Ch. 5**) and are typically associated with neutrophil infiltrates and stromal oedema with variable degrees of fibrosis, collectively referred to as the **ductular reaction**.

Figure 4.6, cont'd
C: Non-biliary cirrhosis: ductular structures near the edge of the nodule and within the fibrotic portal tract. **D:** Multilobular necrosis: the duct-like structures probably reflect progenitor-cell activity in the absence of adequate hepatocellular regeneration. (H&E.)

The ductular reaction can be viewed as a stereotypical periportal response to injury[9] which is exemplified by acute biliary obstruction, but which also occurs in several other pathological settings.

Certain features help in interpreting the diagnostic significance of the ductular reaction. In acute biliary obstruction, the ductular structures are arranged in parallel to the portal–parenchymal interface, associated with the portal oedema and scattered neutrophils previously mentioned (**Fig. 4.6A**). In chronic biliary tract diseases such as primary biliary cirrhosis, the ductular profiles may lie at an angle to the interface or form convoluted tangles (**Fig. 4.6B**). Hepatocellular diseases may also act as a stimulus for the ductular reaction. In a minority of patients with acute hepatitis with much cholestasis, as seen for example in hepatitis A, a ductular reaction may accompany portal infiltrates of lymphocytes and plasma cells.[10] The picture can mimic that of biliary obstruction, and the distinction requires careful consideration of the lobular changes. Ductular reaction is virtually always associated with neutrophils, so that the presence of these cells is not in itself evidence of bile-duct obstruction. Ductular reaction also is seen in some examples of non-biliary cirrhosis in which the ductular structures are not necessarily limited to the margins of portal tracts or the septal–parenchymal interface, but extend to greater distances into the fibrous tissue (**Fig. 4.6C**). However, extensive ductular reaction accompanied by other features of chronic cholestasis suggests cirrhosis of biliary origin.

In panlobular necrosis (seen, for example, in patients with fulminant or subacute viral hepatitis, in severe drug hepatotoxicity or in autoimmune hepatitis), extensive loss of hepatocytes is often associated with an exuberant ductular reaction extending from periportal regions further inward and toward the centres of lobules (**Fig. 4.6D**). Finally, it should be noted that a ductular reaction of varying degree may develop in chronic hepatitis, including chronic hepatitis B and C[11,12] and autoimmune hepatitis (**see Fig. 9.7**). It may be unusually prominent in fibrosing cholestatic hepatitis, which develops in a minority of patients with recurrence of hepatitis B or C after liver transplantation (**see Fig. 16.16**). In any situation in which the relative diagnostic importance of the ductular reaction must be established, immunostains for cytokeratin 7 or 19 are useful for highlighting the ductular structures (**Fig. 4.7 and see Figs 5.24, 5.25**).

Bile-duct loss

Loss of interlobular bile ducts is a key feature of several diseases in childhood and adult life. These are sometimes referred to as **vanishing bile-duct syndromes**. The principal causes in children are syndromatic and non-syndromatic paucity of intrahepatic bile ducts, α_1-antitrypsin deficiency and early-onset sclerosing cholangitis. Some uncommon familial cholestatic syndromes and Langerhans-cell histiocytosis should also be considered. In adults (**see Table 5.3**) the commonest causes are primary biliary cirrhosis, primary sclerosing cholangitis, graft-versus-host disease and chronic liver graft rejection.

In assessing duct loss it is important to bear in mind that not every small portal tract is seen to contain a bile duct in the plane of section. In a study of normal human liver biopsies,[13] 7% of sectioned portal tracts did not contain a bile duct. For confident assessment of duct numbers a biopsy must therefore contain several portal tracts. Loss of ducts is accompanied in many, but not all, cases by the features of chronic cholestasis outlined above. This depends on the extent of duct loss, the underlying aetiology and the degree of fibrosis. A significant ductular reaction develops in some conditions of bile-duct loss (primary biliary cirrhosis, primary sclerosing cholangitis) but not others (Alagille's syndrome in children,[14] chronic liver graft rejection;[15] **see Fig. 1.8**).

Copper-associated protein

Granules of the copper-associated protein metallothionein can be stained by several methods, including orcein and Victoria blue. They are usually positive with periodic acid–Schiff (PAS) staining after diastase digestion. Their most common location is in periportal hepatocytes or, in cirrhotic livers, in hepatocytes at the periphery of nodules. This reflects the inability of the hepatocytes to excrete copper efficiently. Some granules can be seen in cirrhosis of any cause, but large amounts should lead to a suspicion of chronic biliary tract disease or intrahepatic cholestasis.[16] Copper itself is usually demonstrable in the same

Figure 4.7 The ductular reaction with cytokeratin 7 immunohistochemistry.
In this case of primary sclerosing cholangitis numerous bile ductular structures have developed and are more or less parallel to the portal–parenchymal interface. A few periportal cells with less intense staining more closely resemble hepatocytes and represent intermediate hepatobiliary cells (IHBC). Small, round and darkly stained periportal cells are likely progenitor/stem cells (P/SC). (Needle biopsy, specific immunoperoxidase.)

location, and there may be other features of chronic cholestasis such as ductular proliferation, neutrophils, intercellular fibrosis and oedema. A few granules of copper-associated protein are sometimes seen deeper within the acini in prolonged acute cholestasis.

Copper-associated protein also accumulates in Wilson's disease, as discussed in **Chapter 14**. As a rule neither the protein nor copper itself is demonstrable by staining in the early stages of the disease. When cirrhosis develops in Wilson's disease some nodules may be rich in copper-associated protein and copper (although one may be demonstrable without the other), while others are negative. The copper and the protein are usually diffusely distributed throughout a nodule, in contrast to their location in chronic cholestasis.

Hepatocyte swelling

Normal hepatocytes are polygonal in shape, with abundant pale-staining granular cytoplasm rich in glycogen. Moderate swelling is sometimes due to adaptive hyperplasia of the smooth endoplasmic reticulum in response to drugs (**Fig. 4.8, and see Fig. 8.1**). More severe swelling with rounding of the cell outlines, or hepatocellular ballooning, is a feature of cell damage. It may accompany canalicular cholestasis (**see Fig. 5.2**) but is most characteristically found in various forms of hepatitis (**see Fig. 6.2**). This is recognised by disruption of the liver-cell plates and by accompanying inflammatory cell infiltration.

Figure 4.8
Ground-glass and ground-glass-like hepatocytes.
A: Numerous ground-glass cytoplasmic inclusions are seen within hepatocytes in this case of chronic hepatitis B. The inclusions represent hepatitis B virus surface antigen. Some inclusions are separated from the hepatocyte cell membrane by an artefactual empty or white halo. **B:** Hepatocytes around the terminal venule (V) show pseudo-ground-glass change (induction of smooth endoplasmic reticulum) due to medication. Compare with the normal granular-appearing hepatocytes in the lower right-hand field.

C: Liver biopsy from a bone marrow transplant recipient with graft-versus-host disease manifested by bile-duct injury and dysmorphism (arrow). There are also numerous periportal ground-glass-like inclusions. The inclusions resemble glycogen, are positive on PAS stain, may be found in a variety of transplant recipients and are thought to be a result of the many medications used in the post-transplantation clinical setting. (Needle biopsies, H&E.)

Perivenular liver-cell ballooning associated with inflammation and a pericellular network of 'chicken-wire' fibrosis is characteristic of steatohepatitis due to various causes[17] (**see Fig. 7.16**). Following liver transplantation, ballooned hepatocytes can result from perfusion injury, hypoperfusion or hepatitis (**see Fig. 16.2**). In microvesicular steatosis, the cytoplasm of hepatocytes is expanded by minute fat droplets which are sometimes too small to resolve by routine microscopy. The frequent presence of larger fat vacuoles and the clinical context should help to make the diagnosis.

Hepatocyte ground-glass change

Hepatocytes with cytoplasmic 'ground-glass' change are seen in a variety of conditions[18] (**Table 4.4**). The affected liver cells have a pale pink homogeneous appearance resembling frosted glass. The change may involve all or a portion of the hepatocyte cytoplasm or may be in the form of a rounded or crescentic inclusion, sometimes with a surrounding artefactual empty white space. A common example is the hepatitis B surface antigen-containing ground-glass inclusion seen in individuals with chronic hepatitis B (**Fig. 4.8A, and see Fig. 9.13**). Such inclusions are scattered randomly through the lobular parenchyma but sometimes are numerous. Use of certain medications (e.g. barbiturates) and occasionally cholestasis[19] can result in similar appearances but confined to perivenular hepatocytes (**Fig. 4.8B, and see Fig. 8.1**), where it is referred to as 'pseudo-ground-glass' change. Recipients of transplants (liver, cardiac, bone marrow) may also show ground-glass-like inclusions containing an abnormal type of glycogen[20–22] (**Fig. 4.8C**). These have a predilection for periportal hepatocytes, as do the ground-glass inclusions of Lafora's disease (myoclonus epilepsy). Assessment of the clinical setting together with the staining methods shown in **Table 4.4** usually clarifies the cause of the ground-glass change.

Table 4.4 Differential diagnosis of ground-glass hepatocytes

Condition	Staining method(s)
Chronic hepatitis B	Orcein, Victoria blue Immunostain for HBsAg
Medication (e.g. barbiturate)	–
Cyanamide alcohol aversion therapy	Diastase–PAS
Lafora's disease (myoclonus epilepsy)	PAS, colloidal iron
Type IV glycogenosis	PAS
Transplant recipients	PAS

Apoptosis

An occasional apoptotic body (acidophil body) may be seen in normal liver. In cholestasis from any cause, and in donor livers shortly after transplantation, there is often an increase in the number of apoptotic bodies as well as in mitotic figures in hepatocytes. Abundant apoptotic bodies are found in acute hepatitis from any cause. They were first described by Councilman in yellow fever, so that the term 'Councilman body' should strictly speaking be confined to that disease.

Inflammatory cell infiltration

Neutrophils

Neutrophils are most numerous in portal tracts in large bile-duct obstruction, and in any condition in which there is an extensive ductular reaction (see above). In ascending cholangitis they are found in the lumens and walls of bile ducts. In intrahepatic or extra-hepatic sepsis there may be neutrophils around ducts and bile within their lumens. Neutrophils are also seen in the sinusoids. A few neutrophils in a predominantly lymphocytic–plasmacytic portal infiltrate are common in acute hepatitis from any cause, but predominance of neutrophils suggests possible drug-related liver injury.

Diffuse infiltration of the parenchyma by neutrophils is unusual. It may represent a classical acute inflammatory response to extensive tissue destruction from any cause. Localised infiltrates are found in steatohepatitis, especially when alcohol related. However, a mainly lymphocytic infiltrate does not exclude the diagnosis if other features are present (**see Ch. 7**). Focal accumulations of neutrophils (microabscesses) are a feature of cyto-megalovirus infection (**see Fig. 16.12**) and of perfusion injury in liver grafts. They are also seen in many other complications of liver transplantation, though usually in smaller numbers than in cytomegalovirus infection.[23] Clusters of neutrophils may be found within sinusoids in any wedge biopsies taken in the course of surgery (**see Fig. 3.12**), and should not then be taken as indicating specific hepatic pathology.

Eosinophils

Portal infiltrates in many different liver diseases include occasional eosinophils, and their presence does not necessarily imply drug hypersensitivity or toxicity. Portal tracts often show a few eosinophils accompanying lymphocytes and plasma cells in chronic viral and autoimmune hepatitis. They are common in primary biliary cirrhosis and are occasionally abundant.[24] After liver transplantation they are one of the manifestations of cellular rejection.[25] An infiltrate with very prominent eosinophils suggests drug toxicity, systemic conditions with eosinophilia, parasitic disease or eosinophilic gastroenteritis.[26] Focal accumulations of eosinophils are seen in the parenchyma within some granulomas, notably those due to parasites.

Plasma cells

Portal and acinar plasma cell infiltrates are often striking in autoimmune hepatitis, but they may also be seen in acute or chronic viral hepatitis. They are sometimes abundant in hepatitis A. Plasma cells form an important part of the portal infiltrates of primary biliary cirrhosis.

Lymphoid follicles and aggregates

Portal follicles are common and large in many patients with hepatitis C.[27] In this condition they may have easily identifiable germinal centres. Similar follicles are found in primary biliary cirrhosis and autoimmune hepatitis. Less prominent follicles without germinal centres, sometimes referred to as lymphoid aggregates, may be seen in hepatitis B and C as well as in primary biliary cirrhosis and primary sclerosing cholangitis.

Abnormal macrophage pigment

Tan pigment within enlarged sinusoidal Kupffer cells may represent either phagocytic debris following recent necroinflammatory activity (e.g., in acute or chronic hepatitis or in ischaemic injury), biliary material after an episode of cholestasis, or hemosiderin derived from erythrocyte breakdown. The latter pigment is positive on iron stain, while the former pigments usually are DPAS-positive. Granular black haemozoin pigment (derived from haemoglobin breakdown) within sinusoidal Kupffer cells and/or portal macrophages is seen in malaria and in schistosomiasis (**see Ch. 15**). A similar black pigment occasionally is seen in individuals who have received gold salts or total knee or hip titanium–aluminium prosthetic replacements.[28]

References

1   Foschini M, Sarti F, Dina RE, et al. Standardized reporting of histological diagnoses for non-neoplastic liver conditions in needle biopsies. *Virchows Arch* 1995; **426**: 593–596.

2   Yoon J-H, Gores GJ. Death receptor-mediated apoptosis and the liver. *J Hepatol* 2002; **37**: 400–410.

3   Lemasters JJ. Dying a thousand deaths: redundant pathways from different organelles to apoptosis and necrosis. *Gastroenterology* 2005; **129**: 351–360.

4   Kerr JFR, Searle J, Halliday WJ, et al. The nature of piecemeal necrosis in chronic active hepatitis. *Lancet* 1979; **ii**: 827–828.

5   Hiramatsu N, Hayashi N, Katayama K, et al. Immunohistochemical detection of Fas antigen in liver tissue of patients with chronic hepatitis C. *Hepatology* 1994; **19**: 1354–1359.

6   Takahara T, Nakayama Y, Itoh H, et al. Extracellular matrix formation in piecemeal necrosis: immuno-electron microscopic study. *Liver* 1992; **12**: 368–380.

7   Roskams T, Desmet V. Ductular reaction and its diagnostic significance. *Semin Diagn Pathol* 1998; **15**: 259–269.

8   Portmann B, Popper H, Neuberger J, et al. Sequential and diagnostic features in primary biliary cirrhosis based on serial histologic study in 209 patients. *Gastroenterology* 1985; **88**: 1777–1790.

9   Roskams T. Progenitor cell involvement in cirrhotic human liver diseases: from controversy to consensus. *J Hepatol* 2003; **39**: 431–434.

10 Teixeira MR Jr, Weller IVD, Murray AM, et al. The pathology of hepatitis A in man. *Liver* 1982; **2**: 53–60.

11 Fotiadu A, Tzioufa V, Vrettou E, et al. Progenitor cell activation in chronic viral hepatitis. *Liver Int* 2004; **24**: 268–274.

12 Eleazar JA, Memeo L, Jhang JS, et al. Progenitor cell expansion: an important source of hepatocyte regeneration in chronic hepatitis. *J Hepatol* 2004; **41**: 983–991.

13 Crawford AR, Lin X-Z, Crawford JM. The normal adult human liver biopsy: a quantitative reference standard. *Hepatology* 1998; **28**: 323–331.

14 Fabris L, Cadamuro M, Guido M, et al. Analysis of liver repair mechanisms in Alagille syndrome and biliary

atresia reveals a role for Notch signaling. *Am J Pathol* 2007; **171**: 641–653.

15 International Panel. Update of the international Banff schema for liver allograft rejection: working recommendations for the histopathologic staging and reporting of chronic rejection. *Hepatology* 2000; **31**: 792–799.

16 Guarascio P, Yentis F, Cevikbas U, et al. Value of copper-associated protein in diagnostic assessment of liver biopsy. *J Clin Pathol* 1983; **36**: 18–23.

17 Gramlich T, Kleiner DE, McCullough AJ, et al. Pathologic features associated with fibrosis in nonalcoholic fatty liver disease. *Hum Pathol* 2004; **35**: 196–199.

18 Vázquez JJ. Ground glass hepatocytes: light and electron microscopy. Characterization of the different types. *Histol Histopathol* 1990; **5**, 379–386.

19 Popper H, Schaffner F. Pathophysiology of cholestasis. *Hum Pathol* 1970; **1**: 1–24.

20 Lefkowitch JH, Lobritto SJ, Brown RS Jr, et al. Ground-glass, polyglucosan-like hepatocellular inclusions: a 'new' diagnostic entity. *Gastroenterology* 2006; **131**: 713–718.

21 Wisell J, Boitnott J, Haas M, et al. Glycogen pseudoground glass change in hepatocytes. *Am J Surg Pathol* 2006; **30**: 1085–1090.

22 Bejarano PA, Garcia MT, Rodriguez MM, et al. Liver glycogen bodies: ground-glass hepatocytes in transplanted patients. *Virchows Arch* 2006; **449**: 539–545.

23 MacDonald GA, Greenson JK, DelBuono EA, et al. Mini-microabscess syndrome in liver transplant patients. *Hepatology* 1997; **26**: 192–197.

24 Terasaki S, Nakanuma Y, Yamazaki M, et al. Eosinophilic infiltration of the liver in primary biliary cirrhosis: a morphological study. *Hepatology* 1993; **17**: 206–212.

25 Datta Gupta S, Hudson M, Burroughs AK, et al. Grading of cellular rejection after orthotopic liver transplantation. *Hepatology* 1995; **21**: 46–57.

26 Schoonbroodt D, Horsmans Y, Laka A, et al. Eosinohilic gastroenteritis presenting with colitis and cholangitis. *Dig Dis Sci* 1995; **40**: 308–314.

27 Scheuer PJ, Ashrafzadeh P, Sherlock S, et al. The pathology of hepatitis C. *Hepatology* 1992; **15**: 567–571.

28 Brenard R, Dumortier P, Del Natale M, et al. Black pigments in the liver related to gold and titanium deposits. A report of four cases. *Liver Int* 2007; **27**: 408–413.

General reading

Ludwig J, Batts K. Practical Liver Biopsy Interpretation: Diagnostic Algorithms, 2nd edn. Chicago, IL: ASCP Press, 1998.

Odze RD, Goldblum JR (eds). Surgical Pathology of the GI Tract, Liver, Biliary Tract and Pancreas. 2nd Edn. Philadelphia: Saunders Elsevier, 2009.

Roskams T, Desmet VJ. Ductular reaction and its diagnostic significance. *Semin Diagn Pathol* 1998; **15**: 259–269.

Biliary Disease

Introduction

There are many sites along the biliary tree where bile flow may be interrupted, from the bile canaliculi and smallest intrahepatic ducts to the large bile ducts and duodenum (**Fig. 5.1**). Damage or obstruction at these various sites may result in visible bile in histological sections (cholestasis), altered bile-duct morphology, changes within the portal tracts and periportal parenchyma, or combinations of these. Diseases of the larger ducts must be distinguished from diffuse intrahepatic diseases because of different clinical management, and liver biopsy is often helpful in this respect. However, diseases of large bile ducts outside and within the liver share pathological features and may be amenable to similar forms of treatment; for this reason the term 'extrahepatic biliary obstruction' is not used in this chapter. Carcinoma of the main hepatic ducts, for example, may be situated wholly within the liver, yet lead to the changes of large-duct obstruction. This chapter discusses these changes as well as the pathology of primary biliary cirrhosis and primary sclerosing cholangitis, the diagnostic problem of overlap with autoimmune hepatitis and several bile-duct paucity disorders.

Cholestasis

The term *cholestasis* in clinical and pathological usage refers to impairment of bile flow. Under the light microscope, cholestasis (sometimes called *bilirubinostasis*) is defined as the presence of bile pigment within bile canaliculi, hepatocytes and other sites. It is the morphological correlate of clinical jaundice. Cholestasis is an important finding in large bile-duct obstruction or in extensive intrahepatic bile-duct disease, but may also accompany the parenchymal damage in certain types of hepatitis. Pure (bland) cholestasis as an isolated lesion requires consideration of several possible aetiologies (**Table 5.1**), which may not be distinguishable by light microscopy alone. For example, in neonatal and childhood jaundice, cholestasis may result from mutations in bile-salt transport proteins on the canalicular membrane[1] or from mitochondriopathies,[2] problems discussed further in **Chapter 13**. In adults, drug hepatotoxicity, circulating endotoxin in septicaemia[3] and cytokine release from extrahepatic lymphoma[4] are further examples of functional disorders of bile secretory physiology that may lead to intrahepatic cholestasis (discussed further in **Ch. 4**). The pathologist's first priority when cholestasis is present, nevertheless, is careful examination of the portal tracts for possible changes of mechanical large bile-duct obstruction, which are described below.

©2010 Elsevier Ltd
DOI: 10.1016/B978-0-7020-3410-7.00011-3

Figure 5.1 The biliary tree.
The ramifying structures of the biliary system are shown schematically. The large segmental and area ducts have peribiliary glands (PGs). The finer branches are shown in an enlargement at upper left. Boxes at right show examples of biliary disease at the specific levels affected. PBC = primary biliary cirrhosis; PSC = primary sclerosing cholangitis.

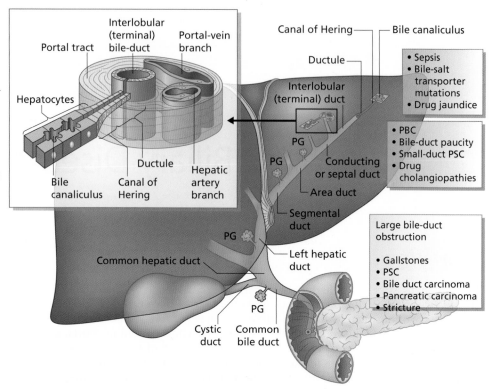

Large bile-duct obstruction

Biopsies from patients with large-duct obstruction are much less often seen than formerly because of improved imaging methods. However, the pathologist needs to be able to recognise the characteristic changes, especially following liver transplantation. From the first weeks of obstruction there is cholestasis in perivenular areas; that is to say, bile is visible under the microscope in the form of bile thrombi (bile plugs) in canaliculi and as yellow-brown pigment in hepatocytes and Kupffer cells (**Fig. 5.2**). The presence of canalicular bile thrombi distinguishes cholestasis from other pigmentations (**see Table 4.1**). Kupffer cells in cholestatic areas are enlarged and pigmented, containing both bile and diastase-resistant periodic acid–Schiff (PAS)-positive material. In recovering obstruction the Kupffer-cell changes persist while bile thrombi become smaller and less numerous. Finally, as in residual acute hepatitis, a few diastase–PAS-positive Kupffer cells may provide the only histological evidence of a recent episode of jaundice.

At first the hepatocytes in areas of cholestasis show little change, but with time they often become swollen. Their nuclei increase in size and number and a few apoptotic bodies and mitoses may be seen, indicating increased cell turnover. Individual hepatocytes or small groups of cells undergo **feathery degeneration**, characterised by rarefied and reticular cytoplasm (**Fig. 5.3**). The lesion is focal and the affected cells are typically surrounded by more or less normal hepatocytes. Feathery degeneration may be difficult to distinguish from the ballooning degeneration of hepatitis (**see Fig. 6.2**)

Table 5.1 Causes of intrahepatic cholestasis

Septicaemia
Drug hepatotoxicity
Bile-salt transporter mutations (e.g. Byler disease)
Extrahepatic lymphoma
Mitochondriopathies (e.g. Navajo neurohepatopathy)
Early large bile-duct obstruction

Figure 5.2
Cholestasis.
Bile is seen in the form of bile thrombi (bile plugs) in dilated canaliculi (C), as well as in Kupffer cells (K). (Needle biopsy, H&E.)

Figure 5.3
Cholestasis.
Small groups of swollen hepatocytes at centre have undergone feathery degeneration. Adjacent hepatocytes appear normal. (Wedge biopsy, H & E.)

or following liver transplantation, but in ballooning the cytoplasm is often granular rather than feathery and the lesion is more widespread in the lobule.

In a minority of patients with obstructed ducts **bile infarcts** form (**Fig. 5.4**). These are substantial areas of hepatocellular degeneration or death containing pale or bile-stained hepatocytes or discrete rounded cells that are difficult to distinguish from macrophages.

Figure 5.4 Large bile-duct obstruction with bile infarct. A bile infarct is seen at the centre of the field near the portal tract. Hepatocyte nuclei are pyknotic within the infarct. Some of the pink strands represent fibrin. (Wedge biopsy, H&E.)

There are variable amounts of bile and fibrin, the latter often abundant. Reticulin fibres become progressively more difficult to demonstrate. Bile eventually leaches out of the infarct to leave a barely pigmented and scarcely stained lesion containing the ghosts of hepatocytes. Small bile infarcts may be found in severe cholestasis from any cause; larger infarcts such as the one shown in **Fig. 5.4**, especially if adjacent to a portal tract, are highly suggestive of bile-duct obstruction. However, because such infarcts are seen in only a minority of patients with obstructed ducts, the diagnosis must usually be established by other criteria.

As a result of these various forms of hepatocellular damage in biliary obstruction, and indeed in cholestasis generally, a certain amount of inflammatory infiltration of the parenchyma is commonly seen after a period of some weeks. This infiltration is usually mild and restricted to the cholestatic areas, unlike the inflammation of an acute hepatitis. When cholestasis resulting from duct obstruction is prolonged, especially in older patients, inflammation and liver-cell damage are occasionally severe enough to raise the alternative possibility of an acute hepatitis. It is then helpful to note that in bile-duct obstruction the liver-cell plates remain for the most part intact, whereas in hepatitis they become irregular as a result of cell loss, swelling and regeneration. Central–portal (zone 3) bridging necrosis is not a feature of biliary obstruction.

Within a few days or weeks of the onset of duct obstruction a characteristic triad of portal changes develops,[5] consisting of portal oedema and swelling (**Fig. 5.5**), infiltration by inflammatory cells, and increased numbers of bile-duct profiles at the margins of the portal tracts (**Figs 5.6, 5.7**). These marginal bile-duct structures are the most consistent finding in the portal tracts and are rarely absent.[5] They may originate from canals of Hering, periportal stem cells or other sources[6] and are an early response to the increased portal tract pressure due to obstruction, circulating mediators[7] and expression of developmental proteins such as Notch receptors and Jagged proteins.[8] The term **ductular reaction** refers to these proliferated bile ductules accompanied by inflammation and stromal changes at the edges of the portal tracts.[9] Usage of 'ductular reaction' is now preferable to 'bile ductular proliferation' or 'typical' and 'atypical' bile ductules, which embody considerable imprecision.[6] The ductular structures may be of normal calibre or dilated, but are

Figure 5.5 Large bile-duct obstruction. The connective tissue of a small portal tract is oedematous. There is little inflammation in this example. (Wedge biopsy, H&E.)

Figure 5.6 Large bile-duct obstruction. A prominent ductular reaction (arrowheads) is present at the edge of an inflamed and oedematous portal tract. The original interlobular duct is marked by an arrow. (Needle biopsy, H&E.)

often flattened with small or imperceptible lumens (**Fig. 5.7**) and variations in nuclear size, staining and location. These structures can be highlighted by immunostaining for cytokeratin 7 or 19 (**see Figs 5.24, 5.25**). Surprisingly, bile is not usually seen within dilated ducts or ductules in uncomplicated obstruction; when it is present, sepsis should be suspected. The differentiation of the ductular reaction of biliary obstruction from that of chronic liver disease has already been discussed in **Chapter 4**.

Figure 5.7
Ductular reaction in large bile-duct obstruction.
The upper left-hand portion of **Fig. 5.6** is shown at higher magnification. The irregular ductular structures at the edge of the portal tract show compressed, narrow lumens and an associated neutrophil infiltrate. (Needle biopsy, H&E.)

Within the oedematous, swollen portal tracts, especially around proliferated bile ducts, an inflammatory infiltrate develops, mediated by the complex interactions of cytokines and cellular adhesion molecules (some produced by biliary epithelium itself[10]) and pro-inflammatory agents such as endotoxin.[3] Neutrophils are prominent owing to the expression of the chemoattractant interleukin-8 by the ductular cells.[11] There may also be other cells including lymphocytes and eosinophils. The presence of a few eosinophils is therefore not in itself sufficient evidence for a diagnosis of drug jaundice. As a result of the proliferative and inflammatory changes of bile-duct obstruction, the outlines of the portal tracts become irregular and the limiting plates of hepatocytes are disrupted to a variable extent. This disruption should be distinguished from interface hepatitis in which the infiltrate is predominantly composed of lymphocytes and plasma cells, and in which the acute inflammatory changes of bile-duct obstruction are not seen.

In a few patients with bile-duct obstruction the portal changes are inconspicuous (**Fig. 5.5**) or even absent. Biliary obstruction should therefore be considered in the differential diagnosis of canalicular cholestasis without portal reaction (so-called 'pure' or 'bland' cholestasis). Conversely, portal changes resembling those of duct obstruction are occasionally found in severe acute hepatitis, when the parenchymal alterations make the diagnosis clear. Sometimes similar portal changes are seen without cholestasis near space-occupying lesions such as metastases,[12] usually together with sinusoidal dilatation. Portal inflammation without cholestasis is also found in patients with disease affecting one or other part of the biliary tree but without current obstruction of the segment biopsied. It is seen in chronic pancreatitis[13] and in patients with acute cholecystitis or choledocholithiasis.[14] Biopsies showing only an increased number of well-differentiated bile ductules at the portal interface, unaccompanied by inflammation or stromal changes, have been noted in patients with idiopathic **isolated ductular hyperplasia** (IDH)[15] (**Fig. 5.8**). These patients have long-standing abnormalities in serum alanine aminotransferase and/or γ-glutamyl transferase, no proven biliary tract disease and an apparently good prognosis (although the cause of this reactive lesion is uncertain).

In a few instances of biliary obstruction, bile escapes from a duct into the connective tissue of a portal tract, giving rise to a *bile extravasate*. This leads to a phagocytic reaction,

Figure 5.8 Isolated ductular hyperplasia.
Well-differentiated hyperplastic bile ductules are present in this biopsy from a patient with persistent liver function test abnormalities unrelated to viral hepatitis or demonstrable biliary disease. The absence of oedema and inflammation help distinguish this lesion from large bile-duct obstruction. (Needle biopsy, H&E.) *Inset*: Immunostain for cytokeratin 7 on a deeper level highlights the bile ductules. (Needle biopsy, specific immunoperoxidase.) (Case kindly provided by Drs Bernard Traub and John B. Herrington, III, Sleepy Hollow, New York, NY, USA.)

with or without foreign-body giant cells (**Fig. 5.9**). Bile extravasates, like large bile infarcts, are almost diagnostic of obstruction but are seen in only a minority of patients. If the extravasate extends beyond the confines of a portal tract into the adjacent parenchyma, the appearances at the periphery of the lesion are very like those of a bile infarct.

Chronic bile-duct obstruction and biliary cirrhosis

When bile duct obstruction persists, the acute inflammatory reaction in the portal tracts is followed by increasing fibrosis. Production of fibrogenic cytokines by bile-duct epithelium contributes to this process.[16] Eventually the tracts are linked by broad fibrous septa. There is a variable degree of acute and chronic inflammatory infiltration, the chronic element less striking than in primary biliary cirrhosis. In some patients the lesion appears to progress more by cholangitis than by obstruction, and cholestasis is therefore not always prominent or even present.

Interference with normal secretion of bile leads to several changes in hepatocytes adjacent to portal tracts and fibrous septa. The cells become swollen and separated by fibrous tissue, inflammatory cells and ductular structures (neocholangioles) derived from hepatocytes or bipotential stem cells.[17] Their cytoplasm is rarefied and may contain visible bile pigment, Mallory bodies, copper and copper-associated protein (**Fig. 5.10**). The last is seen in the form of fine red granules on haematoxylin and eosin (H&E) (**see Fig. 5.27** Inset), staining variably with diastase–PAS and strongly with orcein or Victoria blue. The

Figure 5.9 Large bile-duct obstruction.

Bile extravasate. Bile has escaped from a duct and has evoked a phagocytic reaction. (Needle biopsy, H&E.)

Figure 5.10 Chronic cholestasis.

Hepatocytes near a portal tract (below) are swollen and pale-staining. Many contain Mallory bodies (lower arrow and triple arrow). Bile thrombi are also seen (top arrow). (Wedge biopsy, H&E.)

combination of all these changes is known as **chronic cholestasis** or **cholate stasis (pseudoxanthomatous change, precholestasis)** on the basis that some of the alterations probably result from the accumulation of toxic bile salts. Canalicular cholestasis is sometimes seen between the affected hepatocytes. The hepatocellular changes, ductular proliferation and associated fibrosis in the periportal or periseptal region in effect produce an irregular interface with the parenchyma.[18]

Figure 5.11
Secondary biliary cirrhosis.
Irregular nodules resemble pieces of a jigsaw puzzle. Note the narrow zone of oedema and ductular proliferation at the nodule margin. (Wedge biopsy, H&E.)

The fibrous septa which eventually form in chronic biliary tract disease surround and outline groups of classical hepatic lobules, leaving the normal vascular relationships essentially intact. Islands of parenchyma with characteristic protruding studs resemble the pieces of a jigsaw puzzle or landmasses on a map (**Fig. 5.11**). Spherical nodules are sparse at first, in spite of evidence of liver-cell hyperplasia in the form of thickened liver-cell plates, seen particularly in patients with associated portal hypertension.[19] An occasional rounded parenchymal island may merely represent a tangential section of a complex parenchymal mass such as the one shown in **Fig. 5.11**, rather than a true regeneration nodule of cirrhosis. This is especially common just deep to the liver capsule. A histological diagnosis of cirrhosis should therefore be made with caution, because at a fibrotic, pre-cirrhotic stage considerable resolution can occasionally result if an obstruction is relieved.[20] Eventually, true **secondary biliary cirrhosis** develops, its biliary origin still evident from nodule shape and the regular, broad fibrous septa composed of loose collagen bundles with parallel arrangement (**Fig. 5.12**). A zone of oedema containing proliferated ductules is often diagnostically helpful and may be striking even at low magnification (the 'halo effect') (**Fig. 5.11**). Thus, many different structural characteristics make it possible to diagnose chronic biliary tract disease, even in the absence of cholestasis. Finally, however, an end-stage cirrhosis forms, no longer necessarily recognisable as biliary in origin.

Cholangitis: infection of the biliary tree

In biliary obstruction the inflammatory infiltrate around bile ducts in small portal tracts typically includes neutrophils. There is, therefore, cholangitis in a strictly histological sense, but this does not imply that there must be bacterial infection of the biliary tree or clinical ascending cholangitis. In the latter, neutrophils are more numerous and are found not only around ducts but also in their walls and lumens[21] (**Fig. 5.13**). Paradoxically, interlobular bile ducts are most affected, and larger ducts may appear histologically normal. The wall of a small duct may rupture, leading to abscess formation in the portal

Figure 5.12 Secondary biliary cirrhosis.
Nodules are surrounded by loose bundles of parallel collagen fibres showing little compression. (Wedge biopsy, reticulin.)

Figure 5.13 Acute cholangitis.
Many neutrophil leucocytes are seen in the walls and dilated lumens of the bile ducts, and in the surrounding connective tissue. (Wedge biopsy, H&E.)

tract. Neutrophils are seen in the sinusoids and abscesses may form in the acini. Associated lesions include fibrin thrombi in portal-vein branches, pyelophlebitis and various degrees of parenchymal necrosis,[22] the last probably related to hypoperfusion of the parenchyma. Cholestasis is more often absent than present. Causes of ascending cholangitis include cholecystitis and choledocholithiasis, strictures including those due to primary sclerosing cholangitis, intrahepatic biliary stones,[23] AIDS cholangiopathy,[24,25] pancreatitis, neoplasia of the biliary tree and Caroli's disease. If cholangitis persists or recurs over a period of years, secondary biliary cirrhosis may develop. The histological features are then as described above in the section on bile duct obstruction. Septicaemia uncommonly is associated with a particular form of histological cholangitis principally affecting the canals of Hering.[26] Affected ductules are dilated and filled with inspissated bile. Neutrophils accumulate around and sometimes within them. Larger ducts may be affected, as may the periportal parenchyma in which bile is seen in dilated bile canaliculi. These changes are easily confused with those of large bile-duct obstruction, but in obstruction the inspissated bile in the canals of Hering is not a feature unless there is concomitant sepsis. Sepsis more often gives rise to widespread canalicular cholestasis; the ductular cholestasis pattern (**see Fig. 15.11**) is seen in the minority of septic patients.[26] In the toxic shock syndrome the appearances of the small bile ducts can closely mimic ascending bacterial cholangitis.[27]

Primary sclerosing cholangitis

Primary sclerosing cholangitis (PSC) is characterised by inflammation, strictures and saccular dilatations in the biliary tree. Typically found in adults with ulcerative colitis, it is also seen in neonates and children[28] and in the absence of inflammatory bowel disease. In a few cases the latter is Crohn's disease rather than ulcerative colitis.[29] Any part of the biliary tree may be affected, and involvement of the gallbladder[30] and pancreas[31] has been reported. The gallbladder shows intramural lymphoplasmacytic infiltrates and lymphoid aggregates.[32] Patients do not necessarily have symptoms referable to the liver or abnormal liver function tests.[33] The disease may recur after liver transplantation.[34] Lesions similar to those of primary sclerosing cholangitis have been found in patients given arterial infusion of the anti-cancer drug fluorodeoxyuridine and other[35] chemotherapeutic agents.[36] Obliteration or narrowing of hepatic arteries and portal-vein branches suggests that, in drug-related cases at least, the bile-duct damage may have an ischaemic origin.[37] Systemic vasculitis, liver transplantation-related hepatic artery thrombosis or chronic rejection vasculopathy and, rarely, septic shock[38] are other causes of ischaemic bile-duct injury[39] (ischaemic cholangiopathy).

Final diagnosis of primary sclerosing cholangitis normally rests on cholangiographic demonstration of the characteristic beading of bile ducts, but similar histological features, as described below, may be found in patients with normal cholangiograms. This can be explained on the basis of involvement of the smallest ducts, too small to be seen radiographically.[40] This **small-duct primary sclerosing cholangitis** corresponds approximately to the now obsolete label of 'pericholangitis', when applied to patients without cholangiographic abnormalities. Large- and small-duct forms of the disease frequently coexist.

The features seen on liver biopsy depend in part on the location of strictures in relation to the biopsy site. If the biopsy is taken from a part of the liver unaffected by the primary disease but proximal to a stricture, then the changes, if any, will simply be those of bile-duct obstruction or cholangitis. The presence of chronic inflammation may lead to confusion with chronic hepatitis. If, on the other hand, the biopsy site is affected by the primary disease, there may be one or more features suggesting the diagnosis. These include periduct oedema and concentric fibrosis (**Fig. 5.14**), ductular proliferation, portal inflammation and atrophy or disappearance of the small ducts (**Fig. 5.15**). Loss of ducts is the commonest finding in the smallest portal tracts, while periduct fibrosis is typical of medium-sized tracts.[41] Major bile ducts, as seen for example in explanted livers at transplantation, may be inflamed, ulcerated or dilated. They may also rupture, producing a perihilar **xanthogranulomatous cholangitis**.[42]

Loss of interlobular bile ducts from the smallest portal tracts can be assessed only in biopsy samples of adequate size, that is to say, containing several portal tracts. While interlobular ducts are not necessarily seen in all tracts because of the plane of section, arteries provide a useful guide; from 70–80%[43] to 92%[44] of arteries are normally

Figure 5.14
Primary sclerosing cholangitis.
A bile duct is surrounded by a cuff of oedematous, inflamed fibrous tissue with an 'onion-skin' appearance. (Needle biopsy, H&E.)

Figure 5.15
Primary sclerosing cholangitis.
The inflamed portal tract lacks a bile duct. An aggregate of lymphocytes to the left of a small hepatic arteriole at the centre of the field is likely the former site of the duct. Inflammation extends into the adjacent parenchyma and there is interface hepatitis to the right of the portal tract. (Wedge biopsy, H&E.)

accompanied by a duct lying near the centre of a portal tract. If there is doubt, for instance because ducts are difficult to identify in an inflammatory infiltrate, immunostaining of duct-associated cytokeratins is helpful.[45] Suitable antibodies include AE-1 (Signet) and other antibodies against cytokeratins 7 and 19. In the presence of a ductular reaction, identification and counting of interlobular bile ducts are sometimes difficult.

The concentric fibrosis around medium-sized ducts is not entirely diagnostic, since it is occasionally found in other forms of biliary disease such as hepatolithiasis.[46] It is,

Figure 5.16
Primary sclerosing cholangitis.
The bile duct in a large portal tract has been replaced by a fibrous scar (S). (Wedge biopsy, H&E.)

however, a very helpful finding. The lamellar pattern of the fibrosis gives an 'onion-skin' appearance. The cuff of connective tissue around the duct may be oedematous and pale-staining or sclerotic, depending on the stage of the process. Inflammatory cells are seen in small numbers lying between the layers of collagen. The duct epithelium may show various degrees of atrophy, and sometimes disappears entirely, leaving a characteristic rounded fibro-obliterative scar[47] (**Fig. 5.16**). Staining with diastase–PAS often reveals irregular or regular thickening of the basement membrane material around both scarred and unscarred ducts.[48] In long-standing or severe cases, portal fibrosis gradually increases, fibrous septa form and secondary biliary cirrhosis may develop. In some patients, on the other hand, the lesions remain mild and clinically insignificant for many[29] years.[33] Portal tract fibrogenesis in sclerosing cholangitis and in primary biliary cirrhosis is in part attributed to an increased number of intrahepatic mast cells compared with other chronic liver diseases.[49] In fact, systemic mastocytosis has been associated with cholestasis[50] and a case of PSC.[51]

Parenchymal changes in PSC are usually less striking than the portal ones. Cholestasis may be seen as a result of large-duct obstruction or small-duct loss. In the later stages, the cholestasis is typically of the chronic type, with accumulation of copper and copper-associated protein. Extension of portal tract lymphoplasmacytic infiltrates into the peri-portal parenchyma (interface hepatitis) is common but not as a rule severe (**Fig. 5.15**). However, more severe interface hepatitis may be seen in patients with an unfavourable clinical course[29] or in an overlap syndrome with autoimmune hepatitis. In children, the combination of autoimmune hepatitis and PSC is well recognised.[52] Liver cells may undergo hyperplasia, indicated by thickening of cell plates.

Histological assessment of liver biopsies in patients with an established diagnosis of PSC is important for prognosis. Ludwig and colleagues[40,53,54] have proposed a histological staging system based on essential and non-essential features. The stages correspond approximately to those of primary biliary cirrhosis: they are respectively designated portal, periportal, septal, and cirrhotic.

Figure 5.17 Cholangiocarcinoma in primary sclerosing cholangitis.
Carcinoma has developed in the bile duct at left, still surrounded by periduct fibrosis (F). Invasive glands (arrows) are seen in the adjacent stroma. (Explanted liver, H&E.)

Figure 5.18 Bile duct dysplasia in primary sclerosing cholangitis.
The epithelium of the right portion of the bile duct is crowded, adenomatous and shows nuclear atypia. (Operative specimen, H&E.)

There is an increased risk of carcinoma of the biliary tree in patients with sclerosing cholangitis[55] (**Fig. 5.17**) who may also have dysplasia of interlobular and septal bile ducts[56] (**Fig. 5.18**) and gallbladder,[57] including papillary bile-duct dysplastic lesions.[58] The same risk of carcinoma does not appear to apply to the small duct form of PSC.[59]

The main **differential diagnosis** of PSC is from chronic hepatitis, primary biliary cirrhosis and other forms of chronic biliary tract disease. In **chronic hepatitis** bile-duct numbers are normal, periduct fibrosis is not seen and cholestasis is very uncommon. Stains for copper and copper-associated protein are negative or near-negative unless cirrhosis has developed.[60] **Primary biliary cirrhosis** closely resembles PSC in its later stages, and firm diagnosis usually requires cholangiography and testing for antimitochondrial antibodies. However, the typical granulomatous cholangitis of primary biliary cirrhosis is not a feature of sclerosing cholangitis, although granulomas are very occasionally found in the liver. Substantial chronic inflammation of portal tracts with or without lymphoid follicles favours primary biliary cirrhosis. Conversely, fibrous obliteration of ducts is much more characteristic of sclerosing cholangitis, and there is often dense portal fibrosis with relatively little inflammation. The main difference from **other chronic biliary diseases** is the loss of ducts and interface hepatitis. There is occasionally confusion between the focal duct dilatations of **Caroli's disease** and the cholangiectases which are typically seen in the large and medium-sized bile ducts in primary sclerosing cholangitis.[47,61] **IgG4-associated cholangitis** (IAC), a steroid-sensitive, autoimmune cholangiopathy, also needs consideration since it causes histological changes similar to PSC.[62,63] This condition is part of the spectrum of autoimmune diseases featuring IgG4-positive plasma cells and sclerosis which also includes autoimmune pancreatitis and certain cases of inflammatory pseudotumour.[64] Like PSC, the large ducts in IAC are surrounded by dense lymphoplasmacytic infiltrates (often with lymphoid aggregates and follicles), but in IAC the infiltrates extend deeply into the soft tissues surrounding the ducts with entrapment of nerves and obliterative phlebitis of large-calibre veins. In contrast to other chronic biliary diseases where IgG4-positive plasma cells are absent or sparse, IAC shows numerous IgG4-positive plasma cells on immunostaining (>25–30 per medium power field[62]). A subgroup of more clinically aggressive PSC cases may also show such increased IgG4+ plasma cells.[64a] Liver biopsies in IAC show portal tract infiltrates of lymphocytes, eosinophils and increased IgG4+ plasma cells (>5–10 per high power field).[65,65a] The inflammation is accentuated around portal vein branches and portal connective tissue is widened by storiform fibro-inflammatory nodules.[65a]

Primary biliary cirrhosis

Primary biliary cirrhosis (PBC), generally regarded as an autoimmune disease, is characterised by a chronic non-suppurative destructive cholangitis, which can eventually lead to cirrhosis.[66] For much of its course the term 'cirrhosis' is not strictly applicable, but the name survives despite this inconsistency. PBC typically presents in middle life, but may also be found in the elderly, younger adults and uncommonly in adolescents.[67] Women are about ten times as commonly affected as men. In symptomatic patients the onset is insidious, with itching as the commonest presenting symptom. Jaundice and histological cholestasis are usually absent in the early years of the disease. Characteristic findings on investigation of both symptomatic and asymptomatic patients include raised level serum alkaline phosphatase and the presence of antimitochondrial antibodies (AMAs). The antibodies are specifically the M2 type, directed against inner mitochondrial membrane autoantigens, which are members of the 2-oxo-acid dehydrogenase complex (2-OADC) of enzymes.[68] The most common of these antibodies reacts with the E2 subunit of the pyruvate dehydrogenase complex (PDC-E2). AMAs can be detected in more than 90% of patients. Serum IgM values are typically elevated.[69] Current hypotheses suggest that expression of 2-OADC antigens on bile-duct epithelium together with appropriate class II histocompatibility antigens, production of antimitochondrial antibodies and T-lymphocyte response[70] mediate the bile-duct damage in PBC.[71] Cross-reactivity of human AMAs with bacterial antigens on *Escherichia coli* and other organisms that may infect patients with PBC has been suggested in the 'molecular mimicry' hypothesis.[72] Dysregulation of interleukin-12 signalling may also be involved.[73]

PBC is associated with a wide range of other conditions, many of them regarded as autoimmune in origin. The commonest association is with the sicca complex of dry eyes and mouth.[74] Others include scleroderma, thyroiditis, rheumatoid arthritis, membranous glomerulonephritis and coeliac disease.

Table 5.2 Stages of primary biliary cirrhosis
1. The florid duct lesion; portal hepatitis
2. Ductular reaction and periportal hepatitis
3. Scarring; bridging necrosis, septal fibrosis
4. Cirrhosis

Liver biopsy plays an important part in diagnosis throughout the often-long course of the disease. Four histological stages have been described[53,66,75] (**Table 5.2**). These are not always easy to determine in needle biopsies, partly because the lesions of PBC are unevenly distributed within the liver and partly because the stages overlap. For example, stage 1 bile-duct lesions and granulomas are sometimes seen in an established cirrhosis. From a practical point of view, however, the pathologist is usually able to decide whether the disease appears to be still in stage 1, with lesions more or less restricted to enlarged portal tracts, or whether it has extended to a significant degree into the adjacent parenchyma, with consequent alteration of acinar structure (the progressive lesion; stages 2, 3 or 4). This is of some clinical importance, because stage 1 often lasts for many years and the prognosis is therefore relatively favourable, especially in patients without symptoms referable to the liver. Having established in other patients that the disease has progressed beyond stage 1, the pathologist may also be able to determine with reasonable confidence that cirrhosis has developed. The patient is then at increased risk for hepatocellular carcinoma,[76,77] sometimes preceded by macroregenerative nodule formation.[78] However, other risk factors such as hepatitis C virus infection must be considered in patients with PBC who develop carcinoma.[79] Because different sets of differential diagnoses should be considered for the portal and the progressive lesion, these are considered separately in the following section.

The portal lesion of primary biliary cirrhosis

The bile-duct damage characteristic of early PBC mainly affects the septal and larger interlobular ducts, while the smaller interlobular ducts remain intact until later. The epithelium of the affected ducts becomes irregular and is infiltrated with lymphocytes. The basement membrane becomes disrupted, and the duct may rupture (**Fig. 5.19**). An inflammatory infiltrate is seen around or to one side of the duct. The denser parts of this infiltrate are

Figure 5.19 Primary biliary cirrhosis.

A damaged large interlobular bile duct shows an irregular configuration, partly attenuated epithelium and intra-epithelial inflammatory cells. The surrounding infiltrate is rich in lymphocytes and plasma cells. (Wedge biopsy, H&E.)

mainly composed of lymphocytes, which may form aggregates or follicles with germinal centres (**Fig. 5.20**). Elsewhere there is a mixture of plasma cells (often abundant), eosinophils and neutrophils. The eosinophils contribute to bile-duct damage, granuloma formation and other aspects of the inflammatory response by releasing mediators which are located within their granules.[80] The biochemical and/or histological improvement seen in certain patients treated with ursodeoxycholic acid appears to be attributable in part to inhibition of eosinophil degranulation.[81] Of the various histological features of the disease, interface hepatitis appears to be the most resistant to improvement with ursodeoxycholic acid.[82]

In line with the presence of elevated serum IgM in individuals with PBC is the predominance of IgM-positive plasma cells in the portal tract plasmacytic infiltrates.[83] Specific IgM immunostaining can therefore be diagnostically useful (and contrasts with the IgG-predominant plasma cells seen in autoimmune hepatitis[83,83a]).

Granulomas are present in many patients although they are not necessarily seen in small biopsies; their absence does not therefore exclude the diagnosis. They take a variety of forms,[84] ranging from well-defined granulomas like those of sarcoidosis or tuberculosis (**Fig. 5.21**) to small focal collections of histiocytoid cells. Alternatively, there may be a substantial component of histiocytes or epithelioid cells within the inflammatory infiltrate, without formation of identifiable localised granulomas. A few intra-acinar granulomas may also be present, but large numbers should suggest the diagnosis of other granulomatous diseases (**see Ch. 15**).

Not all liver biopsies from patients in this stage of the disease show the typical bile-duct lesions, so that a firm histological diagnosis cannot always be made. Small portal tracts may merely show 'non-specific' portal inflammation, in which case step sections may make the true diagnosis clear by revealing bile-duct lesions or granulomas. In a small number of patients with the **premature ductopenic variant** of PBC,[85] widespread bile-duct destruction and loss are accelerated at an early stage before the development of fibrosis or cirrhosis, with worse pruritus and clinical evidence of chronic cholestasis than would be anticipated.

Although in the first stage of PBC the lesions are by definition mainly portal, slight disruption of the limiting plate is common. Sinusoids may be infiltrated by lymphocytes,

**Figure 5.20
Primary biliary cirrhosis.**
A lymphoid aggregate and a follicle with a germinal centre (arrow) are seen near an inflamed duct with stratified epithelium. (Wedge biopsy, H&E.)

Figure 5.21
Primary biliary cirrhosis.
A well-formed epithelioid-cell granuloma (G) has formed near a damaged bile duct (arrow). The background infiltrate contains many lymphocytes, plasma cells and scattered eosinophils. (Needle biopsy, H&E.)

Kupffer cells are prominent and there may be focal necrosis[86] and thickening of liver-cell plates. Nodular regenerative hyperplasia, best recognised in reticulin preparations, is common even at this stage,[87,88] and together with portal vein narrowing[89] helps to explain the portal hypertension which frequently precedes the development of significant fibrosis or cirrhosis. Foci of small hepatocytes with basophilic cytoplasm and hyperchromatic nuclei (small-cell dysplasia) or hepatocytes with enlarged, pleomorphic nuclei (large-cell dysplasia) are occasionally found.[90]

Canalicular cholestasis is unusual in early PBC unless there is a complicating factor such as steroid-induced jaundice. Cholestasis of the chronic type (cholate stasis) does not develop until later, although small amounts of copper-associated protein are occasionally seen in periportal hepatocytes.

The **differential diagnosis of early primary biliary cirrhosis** includes other causes of portal inflammation and of bile-duct damage. The differentiation from **primary sclerosing cholangitis** was discussed earlier. In this disease duct atrophy and fibrosis predominate and granulomas are unusual. **Drug injury** occasionally leads to bile-duct damage, but the ducts affected are smaller than those in early PBC; other parenchymal changes (fat, hepatocyte ballooning and apoptosis) are often present and the lesion is seen in the clinical context of an acutely jaundiced patient. Amoxicillin–clavulanic acid hepatotoxicity is an example of PBC-like, eosinophil-rich bile-duct damage.[91] Bile ducts are often abnormal in acute and chronic **viral hepatitis**, especially hepatitis C.[92] In hepatitis the epithelium of the affected ducts may be abnormal in only part of its circumference (**Fig. 6.7**), and is typically stratified and vacuolated.[93] The surrounding infiltrate is almost entirely composed of lymphocytes, with few plasma cells or segmented leucocytes and no granulomas. Large numbers of eosinophils, sometimes seen in PBC,[94] are rare. In doubtful cases the clinical context and laboratory investigations usually make the diagnosis clear. Because in viral hepatitis the duct damage is focal and does not lead to extensive duct loss, the clinical and biochemical picture is not necessarily cholestatic. Other causes of bile-duct damage include **autoimmune hepatitis**,[95] **bile-duct obstruction with suppuration**, **graft-versus-host disease** and **rejection of a grafted liver**. The last two situations are discussed in **Chapter 16**. Two rare causes of bile-duct damage associated with granulomas are **fascioliasis** and **sarcoidosis**, but in general this association strongly supports a diagnosis of PBC.

Figure 5.22
Primary biliary
cirrhosis.
Aggregates of
lymphocytes
(arrows) mark the
former sites of bile
ducts in this
inflamed, fibrotic
liver. The picture is
very typical of the
progressive phase of
the disease. (Needle
biopsy, H&E.)

The progressive lesion of primary biliary cirrhosis

The disease now extends beyond the confines of the portal tracts and there is increasing fibrosis and alteration of acinar architecture. Bile-duct damage is less dramatic and granulomas are fewer, but there is a progressive fall in duct numbers. Duct numbers are best assessed in relation to arteries,[43] as already discussed in relation to PSC. The sites of former ducts are marked by aggregates of lymphocytes (**Fig. 5.22**). These sometimes show compression artefact, with rupture of lymphocyte nuclei. The inflammatory reaction may also obliterate periductal capillaries.[96]

The portal tracts expand progressively as the inflammatory process begins to extend from them into the adjacent parenchyma. At this time two apparently separate processes affect the future course of the disease. The first comprises a combination of biliary and cholestatic features, probably related to bile duct loss, while the second closely resembles the interface hepatitis of chronic hepatitis.[18,97] The earliest and often most obvious biliary feature is a ductular reaction (**Fig. 5.23**). For a time this allows bile to drain from the parenchyma into the main ducts in spite of destruction of the medium-sized ducts.[98] It is almost always associated with an infiltrate of neutrophils, so that it needs to be distinguished from the duct tortuosity and inflammation of mechanical bile-duct obstruction. The ductular reaction of PBC, and indeed of PSC, is often focal, representing a system of bypass channels in relation to a local interruption of bile flow through the duct system. If the ductular structures are partly obscured by inflammation and fibrosis (**Fig. 5.24**), they can be highlighted by immunostaining for cytokeratin 7 or 19 (**Fig. 5.25**).

Loss of bile ducts also leads to the chronic form of cholestasis marked by swelling of hepatocytes, bile staining, Mallory body formation and accumulation of copper (**Fig. 5.26**) and copper-associated protein (**Fig. 5.27**). Bile plugs are sometimes seen in canaliculi in the affected areas around portal tracts and septa, but more widespread canalicular cholestasis often reflects hepatocellular failure or associated sepsis. There may be many lipid-laden macrophages, forming diffuse or localised xanthomas.

**Figure 5.23
Primary biliary
cirrhosis.**

A widened portal
tract shows chronic
inflammation and a
ductular reaction,
but no native bile
duct. The margins of
the tract are blurred
by fibrosis and
interface hepatitis.
(Wedge biopsy,
H&E.)

**Figure 5.24
Stage 3 primary
biliary cirrhosis.**

The portal tract is
chronically inflamed
and fibrotic, without
a readily identified
bile duct. A ductular
reaction is present,
but obscured by the
inflammation and
fibrosis. Cholestasis
is present at the
periphery of the
lobule (arrow).
(Needle biopsy,
H&E.)

In addition to the cholestatic features described above, interface hepatitis of the classical, lymphoplasmacytic type is common in the progressive stage of PBC.[18] The infiltrate is rich in activated T cells.[97,99,100] Because this hepatocellular component is a regular feature of PBC, the finding of interface hepatitis together with the biliary features of PBC should not by itself lead to the diagnosis of an overlap syndrome (see below). Lymphocytes also form bridge-like extensions into the acini, and may be the forerunners of fibrous septa.[101]

Figure 5.25 Stage 3 primary biliary cirrhosis. The ductular reaction is highlighted by cytokeratin 7 immunostaining of a serial section of the same biopsy shown in **Fig. 5.24**. (Needle biopsy, specific immunoperoxidase.)

Figure 5.26 Primary biliary cirrhosis. Heavy accumulation of copper-rich granules is seen in hepatocytes. Note the different colour of the canalicular bile thrombus slightly below centre. (Needle biopsy, rhodanine.)

An increased number of intrahepatic mast cells is also present, which may have contributed to portal tract fibrosis.[49] Necrosis of perivenular hepatocytes has been noted.[86] There is therefore a histological resemblance to hepatitis. Hepatocellular dysplasia of small- or large-cell type may be present.[90]

The combination of cholestatic and hepatitic processes leads to increasing fibrosis. Portal inflammation diminishes, but lymphoid aggregates continue to mark the former

Figure 5.27
Primary biliary cirrhosis.
Granular deposits of copper-associated protein have accumulated in hepatocytes near a fibrous septum (below) at a late stage of the disease. (Needle biopsy, Orcein.) *Inset*: Copper-associated protein in hepatocytes near the portal tract (PT) appears as fine red cytoplasmic granules. (Needle biopsy, H&E.)

Table 5.3 Causes of bile-duct damage and loss	
Loss of ducts	**Little or no loss**
Primary sclerosing cholangitis	Bile-duct obstruction
Primary biliary cirrhosis	Viral hepatitis
Idiopathic ductopenia	Drug jaundice
Graft-versus-host disease	Parasitic duct disease
Chronic rejection of liver grafts	
Sarcoidosis	
Drug jaundice*	

* Note that while many drugs produce bile duct injury without loss, there are also well-described cases where ductopenia and chronic cholestatic disease (sometimes requiring liver transplantation) are sequelae of drug hepatotoxicity.

sites of bile ducts (**Fig. 5.28**). Septa extend from the portal tracts and eventually come to link portal tracts to each other and to terminal hepatic venules.[101] In patients in whom the biliary and cholestatic features predominate, the cirrhosis which ultimately develops is generally of the biliary type. When hepatitic features predominate, the cirrhosis tends to be of post-hepatitis type. All combinations of the two patterns may be seen.[102] Nodules often develop unevenly throughout the liver, so that nodular areas with the appearance of cirrhosis coexist with areas in which the acinar architecture remains preserved.

The **differential diagnosis of the progressive lesion** includes **primary sclerosing cholangitis** and **other forms of chronic biliary disease**, on the one hand, and **chronic hepatitis** on the other.[103] The differentiation from primary PSC was discussed earlier; in the later stages of the two diseases it is often impossible to make the distinction histologically. With respect to other forms of chronic biliary obstruction and chronic hepatitis, the most important observation is that bile duct numbers remain normal in both, whereas they are characteristically reduced in PBC and in PSC (**Table 5.3**). Granulomas favour PBC over chronic hepatitis, as does chronic cholestasis, particularly when it is seen in the absence of cirrhosis.[60] Difficulties remain even after these factors are taken into account, especially if the biopsy specimen is small or fragmented. They can usually be resolved by consideration of

Figure 5.28
Primary biliary cirrhosis.
There is extensive scarring without nodule formation. Aggregates of lymphocytes mark the former sites of bile ducts, as in **Fig. 5.22**. (Post-mortem liver, H&E.)

the clinical context and laboratory investigations; a middle-aged woman with itching, high levels of serum alkaline phosphatase and AMAs is unlikely to be suffering from chronic viral hepatitis. There are, however, unusual cases which present as overlap syndromes, discussed briefly below.

Overlap syndromes, transitional diseases and autoimmune cholangitis

Establishing a clear-cut diagnosis of PBC or PSC is occasionally problematic when an unusually severe degree of lymphoplasmacytic interface hepatitis is superimposed on otherwise typical histopathological features of either disease (**Fig. 5.29**), raising the possibility of an **overlap syndrome**[104] with AIH. Such patients may show a mix of serum autoantibodies (some of which may be merely non-specific markers of immune disease), further clouding the diagnosis. In some instances there appears to be a genetic predilection for the hepatitic component, as in certain cases of PBC where a specific histocompatibility profile is present.[105] Rendering a diagnosis of either PBC/AIH or PSC/AIH overlap syndrome therefore requires close consultation between pathologist and clinician, taking into account and appropriately weighting the biopsy features, serological and biochemical data and cholangiographic findings.[52,104] Use of the clinicopathological scoring systems developed for AIH may be helpful in some cases.[106–108] The diagnostic dilemma of putative 'overlap' cases resides in the current imprecision in defining the individual outermost diagnostic borders of PBC, PSC and AIH,[109] insensitivity of tests used to detect serum mitochondrial antibodies,[69] non-specific generation of various autoantibodies and superimposition of histological features that may cloud the true diagnosis. A pathological diagnosis of overlap syndrome should therefore be made with due restraint whenever possible and only after careful examination of all the biopsy features, including bile-duct morphology, evidence of chronic cholestasis, lobular necroinflammatory changes and interface hepatitis.

Figure 5.29 Overlap syndrome.
Biopsy from a young patient with ulcerative colitis, but clinicopathological and serological features suggesting primary sclerosing cholangitis–autoimmune hepatitis overlap syndrome. The biopsy features of biliary disease include abnormal bile-duct morphology (B), portal oedema and periduct fibrosis (arrow), while the extensive interface hepatitis (arrowheads) suggests an autoimmune component. (Needle biopsy, H&E.)

The interrelatedness of PBC, PSC and AIH as disorders of cellular immunity[110] is further highlighted by descriptions of clinical **transition** from one form to another. Such examples include cases of PBC progressing to AIH,[111,112] AIH progressing to PSC,[113] paediatric PSC patients with autoimmune serological and histopathological features,[114] and transplanted PBC patients who develop AIH in their allografts.[115]

A number of patients with typical biopsy features of PBC but no demonstrable serum AMAs have been described as cases of **autoimmune cholangitis** because of coexistent antinuclear or other autoantibodies, occasional corticosteroid responsiveness and other features that suggest an autoimmune clinical profile.[116] Such cases may reflect problems in the sensitivity of current mitochondrial antibody tests and are now usually considered to be examples of AMA-negative PBC.[69,104]

Other disorders with intrahepatic bile-duct loss

As indicated earlier, the loss of significant numbers of intrahepatic bile ducts (ductopenia) can be seen not only in PBC and PSC but also in several conditions listed in **Table 5.1**. In addition to these, there are patients in whom the pathogenesis of duct loss is poorly understood. Some of these may represent later stages of childhood **non-syndromatic paucity of intrahepatic bile ducts**.[117] In patients with **idiopathic adulthood ductopenia (IAD)** – predominantly males with cholestatic biochemical profiles – duct loss could also be the end result of small-duct PSC or due to bile-duct damage associated with chronic hepatitis C[118] or autoimmune cholangitis.[119] Rarely, IAD is familial.[120] Ductopenia due to the paraneoplastic effects of **Hodgkin's disease** was reported.[121] A group of asymptomatic patients with idiopathic ductopenia and elevated serum γ-glutamyl transferase activity has also been described.[122]

References

1 Jansen PLM, Sturm E. Genetic cholestasis, causes and consequences for hepatobiliary transport. *Liver Int* 2003; **23**: 315–322.

2 Lee WS, Sokol RJ. Mitochondrial hepatopathies: advances in genetics and pathogenesis. *Hepatology* 2007; **45**: 1555–1565.

3 Crawford JM, Boyer JL. Clinicopathology conferences: inflammation-induced cholestasis. *Hepatology* 1998; **28**: 253–260.

4 Turkish A, Levy J, Kato M, et al. Pancreatitis and paraneoplastic cholestasis as presenting manifestations of pancreatic lymphoma: evaluation, management, and clinical course in a child. *J Pediatr Gastroenterol Nutr* 2004; **39**: 552–556.

5 Christoffersen P, Poulsen H. Histological changes in human liver biopsies following extrahepatic biliary obstruction. *Acta Pathol Microbiol Scand* 1970; **212**: 150–157.

6 Roskams TA, Theise ND, Balabaud C, et al. Nomenclature of the finer branches of the biliary tree: canals, ductules, and ductular reactions in human livers. *Hepatology* 2004; **39**: 1739–1745.

7 LeSage G, Glaser S, Alpini G. Regulation of cholangiocyte proliferation. *Liver* 2001; **21**: 73–80.

8 Nijjar SS, Wallace L, Crosby HA, et al. Altered Notch ligand expression in human liver disease. Further evidence for a role of the Notch signaling pathway in hepatic neovascularization and biliary ductular defects. *Am J Pathol* 2002; **160**: 1695–1703.

9 Gaya DR, Thorburn KA, Oien KA, et al. Hepatic granulomas: a 10 year single centre experience. *J Clin Pathol* 2003; **56**: 850–853.

10 Liver transplantation database (LTD) investigators, Sakamoto T, Ezure T, et al. Interleukin-6, hepatocyte growth factor, and their receptors in biliary epithelial cells during a type I ductular reaction in mice: interactions between the periductal inflammatory and stromal cells and the biliary epithelium. *Hepatology* 1998; **28**: 1260–1268.

11 Isse K, Harada K, Nakanuma Y. IL-8 expression by biliary epithelial cells is associated with neutrophilic infiltration and reactive bile ductules. *Liver Int* 2007; **27**: 672–680.

12 Gerber MA, Thung SN, Bodenheimer HC Jr, et al. Characteristic histologic triad in liver adjacent to metastatic neoplasm. *Liver* 1986; **6**: 85–88.

13 Wilson C, Auld CD, Schlinkert R, et al. Hepatobiliary complications in chronic pancreatitis. *Gut* 1989; **30**: 520–527.

14 Flinn WR, Olson DF, Oyasu R, et al. Biliary bacteria and hepatic histopathologic changes in gallstone disease. *Ann Surg* 1977; **185**: 593–597.

15 Sonzogni A, Colloredo G, Fabris L, et al. Isolated idiopathic bile ductular hyperplasia in patients with persistently abnormal liver function tests. *J Hepatol* 2004; **40**: 592–598.

16 Lewindon PJ, Pereira TN, Hoskins AC, et al. The role of hepatic stellate cells and transforming growth factor-beta-1 in cystic fibrosis liver disease. *Am J Pathol* 2002; **160**: 1705–1715.

17 Zhang L, Theise N, Chua M, et al. The stem cell niche of human livers: symmetry between development and regeneration. *Hepatology* 2008; **48**: 1598–1607.

18 Portmann B, Popper H, Neuberger J, et al. Sequential and diagnostic features in primary biliary cirrhosis based on serial histologic study in 209 patients. *Gastroenterology* 1985; **88**: 1777–1790.

19 Weinbren K, Hadjis NS, Blumgart LH. Structural aspects of the liver in patients with biliary disease and portal hypertension. *J Clin Pathol* 1985; **38**: 1013–1020.

20 Hammel P, Couvelard A, O'Toole D, et al. Regression of liver fibrosis after biliary drainage in patients with chronic pancreatitis and stenosis of the common bile duct. *N Engl J Med* 2001; **344**: 418–423.

21 Carpenter HA. Bacterial and parasitic cholangitis. *Mayo Clin Proc* 1998; **73**: 473–478.

22 Shimada H, Nihmoto S, Matsuba A, et al. Acute cholangitis: a histopathologic study. *J Clin Gastroenterol* 1988; **10**: 197–200.

23 Sasaki M, Nakanuma Y, Kim YS. Expression of apomucins in the intrahepatic biliary tree in hepatolithiasis differs from that in normal liver and extrahepatic biliary obstruction. *Hepatology* 1998; **27**: 46–53.

24 Bouche H, Housset C, Dumont JL, et al. AIDS-related cholangitis: diagnostic features and course in 15 patients. *J Hepatol* 1993; **17**: 34–39.

25 Pol S, Romana CA, Richard S, et al. Microsporidia infection in patients with the human immunodeficiency virus and unexplained cholangitis. *N Engl J Med* 1993; **328**: 95–99.

26 Lefkowitch JH. Bile ductular cholestasis: an ominous histopathologic sign related to sepsis and 'cholangitis lenta'. *Hum Pathol* 1982; **13**: 19–24.

27 Ishak KG, Rogers WA. Cryptogenic acute cholangitis – association with toxic shock syndrome. *Am J Clin Pathol* 1981; **76**: 619–626.

28 Wilschanski M, Chait P, Wade JA, et al. Primary sclerosing cholangitis in 32 children: clinical, laboratory and radiographic features, with survival analysis. *Hepatology* 1995; **22**: 1415–1422.

29 Aadland E, Schrumpf E, Fausa O, et al. Primary sclerosing cholangitis: a long-term follow-up study. *Scand J Gastroenterol* 1987; **22**: 655–664.

30 Jeffrey GP, Reed DW, Carrello S, et al. Histological and immunohistochemical study of the gall bladder lesion in primary sclerosing cholangitis. *Gut* 1991; **32**: 424–429.

31 Kawaguchi K, Koike M, Tsuruta K, et al. Lymphoplasmacytic sclerosing pancreatitis with cholangitis: a variant of primary sclerosing cholangitis extensively involving pancreas. *Hum Pathol* 1991; **22**: 387–395.

32 Abraham SC, Cruz-Correa M, Argani P, et al. Lymphoplasmacytic chronic cholecystitis and biliary tract disease in patients with lymphoplasmacytic sclerosing pancreatitis. *Am J Surg Pathol* 2003; **27**: 441–451.

33 Broome U, Glaumann H, Hultcrantz R. Liver histology and follow up of 68 patients with ulcerative colitis and normal liver function tests. *Gut* 1990; **31**: 468–472.

34 Graziadei IW, Wiesner RH, Batts KP, et al. Recurrence of primary sclerosing cholangitis following liver transplantation. *Hepatology* 1999; **29**: 1050–1056.

35 Kemeny MM, Battifora H, Blayney DW, et al. Sclerosing cholangitis after continuous hepatic artery infusion of FUDR. *Ann Surg* 1985; **202**: 176–181.

36 Herrmann G, Lorenz M, Kirkowa-Reimann M, et al. Morphological changes after intra-arterial chemotherapy of the liver. *Hepatogastroenterology* 1987; **34**: 5–9.

37 Ludwig J, Kim CH, Wiesner RH, et al. Floxuridine-induced sclerosing cholangitis: an ischemic cholangiopathy? *Hepatology* 1989; **9**: 215–218.

38 Engler S, Elsing C, Flechtenmacher C, et al. Progressive sclerosing cholangitis after shock: a new variant of vanishing bile duct disorders. *Gut* 2003; **52**: 688–693.

39 Deltenre P, Valla D-C. Ischemic cholangiopathy. *J Hepatol* 2006; **44**: 806–817.

40 Ludwig J. Small-duct primary sclerosing cholangitis. *Semin Liver Dis* 1991; **11**: 11–17.

41 Harrison RF, Hubscher SG. The spectrum of bile duct lesions in end-stage primary sclerosing cholangitis. *Histopathology* 1991; **19**: 321–327.

42 Keaveny AP, Gordon FD, Goldar-Najafi A, et al. Native liver xanthogranulomatous cholangiopathy in primary sclerosing cholangitis: impact on posttransplant outcome. *Liver Transplant* 2004; **10**: 115–122.

43 Nakanuma Y, Ohta G. Histometric and serial section observations of the intrahepatic bile ducts in primary biliary cirrhosis. *Gastroenterology* 1979; **76**: 1326–1332.

44 Crawford AR, Lin X-Z, Crawford JM. The normal adult human liver biopsy: a quantitative reference standard. *Hepatology* 1998; **28**: 323–331.

45 Van Eyken P, Sciot R, Desmet VJ. A cytokeratin immunohistochemical study of cholestatic liver disease: evidence that hepatocytes can express 'bile duct-type' cytokeratins. *Histopathology* 1989; **15**: 125–135.

46 Nakanuma Y, Yamaguchi K, Ohta G, et al. Pathological features of hepatolithiasis in Japan. *Hum Pathol* 1988; **19**: 1181–1186.

47 Ludwig J, MacCarty RL, LaRusso NF, et al. Intrahepatic cholangiectases and large-duct obliteration in primary sclerosing cholangitis. *Hepatology* 1986; **6**: 560–568.

48 Fleming KA. Interlobular bile duct basement membrane thickening – a specific marker for primary sclerosing cholangitis (PSC)? *J Pathol* 1993; **169** Suppl: (Abstract).

49 Farrell DJ, Hines JE, Walls AF, et al. Intrahepatic mast cells in chronic liver diseases. *Hepatology* 1995; **22**: 1175–1181.

50 Safyan EL, Veerabagu MP, Swerdlow SH, et al. Intrahepatic cholestasis due to systemic mastocytosis: a case report and review of literature. *Am J Gastroenterol* 1997; **92**: 1197–1200.

51 Baron TH, Koehler RE, Rodgers WH, et al. Mast cell cholangiopathy: another cause of sclerosing cholangitis. *Gastroenterology* 1995; **109**: 1677–1681.

52 Gregorio GV, Portmann B, Karani J, et al. Autoimmune hepatitis/sclerosing cholangitis overlap syndrome in childhood: a 16-year prospective study. *Hepatology* 2001; **33**: 544–553.

53 Ludwig J, Dickson ER, McDonald GS. Staging of chronic nonsuppurative destructive cholangitis (syndrome of primary biliary cirrhosis). *Virchows Arch Pathol Anat* 1978; **379**: 103–112.

54 Ludwig,J, LaRusso,NF, Wiesner, RH. The syndrome of primary sclerosing cholangitis. In: Popper H, Shaffner F, eds. Progress in Liver Diseases, Vol. IX. Philadelphia, PA: WB Saunders, 1990: 555–566.

55 Bergquist A, Ekbom A, Olsson R, et al. Hepatic and extrahepatic malignancies in primary sclerosing cholangitis. *J Hepatol* 2002; **36**: 321–327.

56 Fleming KA, Boberg KM, Glaumann H, et al. Biliary dysplasia as a marker of cholangiocarcinoma in primary sclerosing cholangitis. *J Hepatol* 2001; **34**: 360–365.

57 Haworth AC, Manley PN, Groll A, et al. Bile duct carcinoma and biliary tract dysplasia in chronic ulcerative colitis. *Arch Pathol Lab Med* 1989; **113**: 434–436.

58 Ludwig J, Wahlstrom HE, Batts KP, et al. Papillary bile duct dysplasia in primary sclerosing cholangitis. *Gastroenterology* 1992; **102**: 2134–2138.

59 Björnsson E, Olsson R, Bergquist A, et al. The natural history of small-duct primary sclerosing cholangitis. *Gastroenterology* 2008; **134**: 975–980.

60 Guarascio P, Yentis F, Cevikbas U, et al. Value of copper-associated protein in diagnostic assessment of liver biopsy. *J Clin Pathol* 1983; **36**: 18–23.

61 Ludwig J. Surgical pathology of the syndrome of primary sclerosing cholangitis. *Am J Surg Pathol* 1989; **13**(Suppl. 1): 43–49.

62 Björnsson E, Chari ST, Smyrk TC, et al. Immunoglobulin G4 associated cholangitis: description of an emerging clinical entity based on review of the literature. *Hepatology* 2007; **45**: 1547–1554.

63 Webster GJM, Pereira SP, Chapman RW. Autoimmune pancreatitis/IgG4-associated cholangitis–overlapping or separate diseases? *J Hepatol* 2009; **51**: 398–402.

64 Zen Y, Fujii T, Sato Y, et al. Pathological classification of hepatic inflammatory pseudotumor with respect to IgG4-related disease. *Mod Pathol* 2007; **20**: 884–894.

64a. Zhang L, Lewis JT, Abraham SC, et al. IgG4+ plasma cell infiltrates in liver explants with primary sclerosing cholangitis. *Am J Surg Pathol* 2010; **34**: 88–94.

65 Umemura T, Zen Y, Hamano H, et al. Immunoglobulin G4-hepatopathy: association of immunoglobulin G4-bearing plasma cells in liver with autoimmune pancreatitis. *Hepatology* 2007; **46**: 463–471.

65a. Deshpande V, Sainani NI, Chung RT, et al. IgG4-associated cholangitis: a comparative histological and immunophenotypic study with primary sclerosing cholangitis on liver biopsy material. *Mod Pathol* 2009; **22**: 1287–1295.

66 Rubin E, Schaffner F, Popper H. Primary biliary cirrhosis. Chronic non-suppurative destructive cholangitis. *Am J Pathol* 1965; **46**: 387–407.

67 Dahlan Y, Smith L, Simmonds D, et al. Pediatric-onset primary biliary cirrhosis. *Gastroenterology* 2003; **125**: 1476–1479.

68 Kaplan MM, Gershwin ME. Primary biliary cirrhosis. *N Engl J Med* 2005; **353**: 1261–1273.

69 Selmi C, Zuin M, Gershwin ME. The unfinished business of primary biliary cirrhosis. *J Hepatol* 2008; **49**: 451–460.

70 Jones DEJ. Pathogenesis of primary biliary cirrhosis. *J Hepatol* 2003; **39**: 639–648.

71 Leung PSC, Coppel RL, Ansari A, et al. Antimitochondrial antibodies in primary biliary cirrhosis. *Semin Liver Dis* 1997; **17**: 61–69.

72 Neuberger J. Antibodies and primary biliary cirrhosis – piecing together the jigsaw. *J Hepatol* 2002; **36**: 126–129.

73 Hirschfield GM, Liu X, Xu C, et al. Primary biliary cirrhosis associated with *HLA, IL12A*, and *IL12RB2* variants. *N Engl J Med* 2009; **360**: 2544–2555.

74 Culp KS, Fleming CR, Duffy J, et al. Autoimmune associations in primary biliary cirrhosis. *Mayo Clin Proc* 1982; **57**: 365–370.

75 Scheuer P. Primary biliary cirrhosis. *Proc R Soc Med* 1967; **60**: 1257–1260.

76 Jones DEJ, Metcalf JV, Collier JD, et al. Hepatocellular carcinoma in primary biliary cirrhosis and its impact on outcomes. *Hepatology* 1997; **26**: 1138–1142.

77 Cavazza A, Caballeria L, Floreani A, et al. Incidence, risk factors, and survival of hepatocellular carcinoma in primary biliary cirrhosis: comparative analysis from two centers. *Hepatology* 2009; **50**: 1162–1168.

78 Terada T, Kurumaya H, Nakanuma Y, et al. Macroregenerative nodules of the liver in primary biliary cirrhosis: report of two autopsy cases. *Am J Gastroenterol* 1989; **84**: 418–421.

79 Floreani A, Baragiotta A, Baldo V, et al. Hepatic and extrahepatic malignancies in primary biliary cirrhosis. *Hepatology* 1999; **29**: 1425–1428.

80 Neuberger J. Eosinophils and primary biliary cirrhosis – stoking the fire? *Hepatology* 1999; **30**: 335–337.

81 Yamazaki K, Suzuki K, Nakamura A, et al. Ursodeoxycholic acid inhibits eosinophil degranulation in patients with primary biliary cirrhosis. *Hepatology* 1999; **30**: 71–78.

82 Degott C, Zafrani ES, Callard P, et al. Histopathological study of primary biliary cirrhosis and the effect of ursodeoxycholic acid treatment on histology progression. *Hepatology* 1999; **29**: 1007–1012.

83 Daniels JA, Torbenson M, Anders RA, et al. Immunostaining of plasma cells in primary biliary cirrhosis. *Am J Clin Pathol* 2009; **131**: 243–249.

83a Moreira RK, Revetta F, Koehler E, Washington MK. Diagnostic utility of IgG and IgM immunohistochemistry in autoimmune liver disease. *World J Gastroenterol* 2010; **16**: 453–457.

84 Nakanuma Y, Ohta G. Quantitation of hepatic granulomas and epithelioid cells in primary biliary cirrhosis. *Hepatology* 1983; **3**: 423–427.

85 Vleggaar FP, van Buuren HR, Zondervan PE, et al. Jaundice in non-cirrhotic primary biliary cirrhosis: the premature ductopenic variant. *Gut* 2001; **49**: 276–281.

86 Nakanuma Y. Necroinflammatory changes in hepatic lobules in primary biliary cirrhosis with less well-defined cholestatic changes. *Hum Pathol* 1993; **24**: 378–383.

87 McMahon RF, Babbs C, Warnes TW. Nodular regenerative hyperplasia of the liver, CREST syndrome and primary biliary cirrhosis: an overlap syndrome? *Gut* 1989; **30**: 1430–1433.

88 Colina F, Pinedo F, Solís A, et al. Nodular regenerative hyperplasia of the liver in early histological stages of primary biliary cirrhosis. *Gastroenterology* 1992; **102**: 1319–1324.

89 Nakanuma Y, Ohta G, Kobayashi K, et al. Histological and histometric examination of the intrahepatic portal vein branches in primary biliary cirrhosis without regenerative nodules. *Am J Gastroenterol* 1982; **77**: 405–413.

90 Nakanuma Y, Hirata K. Unusual hepatocellular lesions in primary biliary cirrhosis resembling but unrelated to hepatocellular neoplasms. *Virchows Arch [A]* 1993; **422**: 17–23.

91 O'Donohue J, Oien KA, Donaldson P, et al. Co-amoxiclav jaundice: clinical and histological features and HLA class II association. *Gut* 2000; **47**: 717–720.

92 Bach N, Thung SN, Schaffner F. The histological features of chronic hepatitis C and autoimmune chronic hepatitis: a comparative analysis. *Hepatology* 1992; **15**: 572–577.

93 Christoffersen P, Poulsen H, Scheuer PJ. Abnormal bile duct epithelium in chronic aggressive hepatitis and primary biliary cirrhosis. *Hum Pathol* 1972; **3**: 227–235.

94 Terasaki S, Nakanuma Y, Yamazaki M, et al. Eosinophilic infiltration of the liver in primary biliary cirrhosis: a morphological study. *Hepatology* 1993; **17**: 206–212.

95 Czaja AJ, Carpenter HA. Autoimmune hepatitis with incidental histologic features of bile duct injury. *Hepatology* 2001; **34**: 659–665.

96 Washington K, Clavien P-A, Killenberg P. Peribiliary vascular plexus in primary sclerosing cholangitis and primary biliary cirrhosis. *Hum Pathol* 1997; **28**: 791–795.

97 Nakanuma Y, Saito K, Unoura M. Semiquantitative assessment of cholestasis and lymphocytic piecemeal necrosis in primary biliary cirrhosis: a histologic and immunohistochemical study. *J Clin Gastroenterol* 1990; **12**: 357–362.

98 Yamada S, Howe S, Scheuer PJ. Three-dimensional reconstruction of biliary pathways in primary biliary cirrhosis: a computer-assisted study. *J Pathol* 1987; **152**: 317–323.

99 Leon MP, Bassendine MF, Gibbs P, et al. Immunogenicity of biliary epithelium: study of the adhesive interaction with lymphocytes. *Gastroenterology* 1997; **112**: 968–977.

100 Dienes HP, Lohse AW, Gerken G, et al. Bile duct epithelia as target cells in primary biliary cirrhosis and primary sclerosing cholangitis. *Virchows Arch* 1997; **431**: 119–124.

101 Nakanuma Y. Pathology of septum formation in primary biliary cirrhosis: a histological study in the non-cirrhotic stage. *Virchows Arch [A]* 1991; **419**: 381–387.

102 Scheuer PJ. Pathologic features and evolution of primary biliary cirrhosis and primary sclerosing cholangitis. *Mayo Clin Proc* 1998; **73**: 179–183.

103 Williamson JM, Chalmers DM, Clayden AD, et al. Primary biliary cirrhosis and chronic active hepatitis: an examination of clinical, biochemical, and histopathological features in differential diagnosis. *J Clin Pathol* 1985; **38**: 1007–1012.

104 Woodward J, Neuberger J. Autoimmune overlap syndromes. *Hepatology* 2001; **33**: 994–1002.

105 Lohse AW, Meyer zum Büschenfelde K-H, Franz B, et al. Characterization of the overlap syndrome of primary biliary cirrhosis (PBC) and autoimmune hepatitis: evidence for it being a hepatitic form of PBC in genetically susceptible individuals. *Hepatology* 1999; **29**: 1078–1084.

106 Hennes EM, Zeniya M, Czaja AJ, et al. Simplified criteria for the diagnosis of autoimmune hepatitis. *Hepatology* 2008; **48**: 169–176.

107 Alvarez F, Berg PA, Biandin FB, et al. International Autoimmune Hepatitis Group report: review of criteria for diagnosis of autoimmune hepatitis. *J Hepatol* 1999; **31**, 929–938.

108 Kaya M, Angulo P, Lindor KD. Overlap of autoimmune hepatitis and primary sclerosing cholangitis: an evaluation of a modified scoring system. *J Hepatol* 2000; **33**: 537–542.

109 Czaja AJ. Overlap syndrome of primary biliary cirrhosis and autoimmune hepatitis: a foray across diagnostic boundaries. *J Hepatol* 2006; **44**: 251–252.

110 Kita H, Mackay IR, Van de Water J, et al. The lymphoid liver: considerations on pathways to autoimmune injury. *Gastroenterology* 2001; **120**: 1485–1501.

111 Poupon R, Chazouilleres O, Corpechot C, et al. Development of autoimmune hepatitis in patients with typical primary biliary cirrhosis. *Hepatology* 2006; **44**: 85–90.

112 Twaddell WS, Lefkowitch JH, Berk PD. Evolution from primary biliary cirrhosis to primary biliary cirrhosis/autoimmune hepatitis overlap syndrome. *Semin Liver Dis* 2008; **28**: 128–134.

113 Abdo AA, Bain VG, Kichian K, Lee SS. Evolution of autoimmune hepatitis to primary sclerosing cholangitis: a sequential syndrome. *Hepatology* 2002; **36**: 1393–1399.

114 Feldstein AE, Perrault J, El-Youssif M, et al. Primary sclerosing cholangitis in children: a long-term follow-up study. *Hepatology* 2003; **38**: 210–217.

115 Jones DE, James OF, Portmann B, et al. Development of autoimmune hepatitis following liver transplantation for primary biliary cirrhosis. *Hepatology* 1999; **30**: 53–57.

116 Brunner G, Klinge O. Ein der chronisch-destruierenden nicht-eitrigen Cholangitis ähnliches Krankheitsbild mit antinjukleären Antikörpern (Immuncholangitis). *Dtsch Med Wochenschr* 1987; **112**: 1454–1458.

117 Bruguera M, Llach J, Rodés J. Nonsyndromic paucity of intrahepatic bile ducts in infancy and idiopathic ductopenia in adulthood: the same syndrome? *Hepatology* 1992; **15**: 830–834.

118 Dural AT, Genta RM, Goodman ZD, et al. Idiopathic adulthood ductopenia associated with hepatitis C virus. *Dig Dis Sci* 2002; **47**: 1625–1626.

119 Ludwig J. Idiopathic adulthood ductopenia: an update. *Mayo Clin Proc* 1998; **73**: 285–291.

120 Burak KW, Pearson DC, Swain MG, et al. Familial idiopathic adulthood ductopenia: a report of five cases in three generations. *J Hepatol* 2000; **32**: 159–163.

121 Crosbie OM, Crown JP, Nolan NPM, et al. Resolution of paraneoplastic bile duct paucity following successful treatment of Hodgkin's disease. *Hepatology* 1997; **26**: 5–8.

122 Moreno A, Carreño CA, González C. Idiopathic biliary ductopenia in adults without symptoms of liver disease. *N Engl J Med* 1997; **336**: 835–838.

General reading

Balistreri WF, Bezerra JA, Jansen P, et al. Intrahepatic cholestasis: summary of an AASLD single-topic conference. *Hepatology* 2005; **42**: 222–235.

Crawford JM. Development of the intrahepatic biliary tree. *Semin Liver Dis* 2002; **22**: 213–226.

Czaja AJ, Bayraktar Y. Non-classical phenotypes of autoimmune hepatitis and advances in diagnosis and treatment. *World J Gastroenterol* 2009; **15**: 2314–2328.

Kim WR, Ludwig J, Lindor KD. Variant forms of cholestatic diseases involving small bile ducts in adults. *Am J Gastroenterol* 2000; **95**: 1130–1138.

LaRusso NF, Chneider BL, Black D, et al. Primary sclerosing cholangitis: summary of a workshop. *Hepatology* 2006; **44**: 746–764.

Li MK, Crawford JM. The pathology of cholestasis. *Semin Liver Dis* 2004; **24**: 21–42.

Portmann BC, Nakanuma Y. Diseases of the bile ducts. In: Burt AD, Portmann BC, Ferrell LD, eds. *MacSween's Pathology of the Liver*, 5th edn. Edinburgh: Churchill Livingstone/Elsevier, 2007: 517–582.

Roberts SK, Ludwig J, LaRusso NF. The pathobiology of biliary epithelia. *Gastroenterology* 1997; **112**: 269–279.

Roskams T, Desmet VJ. Ductular reaction and its diagnostic significance. *Semin Diagn Pathol* 1998; **15**: 259–269.

Roskams TA, Theise ND, Balabaud C, et al. Nomenclature of the finer branches of the biliary tree: canals, ductules, and ductular reactions in human livers. *Hepatology* 2004; **39**: 1739–1745.

Selmi C, Zuin M, Gershwin ME. The unfinished business of primary biliary cirrhosis. *J Hepatol* 2008; **49**: 451–460.

Stapelbroek JM, van Erpecum KJ, Klomp LWJ, Houwen RHJ. Liver disease associated with canalicular transport defects: current and future therapies. *J Hepatol* 2010; **52**: 258–271.

Wagner M, Zollner G, Trauner M. New molectular insights into the mechanisms of cholestasis. *J Hepatol* 2009; **51**: 565–580.

Acute Viral Hepatitis 6

Introduction

Acute hepatitis is not usually an indication for liver biopsy. There are, however, at least three reasons why pathologists sometimes receive liver biopsy samples from patients with acute hepatitis. First, there may be doubt about the clinical diagnosis, or even a mistaken working diagnosis. Second, a diagnosis of hepatitis may be well established but the clinician needs information on the stage of the disease or its severity. Third, the patient may have received a liver transplant and the pathologist is being asked to help decide if symptoms or biochemical abnormalities are due to recurrent (or new) viral hepatitis or to some other cause such as rejection. For all these reasons, a knowledge of the pathology of acute hepatitis is essential. There is a further reason, no less important than the others: without a knowledge of acute hepatitis, the pathologist cannot hope to understand chronic hepatitis and cirrhosis, together the cause of most liver disease in the world. This chapter describes acute viral hepatitis and its immediate sequelae in the immunocompetent patient. The specific problems of diagnosing hepatitis in an immunosuppressed patient after transplantation are reviewed in **Chapter 16**.

The hepatitis viruses are listed in **Table 6.1**. While several other candidates have been extensively investigated in recent years, none has so far been established as a definite cause of viral hepatitis and most episodes of acute and chronic hepatitis can be attributed to one of the viruses listed, to autoimmune hepatitis (**Ch. 9**) or to a hepatotoxic agent (**Ch. 8**). An exception to this statement is fulminant hepatitis, the cause of which cannot currently be established in a substantial minority of patients,[1–3] including children.[4] Occasionally, a virus more often associated with infection of other organs, such as one of the herpes viruses[5–7] or an adenovirus,[8,9] gives rise to a severe hepatitis. These agents are further discussed in **Chapter 15**. Mild acute hepatitis has been reported in patients infected with the SARS virus (severe acute respiratory syndrome-associated coronavirus).[10,11]

Occasionally, mild serum liver test abnormalities and mild histological hepatitis ('bystander hepatitis') with apoptotic bodies, focal necrosis and lymphocytic inflammation are seen in systemic, non-hepatic viral infections such as pulmonary influenza and result from migration to the liver of and collateral damage by CD8 T-lymphocytes.[12,13]

Pathological features

The essential components of the acute phase of hepatitis are inflammatory-cell infiltration and hepatocellular damage. Other features include cholestasis, Kupffer-cell activation, endotheliitis, bile-duct damage, the ductular reaction and hepatocellular regeneration.

©2010 Elsevier Ltd
DOI: 10.1016/B978-0-7020-3410-7.00012-5

Figure 6.1 Acute viral hepatitis. Surviving hepatocytes in the perivenular area in the centre of the field are swollen and the area is infiltrated by inflammatory cells. (Needle biopsy, H&E.)

Table 6.1 The hepatitis viruses

Virus	Type	Spread and disease
Hepatitis A (HAV)	RNA hepatovirus	Faecal–oral, acute
Hepatitis B (HBV)	DNA hepadnavirus	Parenteral, acute or chronic
Hepatitis C (HCV)	RNA hepacivirus	Parenteral or sporadic; acute, more often chronic
Hepatitis D (HDV)	RNA deltavirus, defective	Pathogenic when combined with HBV
Hepatitis E (HEV)	RNA virus	Faecal–oral, epidemic or sporadic acute disease

Hepatocellular damage

Changes seen under the light microscope range from minor degrees of cell swelling to cell death. They are accompanied by the inflammatory infiltration described below, reflecting the important role of cellular immunity in the pathogenesis of most forms of hepatitis. Both hepatocellular damage and inflammation are usually most severe in perivenular areas, giving rise to a characteristic histological pattern (**Fig. 6.1**). A periportal pattern of necrosis and inflammation, sometimes seen in hepatitis A, is less common.

The mildest and probably reversible change is cell swelling. The cytoplasm of affected cells is rarified, granular and sometimes finely vacuolated. The more severe degrees of cell swelling are called ballooning degeneration (**Fig. 6.2**). This differs from the feathery degeneration of cholestasis, in which the cytoplasm has a reticular pattern (**see Fig. 5.3**). Other hepatocytes undergo apoptosis, which is an important method of cell death in hepatitis.[14] Shrinkage and increased staining of the cytoplasm, sometimes called acidophilic change or degeneration, is probably a precursor of apoptosis, in which the hepatocytes shrink further, become very dense and undergo fragmentation. The apoptotic bodies seen lying free in the sinusoids represent the largest fragments or entire unfragmented

Figure 6.2 Acute viral hepatitis. Normal liver-cell plate structure is disrupted. Hepatocytes vary in size and some are ballooned and vacuolated. An apoptotic hepatocyte is seen left of centre. (Needle biopsy, H&E.)

apoptotic cells (**Fig. 6.2**). They are also called acidophil bodies or Councilman bodies, Councilman having first described them in yellow fever.[15] Apoptotic bodies sometimes contain pyknotic nuclear remnants and often appear to bulge beyond the plane of the section. Another form of hepatocellular damage in acute hepatitis is focal (spotty) necrosis, in which liver-cell plates are disrupted or replaced by small groups of lymphocytes and macrophages. Whether these mark a site of necrosis or of apoptosis is not clear; the damage to hepatocytes is deduced from their absence rather than seen. Whatever its mechanism, loss of hepatocytes or liver-cell drop out, coupled with focal regeneration, leads to a characteristic irregularity of the liver-cell plates, which usually allows acute hepatitis to be distinguished from hepatocellular damage secondary to cholestasis. The loss of hepatocytes also leads to condensation of the extracellular matrix, best seen in reticulin preparations (**Fig. 6.3**).

Hepatocyte nuclei show prominent nucleoli and increased variation in size and may be multiple. When syncytial giant hepatocytes are very prominent, the term giant-cell hepatitis is appropriate.[16,17] This is only rarely of proven viral origin and is also more characteristic of acute hepatitis in neonates. In adults, autoimmune hepatitis and hepatitis C virus with or without human immunodeficiency virus co-infection are important associations.[18-22]

Cholestasis in the form of bile thrombi in canaliculi is common in acute hepatitis but rare in chronic hepatitis, which is diagnostically helpful. It is a result of damage to the bile secretory apparatus of the hepatocytes, but may also result from interference with bile flow at the level of the portal tracts.[23] The term cholestatic hepatitis is best kept as a clinical description of patients with a prolonged cholestatic course. Mild hepatocellular siderosis or steatosis is occasionally seen.

The inflammatory infiltrate

Unlike classic acute inflammation, viral hepatitis is characterised by a mainly lymphocytic infiltrate within the parenchyma and portal tracts. In acute hepatitis, the most conspicuous

Figure 6.3 Acute viral hepatitis. The reticulin framework is condensed near the efferent venules (V), but not immediately around the portal tracts (P). (Needle biopsy, reticulin.)

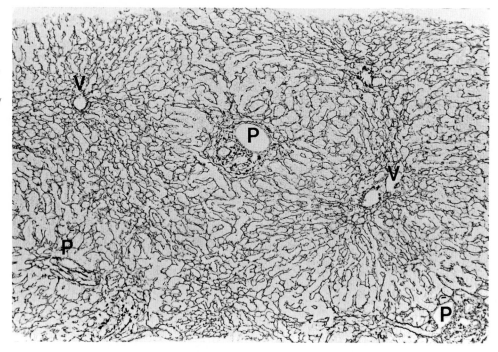

inflammation is usually perivenular. The extent of portal inflammation is very variable and portal tracts may be either normal in size or expanded. The larger conducting tracts are often spared. The edges of small portal tracts may be well defined or blurred by outward extension of the infiltrate. This so-called spillover resembles the interface hepatitis of chronic hepatitis (**Ch. 9**) and may be difficult to distinguish from it. The parenchymal changes, clinical history and virological findings usually make the correct diagnosis clear.

While most of the infiltrating cells in acute hepatitis are small T lymphocytes,[24] plasma cells may also be prominent[25] and there are often a few neutrophils and eosinophils. The plasma cells do not necessarily indicate autoimmune hepatitis, nor do a few eosinophils prove a diagnosis of drug injury. Kupffer cells and other macrophages accumulate and enlarge, many of them forming discrete clumps together with lymphocytes. They may contain tan-brown ceroid pigment, staining with periodic acid–Schiff (PAS) agent after diastase digestion (**Fig. 6.4**). They may also contain stainable iron (**Fig. 6.5**), but this is less common.

Sinusoidal and venular endothelial cells also take part in the hepatitic process. Sinusoidal endothelial cells become swollen and may contain dense iron-positive granules[26] (**Fig. 6.5**). Terminal hepatic venules may show disruption of the endothelium and lymphocytic infiltration.

Portal changes

In contrast to chronic hepatitis the parenchymal changes dominate the picture, but there is always some portal inflammation, affecting most or all of the small portal tracts (**Fig. 6.6**). The density of the infiltrate varies. Interlobular bile ducts may show abnormalities including irregularity, crowding and stratification of the epithelium, cytoplasmic vacuolation and infiltration by lymphocytes (**Fig. 6.7**). These changes, together with lymphoid follicle formation, are most often seen in hepatitis C. Bile-duct loss (ductopenia) is very rare.

Figure 6.4 Acute viral hepatitis. Macrophages contain diastase PAS-positive material. (Needle biopsy, diastase-PAS.)

Figure 6.5 Acute viral hepatitis. Enlarged macrophages are strongly iron-positive. Some endothelial cells also contain dense Perls' stain positive granules. (Section kindly provided by Dr Susan Davies , Cambridge, UK.) (Needle biopsy, Perls' stain.)

Histological variants

The histological changes in acute hepatitis are infinitely variable, but a few patterns deserve special mention. These are confluent necrosis, bridging necrosis, necrosis of entire lobules and periportal necrosis.

Confluent necrosis signifies death of a substantial area of the parenchyma. Focal as opposed to zonal areas of confluent necrosis haphazardly distributed in relation to lobular

Figure 6.6 Acute viral hepatitis. A portal tract is infiltrated by inflammatory cells, mainly lymphocytes. In places the infiltrate extends a short way into the adjacent parenchyma. (Needle biopsy, H&E.)

Figure 6.7 Acute viral hepatitis. Bile-duct epithelium is irregular and infiltrated by lymphocytes. The upper duct profile shows epithelial atrophy and dilatation. (Wedge biopsy, H&E.)

zones are more likely to be due to causes other than acute viral hepatitis; possibilities to be considered include opportunistic infections with herpes simplex or zoster viruses and lymphoma. **Bridging necrosis (Figs 6.8, 6.9, and Fig. 4.2)** is the term given to confluent necrosis linking terminal venules to portal tracts. A possible explanation for this location is that it represents the entire zone 3 of an acinus, a view supported by the curved shape of many bridges. Bridging necrosis is a manifestation of severe acute hepatitis but its distribution even within a single biopsy may be irregular. Necrosis and inflammation linking

Figure 6.8 Acute viral hepatitis: bridging necrosis. Two curved lines of collapse (arrows) extend from a portal tract (P). An efferent venule (V) is seen top centre. (Needle biopsy, H&E.)

Figure 6.9 Acute viral hepatitis: bridging necrosis. Recent collapse following confluent necrosis is seen as condensation of reticulin, mimicking fibrosis. (Needle biopsy, reticulin.)

adjacent portal tracts without involvement of terminal venules should not strictly be called bridging because it almost certainly has different pathogenetic significance; it results from widening of portal tracts, with or without periportal necrosis.

Bridges of confluent necrosis with subsequent collapse may be mistaken for the septa of chronic liver disease. In making the important distinction between them, the pathologist is often helped by stains for elastic tissue. Unlike stains for collagens, these normally give negative results in the parenchyma, but elastic tissue accumulates as septa age.[27]

Figure 6.10 Acute hepatitis: bridging necrosis.
The field is the same as that shown in **Fig. 6.9**. A stain for elastic fibres is positive in two portal tracts (P) but not in the intervening area of collapse. A necrotic bridge (arrow) is also negative. *Inset:* This contrasts with an elastic fibre-rich septum in chronic liver disease. (Needle biopsy, orcein.)

Recent collapse is therefore negative (**Fig. 6.10**), whereas old septa are positive. Substantial amounts of elastic tissue take months or years to accumulate, but small amounts can be detected by sensitive methods such as Victoria blue as early as 1 or 2 months after onset of hepatitis.[28]

In a minority of patients with acute viral hepatitis confluent necrosis extends throughout entire lobules or acini (**panlobular or panacinar necrosis**) or several adjacent ones (**multilobular or multiacinar necrosis**). This is a common feature in patients with fulminant hepatitis. The term 'massive necrosis' is also sometimes used, but can be misleading in so far as a needle biopsy specimen may not be representative of the liver as a whole and can lead to over- or under-estimation of the true extent of liver damage.[29] This throws doubt on the usefulness of liver biopsy as a means of assessing prognosis in severe acute hepatitis. Sometimes multilobular necrosis involves only the subcapsular zone, and a small needle specimen may then give a falsely pessimistic picture (**see Fig. 1.3**). In multilobular necrosis the parenchyma is replaced by collapsed stroma, inflammatory cells and activated macrophages (**Fig. 6.11**). Around the surviving portal tracts, there are prominent duct-like structures, some of which probably represent proliferation of pluripotential progenitor cells[30-32] (**see Fig. 4.6D**). Late-onset hepatic failure is a term used for patients developing encephalopathy between 8 and 24 weeks after onset of symptoms.[33] Study of liver biopsies and explanted livers from these patients has shown a consistent pattern of map-like necrosis together with areas of nodular regeneration.

Periportal necrosis rather than the more usual perivenular necrosis is a feature in some patients with hepatitis A (below).

Individual causes of viral hepatitis

There are more similarities than differences between hepatitis types A, B, C, D and E, but certain patterns are more common in one type than another and are described here. They do not allow the pathologist to identify the cause of the hepatitis on histological

Figure 6.11 Acute viral hepatitis: multilobular necrosis.
Portal tracts (P) can be identified but the parenchyma has been replaced by inflammatory cells, necrotic debris and duct-like structures. (Needle biopsy, H&E.)

appearance alone. The picture may be confused by the presence of more than one virus, or by additional damage resulting from alcohol abuse.

Hepatitis A

Two main patterns are described, occurring separately or together.[34-36] One is a histological picture of perivenular cholestasis with little liver-cell damage or inflammation, easily mistaken for other causes of cholestasis (**Fig. 6.12**). The second is a hepatitis with periportal necrosis and a dense portal infiltrate which includes abundant, often aggregated plasma cells (**Fig. 6.13**). These two patterns may be related, the cholestasis resulting from interruption of bile flow by the periportal necrosis.[22] Other patterns of hepatitis as described above are also found, but fulminant hepatitis with multilobular necrosis is rare. Extensive microvesicular change of hepatocytes, previously described in hepatitis D infection, has been seen also in severe acute hepatitis A (**Fig. 6.14**). Fibrin-ring granulomas have been reported.[37,38] A chronic course[39] is very rare.

Hepatitis B

The histological appearances are broadly similar to those of other forms of viral hepatitis. Some of the differences reported in the literature may well reflect patient selection rather than features specific for hepatitis B virus (HBV) infection. However, lymphocytes and macrophages sometimes lie in close contact with hepatocytes (peripolesis) or even invaginate them deeply (emperipolesis), which probably reflects the immunological nature of the cell damage. In a comparative study, periportal inflammation tended to be more severe in acute hepatitis B than in hepatitis C.[40] Liver cells and their nuclei may show a moderate degree of pleomorphism. In most cases of acute hepatitis, the hepatitis B core and surface antigens (HBcAg and HBsAg) are either not demonstrable or very sparse, but in one study of livers infected with a HBV mutant,[41] HBsAg could be demonstrated by immunostaining

Figure 6.12
Hepatitis A.
Perivenular area showing irregularity of liver-cell plates and cholestasis, but only mild inflammatory infiltration. (Needle biopsy, H&E.)

Figure 6.13
Hepatitis A.
A portal area is heavily infiltrated by lymphocytes and plasma cells, some of which extend into the adjacent parenchyma. The limiting plate is irregular. The picture resembles that of chronic hepatitis with interface hepatitis. (Needle biopsy, H&E.)

in over half of the patients and HBcAg in a minority. The presence of ground-glass hepatocytes (**Ch. 9**) or positive staining of surface material with Victoria blue or orcein indicates chronic disease. Recurrence of HBV infection after liver transplantation is an exception to this rule, both antigens being found in large amounts (**see Ch. 16**). In parenterally transmitted hepatitis, including types B and C, birefringent spicules of talc may be found in portal tracts as a result of intravenous drug abuse.[41]

Figure 6.14
Hepatitis A.
In this patient with a clinical picture of fulminant hepatitis, hepatocytes are swollen and microvesicular. There is cholestasis and a lymphocytic infiltrate. (Needle biopsy, H&E.)

Following clinical recovery of acute hepatitis B, occult infection and mild histological abnormalities including portal inflammation, focal necrosis, apoptosis and fibrosis may persist for at least a decade.[43]

Reactivation of a previously occult or quiescent chronic hepatitis B infection may cause changes closely resembling acute hepatitis. In such instances the presence of (1) portal tract lymphoid aggregates, (2) significant lymphoplasmacytic interface hepatitis, (3) any evidence of fibrosis on connective tissue stains, and (4) substantial positivity of HBsAg in hepatocytes on immunostaining all point to the underlying chronicity of the process.

Hepatitis C

Usually the histological features of hepatitis C are those of any acute hepatitis, but two distinguishing features have been noted. First, there may be prominent infiltration of sinusoids by lymphocytes in the absence of severe liver-cell damage,[44] giving rise to a picture reminiscent of infectious mononucleosis (**Fig. 6.15**). Second, lymphoid follicles and bile-duct damage, features also associated with chronic hepatitis, may be seen within a few weeks or months of onset.[45] There may be cholestasis. The common finding of steatosis in hepatitis C is discussed in **Chapter 9**. Fulminant hepatitis C is very rare in the Western world[3] but may be commoner in parts of Asia.[46]

Hepatitis D (delta hepatitis)

Co-infection or superinfection with the hepatitis D virus (HDV) alters the course of type B hepatitis. It encourages chronicity and enhances severity,[47–49] except after liver transplantation. The antigen, HDAg, can easily be demonstrated immunohistochemically in paraffin sections and is mainly found in hepatocyte nuclei (**Fig. 6.16**). These may have finely granular eosinophilic centres (so-called 'sanded' nuclei[50]). Cytoplasmic and membrane-associated staining is also sometimes seen.

Figure 6.15 Acute hepatitis C.
In this example the main abnormality is infiltration of sinusoids by lymphocytes. (Needle biopsy, H&E.)

Figure 6.16 Delta (HDV) hepatitis.
Some hepatocyte nuclei contain the delta antigen and are stained red. There is a substantial lymphocytic infiltrate. (Needle biopsy, specific immunostain, alkaline phosphatase method.)

Severe acute hepatitis in a patient with markers of HBV infection may be due to super-infection by HDV of a chronic HBV carrier.[51] In an outbreak of HDV infection among Venezuelan Indians, notable features included early small-droplet fatty change, sparse lymphocytes and abundant macrophages in the parenchyma and substantial portal infil-tration.[52] Later in the attack, there was extensive necrosis and collapse. Microvesicular fatty

Figure 6.17
Hepatitis E.
Hepatocytes are vacuolated and one to the left of centre is greatly enlarged and multinucleated. There is a mixed infiltrate and macrophages contain brown ceroid pigment. (Needle biopsy, H&E.)

change and acidophilic necrosis of hepatocytes have been reported from Colombia[53] and North America.[54] In non-immunosuppressed patients with current HDV infection, liver biopsy is likely to show substantial necrosis and inflammation. However, there are HDV-endemic regions where the virus produces little significant disease.[55] Following liver transplantation, on the other hand, HDV without HBV is sometimes demonstrable in the absence of hepatitic changes, indicating that HDV can survive in the absence of HBV. It does not then appear, however, to be capable of causing liver damage.[56]

Hepatitis E

Hepatitis E is the result of enteric infection by an RNA virus with four genotypes.[57,58] The disease has caused epidemics in Asia and has also been found in Africa, North and South America and Europe. In the Western world, it is most often seen in travellers (**Fig. 6.17**) but sporadic disease is sometimes due to local ingestion of virus-contaminated meat.[59] Infection does not appear to lead to chronic disease, but may cause severe decompensation of pre-existing chronic liver disease due to other causes.[60,61] The possibility of post-transplantation chronic hepatitis and cirrhosis due to use of hepatitis E virus-infected donor organs (liver, kidney, pancreas) has been raised in several reports.[62–64]

There is little detailed information on the pathological changes of hepatitis E virus infection in man. In a small number of patients studied, the appearances were like those of hepatitis A, with prominent cholestasis and a predominantly portal and periportal inflammatory infiltrate.[65] Portal lymphoid aggregates and periportal ductular reaction with neutrophilia at the edges of portal tracts are also described.[59] Histological cholestasis has been described in an elderly patient with a prolonged cholestatic clinical course.[66] The liver of a pregnant woman with fatal hepatitis E showed little portal inflammation, much cholestasis and prominent phlebitis, and virus particles were seen in bile ductules by electron microscopy.[67]

Differential diagnosis of acute viral hepatitis

The distinction of acute hepatitis from bile-duct obstruction rests mainly on the finding of typical hepatitic changes in the parenchyma. The portal tract oedema of duct obstruction is absent. Drug-related hepatitis may be indistinguishable from viral hepatitis and should always be suspected if the cause of the hepatitis is in doubt. Features more common in drug-induced than in viral hepatitis include sharply defined perivenular necrosis, granulomas, bile-duct damage, abundant neutrophils or eosinophils and a poorly developed portal inflammatory reaction. Cholestasis may overshadow the hepatitic features. Autoimmune hepatitis may have a clinically acute onset, histologically indistinguishable from viral hepatitis or alternatively with histological features of chronic disease. This is discussed more fully in **Chapter 9**. In steatohepatitis there is usually conspicuous fatty change. Mallory bodies may be present in ballooned hepatocytes and the infiltrate typically includes neutrophils. The key to the diagnosis is the presence of pericellular fibrosis in affected areas. The differentiation of acute from chronic hepatitis is briefly discussed under bridging necrosis in **Chapter 4**. While the parenchymal changes predominate in acute hepatitis, especially in perivenular areas, portal and periportal changes predominate in chronic disease. The distinction is sometimes difficult to make, especially when extensive lobular changes are found during an exacerbation of chronic hepatitis or in reactivated chronic hepatitis B as described earlier.

Fate and morphological sequelae of acute viral hepatitis

Resolution

As far as can be deduced from the available evidence, most examples of hepatitis A, B and E are followed by complete or near-complete resolution and a return of the liver to normal. A chronic course is probably more common when hepatitis B is complicated by delta infection than otherwise, and in hepatitis C the risk of chronicity is high. Even in patients whose hepatitis resolves, some residual changes may persist for many months after clinical recovery (**Figs 6.18, 6.19**).

Scarring

Localised collapse, scarring and regeneration following severe hepatitis with bridging or panlobular necrosis sometimes produce a histological picture indistinguishable from cirrhosis.

Fatal outcome or need for liver transplantation

Necrosis is usually severe. Regenerative hyperplasia of surviving hepatocytes or progenitor cells may be seen.

Chronic hepatitis

Most individuals with hepatitis C virus infection develop chronic hepatitis. This has substantial impact on daily liver biopsy practice. Chronic hepatitis also develops in many patients with hepatitis B.

Figure 6.18 Acute viral hepatitis: residual changes. Short septa extend from the mildly inflamed portal tract to the left. Minimal inflammation and irregular liver-cell plates are seen around the efferent venule below right. (Needle biopsy, H&E.)

Figure 6.19 Acute viral hepatitis: residual changes. Slender septa link portal tracts (left and right), but the perivenular area (centre) is unaffected and architectural relationships are preserved. (Needle biopsy, reticulin.)

Cirrhosis

Cirrhosis resulting from infection with a hepatitis virus almost always follows a period of chronic hepatitis, with repeated or continuous hepatocellular necrosis and regeneration. Occasionally it may follow directly after a single episode of severe acute hepatitis.

Hepatocellular carcinoma

This may develop on the basis of cirrhosis in patients infected with HBV or HCV. Occasionally, however, hepatocellular carcinoma is found in the absence of cirrhosis, usually after a prolonged period of chronic liver disease.[68]

References

1 Ben Ari Z, Samuel D, Zemel R, et al. Fulminant non-A-G viral hepatitis leading to liver transplantation. *Arch Intern Med* 2000; **160**: 388–392.

2 Petrovic LM, Arkadopoulos N, Demetriou AA. Activation of hepatic stellate cells in liver tissue of patients with fulminant liver failure after treatment with bioartificial liver. *Hum Pathol* 2001; **32**: 1371–1375.

3 Schiødt FV, Davern TJ, Shakil AO, et al. Viral hepatitis-related acute liver failure. *Am J Gastroenterol* 2003; **98**: 448–453.

4 Kirsch R, Yap J, Roberts EA, Cutz E. Clinicopathologic spectrum of massive and submassive hepatic necrosis in infants and children. *Hum Pathol* 2009; **40**: 516–526.

5 Peters DJ, Greene WH, Ruggiero F, et al. Herpes simplex-induced fulminant hepatitis in adults: a call for empiric therapy. *Dig Dis Sci* 2000; **45**: 2399–2404.

6 Pinna AD, Rakela J, Demetris AJ, et al. Five cases of fulminant hepatitis due to herpes simplex virus in adults. *Dig Dis Sci* 2002; **47**: 750–754.

7 Collin L, Moulin P, Jungers M, et al. Epstein–Barr virus (EBV)-induced liver failure in the absence of extensive liver-cell necrosis: a case for cytokine-induced liver dysfunction? *J Hepatol* 2004; **41**: 174–175.

8 Wang WH, Wang HL. Fulminant adenovirus hepatitis following bone marrow transplantation. A case report and brief review of the literature. *Arch Pathol Lab Med* 2003; **127**: e246–e248

9 Longerich T, Haferkamp K, Tox U, et al. Acute liver failure in a renal transplant patient caused by adenoviral hepatitis superimposed on a fibrosing cholestatic hepatitis B. *Hum Pathol* 2004; **35**: 894–897.

10 Chau TN, Lee KC, Yao H, et al. SARS-associated viral hepatitis caused by a novel coronavirus: report of three cases. *Hepatology* 2004; **39**: 302–310.

11 Ng W-F, To K-F, Lam WWL, et al. The comparative pathology of severe acute respiratory syndrome and avian influenza A subtype H5N1: a review. *Hum Pathol* 2006; **37**: 381–390.

12 Polakos NK, Cornejo JC, Murray DA, et al. Kupfer cell-dependent hepatitis occurs during influenza infection. *Am J Pathol* 2006; **168**: 1169–1178.

13 Adams DH, Hubscher SG. Systemic viral infections and collateral damage in the liver. *Am J Pathol* 2006; **168**: 1057–1059.

14 Lau JYN, Xie X, Lai MMC, Wu PC. Apoptosis and viral hepatitis. *Semin Liver Dis* 1998; **18**: 169–176.

15 Klotz O, Belt TH. The pathology of the liver in yellow fever. *Am J Pathol* 1930; **6**: 663–689.

16 Phillips MJ, Blendis LM, Poucell S, et al. Syncytial giant-cell hepatitis. Sporadic hepatitis with distinctive pathological features, a severe clinical course and paramyxoviral features. *N Engl J Med* 1991; **324**: 455–460.

17 Fimmel CJ, Guo L, Compans RW, et al. A case of syncytial giant cell hepatitis with features of a paramyxoviral infection. *Am J Gastroenterol* 1998; **93**: 1931–1937.

18 Devaney K, Goodman ZD, Ishak KG. Postinfantile giant-cell transformation in hepatitis. *Hepatology* 1992; **16**: 327–333.

19 Lau JYN, Koukoulis G, Mieli-Vergani G, et al. Syncytial giant-cell hepatitis – a specific disease entity? *J Hepatol* 1992; **15**: 216–219.

20 Protzer U, Dienes HP, Bianchi L, et al. Post-infantile giant cell hepatitis in patients with primary sclerosing cholangitis and autoimmune hepatitis. *Liver* 1996; **16**: 274–282.

21 Ben Ari Z, Broida E, Monselise Y, et al. Syncytial giant-cell hepatitis due to autoimmune hepatitis type II (LKM1+) presenting as subfulminant hepatitis. *Am J Gastroenterol* 2000; **95**: 799–801.

22 Micchelli STL, Thomas D, Boitnott JK, et al. Hepatic giant cells in hepatitis C virus (HCV) mono-infection and HCV/HIV co-infection. *J Clin Pathol* 2008; **61**: 1058–1061.

23 Sciot R, Van Damme B, Desmet VJ. Cholestatic features in hepatitis A. *J Hepatol* 1986; **3**: 172–181.

24 Volpes R, van den Oord JJ, Desmet VJ. Memory T cells represent the predominant lymphocyte subset in acute and chronic liver inflammation. *Hepatology* 1991; **13**: 826–829.

25 Mietkiewski JM, Scheuer PJ. Immunoglobulin-containing plasma cells in acute hepatitis. *Liver* 1985; **5**: 84–88.

26 Bardadin KA, Scheuer PJ. Endothelial cell changes in acute hepatitis. A light and electron microscopic study. *J Pathol* 1984; **144**: 213–220.

27 Scheuer PJ, Maggi G. Hepatic fibrosis and collapse: histological distinction by orcein staining. *Histopathology* 1980; **4**: 487–490.

28 Thung SN, Gerber MA. The formation of elastic fibers in livers with massive hepatic necrosis. *Arch Pathol Lab Med* 1982; **106**: 468–469.

29 Hanau C, Munoz SJ, Rubin R. Histopathological heterogeneity in fulminant hepatic failure. *Hepatology* 1995; **21**: 345–351.

30 Demetris AJ, Seaberg EC, Wennerberg A, et al. Ductular reaction after submassive necrosis in humans. Special emphasis on analysis of ductular hepatocytes. *Am J Pathol* 1996; **149**: 439–448.

31 Roskams T, De Vos R, van Eyken P, et al. Hepatic OV-6 expression in human liver disease and rat experiments: evidence for hepatic progenitor cells in man. *J Hepatol* 1998; **29**: 455–463.

32 Zhang L, Theise N, Chua M, Reid LM. The stem cell niche of human livers: symmetry between development and regeneration. *Hepatology* 2008; **48**: 1598–1607.

33 Ellis AJ, Saleh M, Smith H, et al. Late-onset hepatic failure: clinical features, serology and outcome following transplantation. *J Hepatol* 1995; **23**: 363–372.

34 Teixeira MR Jr, Weller IVD, Murray AM, et al. The pathology of hepatitis A in man. *Liver* 1982; **2**: 53–60.

35 Abe H, Beninger PR, Ikejiri N, et al. Light microscopic findings of liver biopsy specimens from patients with hepatitis type A and comparison with type B. *Gastroenterology* 1982; **82**: 938–947.

36 Okuno T, Sano A, Deguchi T, et al. Pathology of acute hepatitis A in humans. Comparison with acute hepatitis B. *Am J Clin Pathol* 1984; **81**: 162–169.

37 Ponz E, Garcia–Pagan JC, Bruguera M, et al. Hepatic fibrin-ring granulomas in a patient with hepatitis A. *Gastroenterology* 1991; **100**: 268–270.

38 Ruel M, Sevestre H, Henry-Biabaud E, et al. Fibrin ring granulomas in hepatitis A. *Dig Dis Sci* 1992; **37**: 1915–1917.

39 Inoue K, Yoshiba M, Yotsuyanagi H, et al. Chronic hepatitis A with persistent viral replication. *J Med Virol* 1996; **50**: 322–324.

40 Chu CW, Hwang SJ, Luo JC, et al. Comparison of clinical, virologic and pathologic features in patients with acute hepatitis B and C. *J Gastroenterol Hepatol* 2001; **16**: 209–214.

41 Uchida T, Shimojima S, Gotoh K, et al. Pathology of livers infected with 'silent' hepatitis B virus mutant. *Liver* 1994; **14**: 251–256.

42 Molos MA, Litton N, Schubert TT. Talc liver. *J Clin Gastroenterol* 1987; **9**: 198–203.

43 Yuki N, Nagaoka T, Yamashiro M, et al. Long-term histologic and virologic outcomes of acute self-limited hepatitis B. *Hepatology* 2003; **37**: 1172–1179.

44 Bamber M, Murray A, Arborgh BA, et al. Short incubation non-A, non-B hepatitis transmitted by factor VIII concentrates in patients with congenital coagulation disorders. *Gut* 1981; **22**: 854–859.

45 Kobayashi K, Hashimoto E, Ludwig J, et al. Liver biopsy features of acute hepatitis C compared with hepatitis A, B and non-A, non-B, non-C. *Liver* 1993; **13**: 69–73.

46 Chu CM, Sheen IS, Liaw YF. The role of hepatitis C virus in fulminant viral hepatitis in an area with endemic hepatitis A and B. *Gastroenterology* 1994; **107**: 189–195.

47 Govindarajan S, De-Cock KM, Redeker AG. Natural course of delta superinfection in chronic hepatitis B virus-infected patients: histopathologic study with multiple liver biopsies. *Hepatology* 1986; **6**: 640–644.

48 Verme G, Amoroso P, Lettieri G, et al. A histological study of hepatitis delta virus liver disease. *Hepatology* 1986; **6**: 1303–1307.

49 Lin H-H, Liaw Y-F, Chen T-J, et al. Natural course of patients with chronic type B hepatitis following acute hepatitis delta virus superinfection. *Liver* 1989; **9**: 129–134.

50 Moreno A, Ramón Y, Cahal S, et al. Sanded nuclei in delta patients. *Liver* 1989; **9**: 367–371.

51 Smedile A, Farci P, Verme G, et al. Influence of delta infection on severity of hepatitis B. *Lancet* 1982; **ii**: 945–947.

52 Popper H, Thung SN, Gerber MA, et al. Histologic studies of severe delta agent infection in Venezuelan Indians. *Hepatology* 1983; **3**: 906–912.

53 Buitrago B, Popper H, Hadler SC, et al. Specific histologic features of Santa Marta hepatitis: a severe form of hepatitis delta-virus infection in northern South America. *Hepatology* 1986; **6**: 1285–1291.

54 Lefkowitch JH, Goldstein H, Yatto R, et al. Cytopathic liver injury in acute delta virus hepatitis. *Gastroenterology* 1987; **92**: 1262–1266.

55 Rizzetto M. Hepatitis D: thirty years after. *J Hepatol* 2009; **50**: 1043–1050.

56 Davies SE, Lau JYN, O'Grady JG, et al. Evidence that hepatitis D virus needs hepatitis B virus to cause hepatocellular damage. *Am J Clin Pathol* 1992; **98**: 554–558.

57 Aggarwal R, Krawczynski K, Hepatitis E. An overview and recent advances in clinical and laboratory research. *J Gastroenterol Hepatol* 2000; **15**: 9–20.

58 Purcell RH, Emerson SU. Hepatitis E: an emerging awareness of an old disease. *J Hepatol* 2008; **48**: 494–503.

59 Malcolm P, Dalton H, Hussaini HS, et al. The histology of acute autochthonous hepatitis E virus infection. *Histopathology* 2007; **51**: 190–194.

60 Hamid SS, Atiq M, Shehzad F, et al. Hepatitis E virus superinfection in patients with chronic liver disease. *Hepatology* 2002; **36**: 474–478.

61 Ramachandran J, Eapen CE, Kang G, et al. Hepatitis E superinfection produces severe decompensation in patients with chronic liver disease. *J Gastroenterol Hepatol* 2004; **19**: 134–138.

62 Kamar N, Selves J, Mansuy J-M, et al. Hepatitis E virus and chronic hepatitis in organ-transplant recipients. *N Engl J Med* 2008; **358**: 811–817.

63 Kamar N, Mansuy J-M, Cointault O, et al. Hepatitis E virus-related cirrhosis in kidney- and kidney–pancreas-transplant recipients. *Am J Transplant* 2008; **8**: 1744–1748.

64 Aggarwal R. Hepatitis E: does it cause chronic hepatitis? *Hepatology* 2008; **48**: 1328–1330.

65 Dienes HP, Hütteroth T, Bianchi L, et al. Hepatitis A-like non-A, non-B hepatitis: light and electron microscopic observations of three cases. *Virchows Arch [A]* 1986; **409**: 657–667.

66 Mechnik L, Bergman N, Attali M, et al. Acute hepatitis E virus infection presenting as a prolonged cholestatic jaundice. *J Clin Gastroenterol* 2001; **33**: 421–422.

67 Asher LVS, Innis BL, Shrestha MP, et al. Virus-like particles in the liver of a patient with fulminant hepatitis and antibody to hepatitis E virus. *J Med Virol* 1990; **31**: 229–233.

68 Grando-Lemaire V, Guettier C, Chevret S, Beaugrand M, Trinchet JC. Hepatocellular carcinoma without cirrhosis in the West: epidemiological factors and histopathology of the non-tumorous liver. Groupe d'Etude et de Traitement du Carcinome Hepatocellulaire. *J Hepatol* 1999; **31**: 508–513.

General reading

Aggarwal R, Krawczynski K. Hepatitis E. An overview and recent advances in clinical and laboratory research. *J Gastroenterol Hepatol* 2000; **15**: 9–20.

Jaeschke H, Gujral J, Bajt M. Apoptosis and necrosis in liver disease. *Liver Int* 2004; **24**: 85–89.

Lavanchy D. Hepatitis B virus epidemiology, disease burden, treatment and current and emerging prevention and control measures. *J Viral Hepatol* 2004; **11**: 97–107.

Penin F, Dubuisson J, Rey FA, et al. Structural biology of hepatitis C virus. *Hepatology* 2004; **39**: 5–19.

Purcell RH, Emerson SU. Hepatitis E: an emerging awareness of an old disease. *J Hepatol* 2008; **48**: 494–503.

Schmid R. History of viral hepatitis: a tale of dogmas and misinterpretations. *J Gastroenterol Hepatol* 2001; **16**: 718–722.

Theise ND, Bodenheimer HC, Ferrell LD Jr. Acute and chronic viral hepatitis. In: Burt AD, Portmann BC, Ferrell LD, eds. MacSween's Pathology of the Liver, 5th edn. Edinburgh: Churchill Livingstone/Elsevier, 2007: 399–442.

Steatosis, Steatohepatitis and Related Conditions

Steatosis

Steatosis (fatty change, fatty liver) is the accumulation of abnormal amounts of lipid in hepatocytes. Most steatosis is of the macrovesicular type, in which a single large fat vacuole or several smaller ones occupy the greater part of the cell, pushing the nucleus to the periphery (**Fig. 7.1**). The less common and often more serious type is microvesicular steatosis (**Fig. 7.2**). The fat in this type is finely divided and the nucleus remains central. The two types of steatosis are sometimes found together, though one type usually predominates.

Macrovesicular steatosis

Macrovesicular steatosis is common. It is frequently apparent by non-invasive imaging and may be accompanied by moderate abnormalities of serum aminotransferases, alkaline phosphatase and γ-glutamyl transpeptidase. Liver tests may be normal.[1] There are many causes of macrovesicular steatosis, of which the most common are listed in **Table 7.1**. It is usually not possible to determine the cause of uncomplicated large-droplet steatosis from histological examination alone.

The lipid in macrovesicular steatosis accumulates in hepatocytes because of increased triglyceride synthesis or decreased excretion.[2] Increased synthesis results from availability of excess free fatty acids and fatty acid precursors and from reduced fatty acid oxidation. Reduced excretion is a result of diminished apoprotein production, seen for example in protein malnutrition and alcohol abuse. Macrovesicular steatosis provides the background on which the important lesions of alcoholic and non-alcoholic steatohepatitis develop.[3]

Most steatosis is **perivenular**. Alcohol use, adult obesity, diabetes and corticosteroid therapy typically show this location. Increasing amounts of steatosis extend to progressively involve mid-zonal and periportal regions (acinar zones 2 and 1, respectively). In contrast, **periportal steatosis** is more common in children with

Table 7.1 Common causes of macrovesicular steatosis
Obesity and diabetes mellitus
Protein-calorie malnutrition
Total parenteral nutrition
Drugs and toxins (e.g. alcohol, corticosteroids)
Metabolic disorders (e.g. Wilson's disease)
Infections (e.g. hepatitis C)

**Figure 7.1
Macrovesicular
steatosis.**
There are large
fat vacuoles in
perivenular
hepatocytes,
displacing the nuclei
to the edges of the
cells. (Needle biopsy,
H&E.)

**Figure 7.2
Microvesicular
steatosis.**
Swollen hepatocytes
near an efferent
venule (right)
contain numerous
small vacuoles.
The nuclei have
maintained their
central position.
Some large fat
vacuoles are also
present. (Needle
biopsy, H&E.)

non-alcoholic fatty liver disease (discussed later), in patients on parenteral nutrition, in kwashiorkor and protein-calorie malnutrition, and it is sometimes seen in AIDS (**Fig. 7.3**). In **focal fatty change**[4] more or less rounded foci of steatosis are seen in an otherwise normal liver and may be mistaken for neoplasms on imaging.

The histological **grade** of steatosis should be reported based on the percentage of hepatocytes which contain lipid vacuoles. One commonly used scoring system includes

Figure 7.3
Periportal
steatosis.
Liver biopsy from a
patient with AIDS
and portal tract
infiltration by
large-cell lymphoma.
Periportal
hepatocytes contain
large fat vacuoles.
(Needle biopsy,
H&E.)

grades of minimal (<5%), mild (5–30%), moderate (30–60%) and marked (>60%). Provision of a numerical assessment to the nearest percentile is also recommended (e.g. 'marked macrovesicular steatosis is present involving approximately 90% of the parenchyma'). Periodic acid–Schiff and trichrome stains can be helpful in the assessment, providing contrast of the large lipid vacuoles against the more darkly stained background cytoplasm of hepatocytes. Digitised computer image analysis[5] is an alternative method of grading but from a practical standpoint is better suited to research settings.[6]

Occasionally lipid-laden hepatocytes rupture and the fat is then taken up by macrophages. The resulting lesion is a **lipogranuloma (Fig. 7.4)**. Lipogranulomas are situated within the lobules, often near terminal venules. Serial sectioning may be needed to identify the fat in the centre of the lesion. Lipogranulomas may undergo fibrosis, but this does not appear to contribute to progressive liver disease and must be distinguished from the more important pericellular fibrosis characteristic of steatohepatitis (see below). Globules within portal tracts are usually the result of uptake of ingested or injected mineral oils by macrophages, rather than uptake of lipids[7] **(Fig. 7.5)**. **Lipopeliosis** – the formation of large intrasinusoidal fat cysts following release of lipid from hepatocytes after transplantation – is described in **Chapter 16**.

The differential diagnosis of macrovesicular steatosis includes microvesicular steatosis. The presence of several fat vacuoles in one hepatocyte has to be distinguished from true microvesicular steatosis (below) in which vacuoles are generally less than 1 μm in diameter and may even be invisible in paraffin sections by light microscopy. The distinction is clinically important. The location of the nucleus helps to differentiate the two conditions. A second differential diagnosis is from **stellate cell hyperplasia (Fig. 7.6)** in which the vacuoles are not in hepatocytes but in perisinusoidally located stellate cells.[8] Their nuclei are compressed into a crescentic shape by the vitamin A-rich globules. Stellate cell hyperplasia may be unexplained, but should lead to investigation of possible overuse of vitamin A or other retinoids.

**Figure 7.4
Lipogranuloma.**
A lipogranuloma has formed near the terminal venule (V) in this moderately steatotic liver. *Inset*: The lipogranuloma contains large lipid vacuoles and aggregated Kupffer cells with scattered lymphocytes and a few eosinophils. (Needle biopsy, H&E.)

**Figure 7.5
Mineral oil globules.**
A row of vacuoles within macrophages is seen to the right of a portal venule. (Needle biopsy, H&E.)

Figure 7.6 Stellate cell hyperplasia. Stellate cells with single or multiple lipid vacuoles lie in the space of Disse between hepatocytes (arrows). Stellate-cell nuclei are small, intensely basophilic and indented by the cytoplasmic vacuoles. Hepatocyte nuclei are larger, less dense and rounded. (Needle biopsy, H&E.)

Microvesicular steatosis

In this serious and sometimes fatal condition, finely divided fat accumulates in hepatocyte cytoplasm as a result of mitochondrial damage leading to impaired β-oxidation.[9] Causes include acute fatty liver of pregnancy (**Ch. 15**), hepatotoxic drugs such as valproate and nucleoside analogues (**Ch. 8**), mitochondrial DNA depletion and deletion syndromes,[10] foamy degeneration in the alcoholic (see below) and total parenteral nutrition (**Table 7.2**). Another cause, Reye's syndrome, has declined sharply in incidence in recent years. In neonates and children, mitochondrial hepatopathies may need consideration.[10] Viral infections occasionally give rise to similar changes.[11]

Table 7.2 Main causes of microvesicular steatosis
Acute fatty liver of pregnancy
Alcoholic foamy degeneration
Drugs (e.g. nucleoside analogues, valproate)
Toxins (e.g. in Jamaican vomiting disease)
Total parenteral nutrition
Inborn errors of metabolism (e.g. urea cycle disorders)
Reye's syndrome
Infections

Histologically, the cytoplasmic lipid is seen to be very finely divided and is not always obvious in paraffin sections. It can be stained with oil red O in frozen sections. The affected hepatocytes are often swollen. Their nuclei remain central (see **Fig. 7.2**).

The differential diagnosis is from macrovesicular steatosis and from conditions in which hepatocytes are swollen for other reasons, such as hepatitis. As discussed in **Chapter 13**, phospholipids and sphingolipids accumulate in various metabolic disorders. Cholesterol esters accumulate in hepatocytes in Wolman's disease and cholesterol ester storage disease, and glycogen accumulates in glycogen storage disease.

Alcoholic and non-alcoholic fatty liver disease

The terms **alcoholic fatty liver disease** (AFLD) and **non-alcoholic fatty liver disease** (NAFLD) are used to describe the complete range of changes from uncomplicated macrovesicular steatosis to steatohepatitis and cirrhosis seen, respectively, in alcohol abuse and in obesity, diabetes, hyperlipidaemia and the metabolic syndrome. Insulin resistance, central (truncal) obesity, type 2 diabetes, hyperlipidaemia and systemic hypertension constitute the *metabolic syndrome*. NAFLD is considered the hepatic expression of the metabolic syndrome.[12] The recent upsurge in obesity and diabetes in industrialised countries and in other populations has brought NAFLD to increased attention in clinical and basic science. In the United States, NAFLD is currently the leading cause of abnormal serum aminotransferases and chronic liver disease.[13,14] A similar impact is likely in other Western countries and in other populations where the risk factors for NAFLD are prevalent. Emphasis on the histological evaluation of macrovesicular steatosis and related changes in liver biopsy, explant and postmortem specimens has consequently grown.

Systematic histological approach to fatty liver disease

Histological evaluation in AFLD and NAFLD should take into account not only the presence of large-droplet steatosis, but also evidence of hepatocellular damage, inflammation, fibrosis and siderosis which may also be present. The diagnosis of steatohepatitis should be rendered based on specific histological criteria (described in detail below). In AFLD and NAFLD there may be relatively inconspicuous *apoptotic bodies*.[15-17] *Focal lobular inflammation* (usually clusters of lymphocytes and activated Kupffer cells) may be seen but does not constitute steatohepatitis. Uncomplicated steatosis in the majority of cases is not associated with significant portal tract inflammation. However, focal *minimal or mild portal lymphocytic infiltrates* are sometimes present in either condition.[18,19] These must be distinguished from the portal inflammation seen in chronic hepatitis which is denser, regularly involves most or all portal tracts, includes plasma cells and eosinophils in addition to lymphocytes and may also be accompanied by interface hepatitis and lymphoid aggregates or follicles. Any histological doubt on this issue should be resolved by discussion with the clinician and investigations to exclude causes of chronic hepatitis when necessary. Some adult and paediatric patients with NAFLD show positive serum *anti-nuclear and/or anti-smooth muscle antibodies*,[20-22] raising a clinical suspicion of autoimmune hepatitis (AIH). However, these autoantibodies are usually low-titer and are considered non-specific. The characteristic portal lymphoplasmacytic inflammation, interface hepatitis and regenerative rosettes of AIH are typically absent in such instances. Rarely, anti-mitochondrial antibody may be positive.[23,24]

A connective tissue stain is important to evaluate the extent of any fibrosis and its distribution in the steatotic liver. When there is fibrosis in AFLD and NAFLD, it is usually present as a feature of steatohepatitis and is seen in centrilobular regions (acinar zone 3), as described below. Alternatively (and less frequently), there may be portal and periportal fibrosis. This distribution is more common in paediatric NAFLD[25] and in morbidly obese individuals.[26]

An iron stain should also be reviewed for *siderosis*. Mild iron overload in Kupffer cells and/or hepatocytes may be seen in alcoholic patients because of altered intestinal iron absorption and in NAFLD[27,28] due to **dysmetabolic hepatic iron overload (DHIO)**[29] (**Fig. 7.7**). Significant hepatocellular siderosis should always prompt consideration of possible primary (genetic) iron overload.

Several systems have been used to assess steatosis,[30] inflammation and hepatocellular damage in NAFLD.[31] A useful approach was provided by Matteoni and colleagues,[32] who characterised steatotic changes in NAFLD according to four types: NAFLD type 1 (simple steatosis); NAFLD type 2 (steatosis with inflammation); NAFLD type 3 (steatosis with

Figure 7.7 Dysmetabolic hepatic iron overload. This case of non-alcoholic fatty liver disease with marked steatosis is associated with mild siderosis of periportal hepatocytes (long arrows) and sinusoidal Kupffer cells (short arrow). (Needle biopsy, Prussian blue iron stain.)

hepatocellular ballooning degeneration); and NAFLD type 4 (non-alcoholic steatohepatitis or NASH) (**Fig. 7.8**). Increased morbidity and mortality was associated with types 3 and 4. Swollen and ballooned hepatocytes in livers with macrovesicular steatosis are an indication for further careful examination to exclude frank steatohepatitis. The pattern of portal/periportal fibrosis with chronic inflammation (paediatric NAFLD, morbid obesity) might be considered to be NAFLD type 5 (**Fig. 7.9**).

Diabetes mellitus

In patients with diabetes mellitus, glycogen vacuolation of hepatocyte nuclei is common[33] (**Fig. 7.10**). These 'glycogen nuclei' are also seen in Wilson's disease (**Ch. 14**), in non-alcoholic steatohepatitis and in biopsies from children and adolescents less than 14–15 years of age. Hepatomegaly in diabetics is not always attributable to steatosis: rarely, diabetics who are poorly controlled may develop Mauriac's syndrome, with abnormal serum liver tests and massive accumulation of glycogen in hepatocytes (**glycogenic hepatopathy**[34]) giving rise to a picture closely resembling inherited glycogen storage disease (**see Fig. 13.12**). Some diabetics with **diabetic hepatosclerosis**[35] (**Fig. 7.11**) show an increase in perisinusoidal type IV collagen[36] without a zonal predilection.

Steatohepatitis, alcoholic and non-alcoholic

In some patients with steatosis an inflammatory and fibrosing lesion, steatohepatitis, develops. This may then lead to cirrhosis. Some patients later develop hepatocellular carcinoma. Most patients with steatohepatitis are alcohol abusers or are overweight, diabetic, or have a combination of attributes of the metabolic syndrome. The terms alcoholic

**Figure 7.8
Non-alcoholic
fatty liver disease
(NAFLD) types
1–4.**
A: NAFLD type 1
(simple steatosis).
B: NAFLD type 2
(steatosis with focal
inflammation).

Figure 7.8, cont'd
C: NAFLD type 3 (steatosis with ballooned hepatocytes). Swollen hepatocytes with rarefied cytoplasm are seen at right. **D:** NAFLD type 4 (non-alcoholic steatohepatitis or NASH). The terminal venule (V) is surrounded by fibrosis and inflammation. Perivenular hepatocytes are swollen and show cytoplasmic Mallory bodies (arrows). (Needle biopsies, H&E.)

**Figure 7.9
Steatosis with mild periportal fibrosis and chronic inflammation.**
This biopsy from an obese child shows large-droplet steatosis with mild periportal fibrosis and chronic inflammation (at right). This pattern in children with non-alcoholic fatty liver disease is referred to as NASH type 2. Note the absence of liver-cell ballooning, Mallory bodies, inflammation or fibrosis near the terminal venule at lower left. (Needle biopsy, H&E.)

**Figure 7.10
Diabetes mellitus.**
Glycogen vacuolation is seen in the nuclei of most periportal hepatocytes. (Needle biopsy, H&E.)

Figure 7.11 Diabetic hepatosclerosis. A: Increased perisinusoidal collagen is evident (arrows). (H&E.) **B:** The increased perisinusoidal collagen shows no zonal preference. (Trichrome stain.) (Photomicrographs kindly provided by Dr Elizabeth Brunt, St Louis, MO, USA.)

steatohepatitis (ASH) and non-alcoholic steatohepatitis (NASH) are used accordingly. In a minority of patients NASH is associated with other factors, listed later in this chapter. The risk of developing steatohepatitis and cirrhosis in the alcoholic rises with the amount of alcohol consumed daily,[37] but genetic and other factors are also influential. Although simple steatosis in individuals with NAFLD has previously been considered a clinically benign and non-progressive condition, recent studies indicate the potential over time for progression to steatohepatitis, cirrhosis and hepatocellular carcinoma.[14]

Pathological features of steatohepatitis

The changes in ASH and NASH are very similar, and the two conditions cannot usually be distinguished on histological grounds alone.[38] The main pathological features comprise hepatocellular damage, inflammation and fibrosis (**Table 7.3**). The following description is of the fully developed lesion.

Hepatocellular damage is generally most severe in, or even restricted to, perivenular areas (**Fig. 7.12**). It takes the form of cell swelling and clearing of the cytoplasm, together with the appearance of Mallory bodies (Mallory's hyalin, Mallory–Denk bodies[39]). The affected cells often do not contain obvious fat vacuoles, but these are visible in other parts of the parenchyma. The Mallory bodies consist of clumps and skeins of dense eosinophilic material, which sometimes forms a ring around the nucleus. When they are difficult to identify,

Table 7.3 Main pathological features of steatohepatitis

Steatosis
Hepatocyte ballooning
Hepatocyte apoptosis
Mallory body formation

Inflammatory in?ltration
  Neutrophils
  Lymphocytes
  Sinusoidal cells

Fibrosis
  Pericellular
  Other

Figure 7.12 Alcoholic steatohepatitis. Inflammatory cells, mainly neutrophils, are clustered around and within hepatocytes, some of which contain densely stained Mallory bodies (arrows). Many hepatocytes contain large fat vacuoles. (Needle biopsy, H&E.)

Figure 7.13 Mallory bodies. The Mallory bodies in this example of steatohepatitis stain strongly for ubiquitin (arrows). (Needle biopsy, specific immunostain for ubiquitin.)

positive immunostaining for p62 or ubiquitin is helpful[39,40] (**Fig. 7.13**). Swollen hepatocytes in steatohepatitis have reduced or absent filaments of keratins 8 and 18 (K8 and K18),[41] demonstrable by using specific K8 and K18 immunostains.[42] This feature can be used to distinguish steatohepatitic swelling from certain other causes of ballooning such as that seen in viral hepatitis where keratin 8/18 staining is preserved.[42] This can be demonstrated with specific immunostains.[42] Hepatocytes may also contain megamito-chondria, which are rounded or elongated eosinophilic bodies from 2 µm to 10 µm across

**Figure 7.14
Alcoholic
steatohepatitis.**
Two bright red giant
mitochondria are
marked with arrows.
Collagen fibres,
stained blue, are
seen around
ballooned
hepatocytes. (Needle
biopsy, CAB.)

(**Fig. 7.14**). These can be distinguished from Mallory bodies by their more definite outline and by red staining with chromotrope–aniline blue (CAB); Mallory bodies usually stain blue with the latter. Megamitochondria can be found in both ASH and NASH as well as in the livers of alcohol abusers in the absence of steatohepatitis.[43–46] Crystalline intra-mitochondrial inclusions can be seen on transmission electron microscopy in the giant mitochondria of NASH.[46]

The inflammatory infiltrate is characteristically rich in neutrophils but lymphocytes are also present. These are mainly T cells of CD4 and CD8 phenotype, and are found both in areas of steatohepatitis and in portal tracts.[47] Neutrophils surround or even infiltrate bal-looned, Mallory body-containing hepatocytes (**Fig. 7.15**). Macrophages and other sinu-soidal cells take part in the process. Kupffer cells may contain fat vacuoles.[47] Both macrophages and sinusoidal endothelial cells may contain stainable iron.[29]

Fibrosis is an integral part of the lesion of steatohepatitis. The most characteristic form of fibrosis is pericellular ('chicken-wire' fibrosis). Delicate or thicker strands of collagen surround ballooned hepatocytes to form a network which is well seen with trichrome stains (**Fig. 7.16**) and less easy to detect in reticulin preparations. The location corresponds to that of the cell damage and inflammation. In severe steatohepatitis, the fibrosis extends to the portal tracts as well as between perivenular areas, forming fibrous bridges often accompanied by a ductular reaction (**Fig. 7.17**). The evolution of such bridging fibrosis is similar to that seen in NASH.[48] Portal fibrosis is sometimes seen in the absence of the pericellular component.

These are the histological features of a classic, fully developed steatohepatitis. Like all pathological processes, however, steatohepatitis is an evolving lesion, which also varies in severity. For these reasons liver biopsy may show less obvious changes, not readily recog-nised as part of the spectrum. Mallory bodies may be absent or not demonstrable in the biopsy sample. The inflammatory infiltrate may be predominantly lymphocytic, and peri-cellular fibrosis may be slight or undetectable. In a small minority of patients the only indication of a probable steatohepatitis is finding a few swollen, Mallory body-containing hepatocytes without associated inflammation. This should always be reported and regarded

Figure 7.15
Alcoholic
steatohepatitis.
Hepatocytes contain
abundant Mallory
bodies and
neutrophils. (Needle
biopsy, H&E.)

Figure 7.16
Pericellular fibrosis.
Collagen fibres,
stained blue, form a
meshwork in this
example of
steatohepatitis.
(Needle biopsy,
CAB.)

as a sign that the patient may be at risk of progressive disease, which is more important from the point of view of patient management than the definition of minimal diagnostic criteria. Another feature of probable significance is the finding of pericellular fibrosis without any of the other changes of steatohepatitis, possibly the result of past steatohepatitis.

Figure 7.17 Fibrosis in alcoholic steatohepatitis. Abundant collagen (C) has been laid down in a perivenular area, linked to a portal tract (P) by a fibrous bridge with ductular reaction (arrows). (Needle biopsy, Martius scarlet blue.)

Non-alcoholic steatohepatitis

NASH has assumed increasing importance in recent years and the diagnosis is now a major clinical consideration when liver function tests are abnormal but viral markers are negative. The main clinical associations are listed in **Table 7.4**. It is important to note that, while obesity, diabetes and the metabolic syndrome are common associations with NASH, patients are not all obese,[49] and hyperlipidaemia and other disorders of lipid metabolism may need to be investigated. Certain drugs (amiodarone,[50] calcium channel blockers,[51] tamoxifen[52]) and toxins[53] and rare disorders such as Weber–Christian disease[54] (nodular panniculitis) are other possible causes. NASH can affect men, women and also children.[25] In **paediatric NASH**, a histological picture of steatosis, portal fibrosis with or without fibrous septa and a mainly lymphocytic infiltrate (**Fig. 7.9**) is more common than the typical perivenular lesion of adult NASH; in the paediatric population this is referred to as NASH type 2.[25]

There is an extensive literature on the pathogenesis of NASH, some of it cited under General reading at the end of this chapter. The exact mechanisms have not been fully elucidated, but many of the important factors involved have been defined. These include insulin resistance,[55] excess of free fatty acids in hepatocytes, lipid peroxidation[56] and oxidative stress.[57] Venous obstruction may be important in the progression to cirrhosis.[58] An element of genetic predisposition is likely[59,60] and NASH has been reported in kindreds.[61] Some of the above factors, such as excess of free fatty acids and oxidative stress, are common to NASH and ASH and help to explain their similarity.

The histological lesion in NASH (**Fig. 7.18**) is as described above under 'Pathological features of steatohepatitis', but may not be as severe as that in ASH. The presence of abundant neutrophils and Mallory bodies should therefore lead to a suspicion of alcohol abuse.

Table 7.4 Main causes and associations of non-alcoholic steatohepatitis
Obesity
Diabetes mellitus
Metabolic syndrome
Hyperlipidaemia
Gastrointestinal surgery for obesity
Drugs and chemicals (e.g. amiodarone, tamoxifen, petrochemicals[53])

Figure 7.18 Non-alcoholic steatohepatitis. There is steatosis, hepatocellular ballooning and infiltration by neutrophils, as in the alcoholic counterpart. (Needle biopsy, H&E.)

Glycogen vacuolation of nuclei is common in NASH.[38] Occasionally the lobular changes appear to be periportal rather than perivenular,[62] but this may reflect the difficulty of accurate localisation in two-dimensional sections. The pericellular fibrosis of NASH is very like that of ASH and is illustrated in **Fig. 8.8**. It is associated with hepatocellular injury, as shown by ballooning degeneration and Mallory body formation.[63] As described earlier, in some patients fibrosis is confined to the portal areas.[26,64] Hepatocytes damaged by pathogenetic factors active in NASH may show impaired regeneration ('replicative senescence'), and such affected liver cells may display positive nuclear staining for the cell cycle inhibitor p21 on immunostaining.[48] In this setting, activation of periportal progenitor/stem cells to form a ductular reaction in tandem with fibrosis contribute to the bridging fibrosis and architectural obscuration seen in NASH as it progresses towards cirrhosis.[48] Even in later stages of ASH and NASH, some portal tracts may be spared and this can be a diagnostically helpful finding, further pointing to the centrilobular regions as the site of the initiating insult. The presence of spared portal tracts at the centres of cirrhotic nodules surrounded by fibrous septa bridging between central veins may render an appearance of 'reverse lobulation'.

Progression of the lesion to cirrhosis is variable but often slow.[65] Like other forms of cirrhosis it carries the risk of liver failure and hepatocellular carcinoma.[66-68] Clinical features associated with NASH are also common in patients with cryptogenic cirrhosis, suggesting that the latter is frequently the end result of NASH.[69-72]

A scoring system for NASH has been devised, allowing semi-quantitative assessment and reporting of liver biopsy changes.[73-75] Separate scores are allotted for the severity of the hepatocyte damage and inflammation on the one hand, and for fibrosis and cirrhosis on the other (**Table 7.5**). As in the case of scoring in chronic viral hepatitis (**Ch. 9**), the resulting numbers must be regarded as categories rather than measurements.

Histological differential diagnosis

The histological differential diagnosis of steatohepatitis includes other forms of hepatitis. In viral and autoimmune hepatitis the infiltrating cells are lymphocytes and plasma cells rather than neutrophils. In acute viral hepatitis there is collapse of the reticulin framework

Table 7.5 A scoring system for steatohepatitis

Necroinflammatory grading	
Grade 1 (mild)	Steatosis (mainly macrovesicular) involving up to 66% of lobules; occasional ballooned perivenular hepatocytes; scattered neutrophils with or without lymphocytes; no or mild chronic portal inflammation
Grade 2 (moderate)	Steatosis of any degree; obvious ballooning (mainly perivenular); intralobular neutrophils, may be associated with perivenular pericellular fibrosis if evident; mild to moderate portal and intralobular chronic inflammation
Grade 3 (severe)	Panlobular steatosis; obvious perivenular ballooning and disarray; marked lobular inflammation; neutrophils may be concentrated in perivenular areas of ballooning and in areas of pericellular fibrosis if evident; portal inflammation mild or moderate
Fibrosis staging	
Stage 1	Pericellular fibrosis in perivenular areas, focal or extensive
Stage 2	As above, plus focal or extensive periportal fibrosis
Stage 3	Bridging fibrosis, focal or extensive
Stage 4	Cirrhosis

Adapted from Brunt et al.[73] with permission from Nature Publishing Group.

but the 'chicken-wire' pattern of pericellular fibrosis is not seen. There may be steatosis in patients with chronic hepatitis C, particularly genotype 3 infection[76] (**Ch. 9**). Chronic hepatitis C accompanied by steatohepatitis is sometimes seen because of virus-related or co-morbid conditions associated with insulin resistance.[77] The fibrosis of venous outflow obstruction is usually linear and parasinusoidal rather than pericellular, but sometimes the hepatic fibrosis of long-standing cardiac disease can resemble that of steatohepatitis. The presence of congestion and absence of other features of steatohepatitis should make the diagnosis clear.

In chronic cholestasis with or without cirrhosis, hepatocytes near fibrous septa are typically ballooned and may contain Mallory bodies as well as bilirubin. Neutrophils are also seen. The correct diagnosis is made by attention to the location of the lesion, the general absence of steatosis, the presence of copper and copper-associated protein in the affected periportal hepatocytes, and to clinical circumstances. Amiodarone hepatotoxicity shows a similar periportal predilection of Mallory bodies and inflammation, often with little or no steatosis.[78] Ballooning and Mallory bodies are also features of Wilson's disease; again, confusion with steatohepatitis is unlikely.

Because steatohepatitis is common in some populations, it is quite often found together with the changes of another liver disease in the same biopsy. Documented diseases coexisting with steatohepatitis include chronic hepatitis, primary biliary cirrhosis, iron storage disorders, drug-induced liver injury and metabolic disorders.[79] The pathologist should therefore consider whether all the changes seen in a biopsy can be explained by steatohepatitis alone.

Other alcohol-related liver lesions

The pathological features of ASH have been described earlier. A wide variety of other changes may be found in liver biopsies from drinkers (**Table 7.6**). In some alcohol abusers

Table 7.6 Liver lesions in the alcoholic

Steatosis
  Macrovesicular
  Microvesicular (foamy degeneration)

Steatohepatitis

Megamitochondria

Siderosis

Fibrosis
  Pericellular
  Perivenular
  Portal

Cirrhosis

Hepatocellular carcinoma

Effects of non-hepatic alcohol-related diseases

the liver is histologically normal or shows only mild macrovesicular steatosis. Portal tracts may contain lymphocytic infiltrates in the absence of other features of hepatitis.[80]

Alcoholic foamy degeneration

Alcoholic foamy degeneration[81] is a relatively rare, potentially life-threatening condition characterised by extensive microvesicular steatosis in perivenular areas. Macrovesicular fat may be seen elsewhere. There may be cholestasis, fine fibrosis and scanty Mallory bodies, but inflammation is minimal or absent and the condition is thus distinct from ASH. Biochemical and histological features of cholestasis have been described.[82]

Fibrosis

Fibrosis is occasionally seen in drinkers in the absence of severe steatosis or steatohepatitis. When the fibrosis is portal (**Fig. 7.19**), the possibility of associated biliary disease, alcoholic pancreatitis or coexisting viral hepatitis should be considered. Perivenular fibrosis may be found with or without steatosis or steatohepatitis. Pericellular fibrosis is an important component of steatohepatitis as already noted, and should always be looked for with the help of a collagen stain. When it is found in the absence of the other features of steatohepatitis it may represent the remnant of a previous episode of this lesion. As such, it is a warning that the patient may be at risk of progressive disease if the cause is not removed.

Figure 7.19 Portal fibrosis in an alcoholic.
A small portal tract has undergone fibrosis to produce a stellate outline. (Needle biopsy, H&E.)

Fetal alcohol syndrome

In the fetal alcohol syndrome, children of mothers abusing alcohol during pregnancy have fatty livers together with perisinusoidal and portal fibrosis.[83]

Cirrhosis

Cirrhosis in the alcoholic develops as a result of increasing fibrosis in steatohepatitis, together with nodular regeneration of the surviving parenchyma. There may also be other routes to cirrhosis, not involving steatohepatitis, but these are difficult to prove. Because steatohepatitis tends to involve all lobules, the cirrhosis is usually micronodular at first (see Figs 10.12, 10.13). As the regeneration nodules enlarge, the cirrhosis remodels to a macronodular pattern and the original cause of the cirrhosis becomes more difficult or even impossible to establish on histological grounds. Venous occlusion is common,[84,85] and may be missed unless stains for collagen or elastic tissue are examined. Hepatocellular carcinoma may develop within the cirrhotic liver.

Other lesions

Alcohol-related lesions affecting organs other than the liver may cause liver changes. Chronic alcoholic pancreatitis has already been cited as a cause of portal fibrosis.[86] In patients with alcoholic cardiomyopathy the changes of right-sided heart failure may be found.

Finally, alcohol-related liver disease may coexist with other, non-alcohol-related liver diseases such as chronic hepatitis C. Alcohol consumption appears to accelerate the progression of fibrosis in hepatitis C.[87]

References

1 Fracanzani AL, Valenti L, Bugianesi E, et al. Risk of severe liver disease in nonalcoholic fatty liver disease with normal aminotransferase levels: a role for insulin resistance and diabetes. *Hepatology* 2008; **48**: 792–798.

2 Burt AD, Mutton A, Day CP. Diagnosis and interpretation of steatosis and steatohepatitis. *Semin Diagn Pathol* 1998; **15**: 246–258.

3 Day CP, James OFW. Steatohepatitis: a tale of two 'hits'? *Gastroenterology* 1998; **114**: 842–845.

4 Wanless IR. Benign liver tumors. *Clin Liver Dis* 2002; **6**: 513–526.

5 Franzén LE, Ekstedt M, Kechagias S, et al. Semiquantitative evaluation overestimates the degree of steatosis in liver biopsies: a comparison to stereological point counting. *Mod Pathol* 2005; **18**: 912–916.

6 Turlin B, Ramm GA, Purdie DM, et al. Assessment of hepatic steatosis: comparison of quantitative and semiquantitative methods in 108 liver biopsies. *Liver Int* 2009; **29**: 530–535.

7 Wanless IR, Geddie WR. Mineral oil lipogranulomata in liver and spleen. A study of 465 autopsies. *Arch Pathol Lab Med* 1985; **109**: 283–286.

8 Levine PH, Delgado Y, Theise ND, et al. Stellate-cell lipidosis in liver biopsy specimens. Recognition and significance. *Am J Clin Pathol* 2003; **119**: 254–258.

9 Fromenty B, Berson A, Pessayre D. Microvesicular steatosis and steatohepatitis: role of mitochondrial dysfunction and lipid peroxidation. *J Hepatol* 1997; **26**(Suppl. 1): 13–22.

10 Lee WS, Sokol RJ. Mitochondrial hepatopathies: advances in genetics and pathogenesis. *Hepatology* 2007; **45**: 1555–1565.

11 Aita K, Jin Y, Irie H, et al. Are there histopathologic characteristics particular to fulminant hepatic failure caused by human herpesvirus-6 infection? A case report and discussion. *Hum Pathol* 2001; **32**: 887–889.

12 Marchesini G, Bugianesi E, Forlani G, et al. Nonalcoholic fatty liver, steatohepatitis, and the metabolic syndrome. *Hepatology* 2003; **37**: 917–923.

13 Charlton M. Cirrhosis and liver failure in nonalcoholic fatty liver disease: molehill or mountain? *Hepatology* 2008; **47**: 1431–1433.

14 Ekstedt M, Franzen LE, Mathiesen UL, et al. Long-term follow-up of patients with NAFLD and elevated liver enzymes. *Hepatology* 2006; **44**: 865–873.

15 Natori S, Rust C, Stadheim LM, et al. Hepatocyte apoptosis is a pathologic feature of human alcoholic hepatitis. *J Hepatol* 2001; **34**: 248–253.

16 Ziol M, Tepper M, Lohez M, et al. Clinical and biological relevance of hepatocyte apoptosis in alcoholic hepatitis. *J Hepatol* 2001; **34**: 254–260.

17 Feldstein AE, Canbay A, Angulo P, et al. Hepatocyte apoptosis and Fas expression are prominent features of human nonalcoholic steatohepatitis. *Gastroenterology* 2003; **125**: 437–443.

18 Colombat M, Charlotte F, Ratziu V, Poynard T. Portal lymphocytic infiltrate in alcoholic liver disease. *Hum Pathol* 2002; **33**: 1170–1174.

19 Brunt EM, Kleiner DE, WIlson LA, et al. Portal chronic inflammation in nonalcoholic fatty liver disease (NAFLD): a histologic marker of advanced NAFLD – clinicopathologic correlations from the Nonalcoholic Steatohepatitis Clinical Research Network. *Hepatology* 2009; **49**: 809–820.

20 Adams LA, Lindor KD, Angulo P. The prevalence of autoantibodies and autoimmune hepatitis in patients with nonalcoholic fatty liver disease. *Am J Gastroenterol* 2004; **99**: 1316–1320.

21 Cotler SJ, Kanji K, Keshavarzian A, et al. Prevalence and significance of autoantibodies in patients with non-alcoholic steatohepatitis. *J Clin Gastroenterol* 2004; **38**: 801–804.

22 Patton HM, Lavine JE, Van Natta ML, et al. Clinical correlates of histopathology in pediatric nonalcoholic steatohepatitis. *Gastroenterology* 2008; **135**: 1961–1971.

23 Loria P, Lonardo A, Leonardi F, et al. Non-organ-specific autoantibodies in nonalcoholic fatty liver disease: prevalence and correlates. *Dig Dis Sci* 2003; **48**: 2173–2181.

24 Czaja AJ, Carpenter HA, Santrach PJ, et al. Genetic predisposition for immunologic features in chronic liver diseases other than autoimmune hepatitis. *J Hepatol* 1996; **24**: 52–59.

25 Schwimmer JB, Behling C, Newbury R, et al. Histopathology of pediatric nonalcoholic fatty liver disease. *Hepatology* 2005; **42**: 641–649.

26 Abrams GA, Kunde SS, Lazenby AJ, et al. Portal fibrosis and hepatic steatosis in morbidly obese subjects: a spectrum of nonalcoholic fatty liver disease. *Hepatology* 2004; **40**: 475–483.

27 Deugnier Y, Brissot P, Loréal O. Iron and the liver: update 2008. *J Hepatol* 2008; **48**: S113–S123.

28 Aigner E, Theurl I, Haufe H, et al. Copper availability contributes to iron perturbations in human nonalcoholic fatty liver disease. *Gastroenterology* 2008; **135**: 680–688.

29 Turlin B, Mendler MH, Moirand R, et al. Histologic features of the liver in insulin resistance-associated iron overload. A study of 139 patients. *Am J Clin Pathol* 2001; **116**: 263–270.

30 Chalasani N, Wilson L, Kleiner DE, et al. Relationship of steatosis grade and zonal location to histological features of steatohepatitis in adult patients with non-alcoholic fatty liver disease. *J Hepatol* 2008; **48**: 829–834.

31 Kleiner DE, Brunt EM, Van Natta M, et al. Design and validation of a histological scoring system for nonalcoholic fatty liver disease. *Hepatology* 2005; **41**: 1313–1321.

32 Matteoni CA, Younossi ZM, Gramlich T, et al. Nonalcoholic fatty liver disease: a spectrum of clinical and pathological severity. *Gastroenterology* 1999; **116**: 1413–1419.

33 Abraham S, Furth EE. Receiver operating characteristic analysis of glycogenated nuclei in liver biopsy specimens: quantitative evaluation of their relationship with diabetes and obesity. *Hum Pathol* 1994; **25**: 1063–1068.

34 Torbenson M, Chen Y-Y, Brunt E, et al. Glycogenic hepatopathy. An underrecognized hepatic complication of diabetes mellitus. *Am J Surg Pathol* 2006; **30**: 508–513.

35 Harrison SA, Brunt EM, Goodman ZD, et al. Diabetic hepatosclerosis: a novel entity or a rare form of nonalcoholic fatty liver disease? *Arch Pathol Lab Med* 2006; **130**: 27–32.

36 Latry P, Bioulac-Sage P, Echinard E, et al. Perisinusoidal fibrosis and basement membrane-like material in the livers of diabetic patients. *Hum Pathol* 1987; **18**: 775–780.

37 David K, Kowdley KV, Unalp A, et al. Quality of life in adults with nonalcoholic fatty liver disease: baseline data from the Nonalcoholic Steatohepatitis Clinical Research Network. *Hepatology* 2009; **49**: 1904–1912.

38 Itoh S, Yougel T, Kawagoe K. Comparison between nonalcoholic steatohepatitis and alcoholic hepatitis. *Am J Gastroenterol* 1987; **82**: 650–654.

39 Zatloukal K, French SW, Stumptner C, et al. From Mallory to Mallory–Denk bodies: what, how and why? *Exp Cell Res* 2007; **313**: 2033–2049.

40 Banner BF, Savas L, Zivny J, et al. Ubiquitin as a marker of cell injury in nonalcoholic steatohepatitis. *Am J Clin Pathol* 2000; **114**: 860–866.

41 Strnad P, Stumptner C, Zatloukal K, et al. Intermediate filament cytoskeleton of the liver in health and disease. *Histochem Cell Biol* 2008; **129**: 735–749.

42 Lackner C, Gogg-Kamerer M, Zatloukal K, et al. Ballooned hepatocytes in steatohepatitis: the value of keratin immunohistochemistry for diagnosis. *J Hepatol* 2008; **48**: 821–828.

43 Caldwell SH, Swerdlow RH, Khan EM, et al. Mitochondrial abnormalities in non-alcoholic steatohepatitis. *J Hepatol* 1999; **31**: 430–434.

44 Sanyal AJ, Campbell-Sargent C, Mirshahi F, et al. Nonalcoholic steatohepatitis: association of insulin resistance and mitochondrial abnormalities. *Gastroenterology* 2001; **120**: 1183–1192.

45 Le TH, Caldwell SH, Redick JA, et al. The zonal distribution of megamitochondria with crystalline inclusions in nonalcoholic steatohepatitis. *Hepatology* 2004; **39**: 1423–1429.

46 Caldwell SH, de Freitas AR, Park SH, et al. Intramitochondrial crystalline inclusions in nonalcoholic steatohepatitis. *Hepatology* 2009; **49**: 1888–1895.

47 Lefkowitch JH, Haythe JH, Regent N. Kupffer cell aggregation and perivenular distribution in steatohepatitis. *Mod Pathol* 2002; **15**: 699–704.

48 Richardson MM, Jonsson JR, Powell EE, et al. Progressive fibrosis in nonalcoholic steatohepatitis: association with altered regeneration and a ductular reaction. *Gastroenterology* 2007; **133**: 80–90.

49 Bacon BR, Farahvash MJ, Janney CG, et al. Nonalcoholic steatohepatitis: an expanded clinical entity. *Gastroenterology* 1994; **107**: 1103–1109.

50 Simon JB, Manley PN, Brien JF, et al. Amiodarone hepatotoxicity simulating alcoholic liver disease. *N Engl J Med* 1984; **311**: 167–172.

51 Babany G, Uzzan F, Larrey D, et al. Alcohol-like liver lesions induced by nifedipine. *J Hepatol* 1989; **9**: 252–255.

52 Pinto HC, Baptista A, Camilo ME, et al. Tamoxifen-associated steatohepatitis – report of three cases. *J Hepatol* 1995; **23**: 95–97.

53 Cotrium HP, De Freitas LAR, Freitas C, et al. Clinical and histopahological features of NASH in workers exposed to

chemicals with or without associated metabolic conditions. *Liver Int* 2004; **24**: 131–135.

54 Wasserman JM, Thung SN, Berman R, et al. Hepatic Weber–Christian disease. *Semin Liver Dis* 2001; **21**: 115–118.

55 De Alwis NMW, Day CP. Non-alcoholic fatty liver disease: the mist gradually clears. *J Hepatol* 2008; **48**: S104–S112.

56 MacDonald GA, Bridle KR, Ward PJ, et al. Lipid peroxidation in hepatic steatosis in humans is associated with hepatic fibrosis and occurs predominately in acinar zone 3. *J Gastroenterol Hepatol* 2001; **16**: 599–606.

57 Seki S, Kitada T, Yamada T, et al. In situ detection of lipid peroxidation and oxidative DNA damage in non-alcoholic fatty liver diseases. *J Hepatol* 2002; **37**: 56–62.

58 Wanless IR, Shiota K. The pathogenesis of nonalcoholic steatohepatitis and other fatty liver diseases: a four-step model including the role of lipid release and hepatic venular obstruction in the progression to cirrhosis. *Semin Liver Dis* 2004; **24**: 99–106.

59 Valenti L, Fracanzani AL, Dongiovanni P, et al. Tumor necrosis factor alpha promoter polymorphisms and insulin resistance in nonalcoholic fatty liver disease. *Gastroenterology* 2002; **122**: 274–280.

60 Namikawa C, Shu-Ping Z, Vyselaar JR, et al. Polymorphisms of microsomal triglyceride transfer protein gene and manganese superoxide dismutase gene in non-alcoholic steatohepatitis. *J Hepatol* 2004; **40**: 781–786.

61 Struben VM, Hespenheide EE, Caldwell SH. Nonalcoholic steatohepatitis and cryptogenic cirrhosis within kindreds. *Am J Med* 2000; **108**: 9–13.

62 Nagore N, Scheuer PJ. The pathology of diabetic hepatitis. *J Pathol* 1988; **156**: 155–160.

63 Gramlich T, Kleiner DE, McCullough AJ, et al. Pathologic features associated with fibrosis in nonalcoholic fatty liver disease. *Hum Pathol* 2004; **35**: 196–199.

64 Adler M, Schaffner F. Fatty liver hepatitis and cirrhosis in obese patients. *Am J Med* 1979; **67**: 811–816.

65 Fassio E, Álvarez E, Domínguez N, et al. Natural history of nonalcoholic steatohepatitis: a longitudinal study of repeat liver biopsies. *Hepatology* 2004; **40**: 820–826.

66 Shimada M, Hashimoto E, Taniai M, et al. Hepatocellular carcinoma in patients with non-alcoholic steatohepatitis. *J Hepatol* 2002; **37**: 154–160.

67 Hui JM, Kench JG, Chitturi S, et al. Long-term outcomes of cirrhosis in nonalcoholic steatohepatitis compared with hepatitis C. *Hepatology* 2003; **38**: 420–427.

68 Hashimoto E, Yatsuji S, Tobari M, et al. Hepatocellular carcinoma in patients with nonalcoholic steatohepatitis. *J Gastroenterol* 2009; **44**(Suppl XIX): 89–95.

69 Caldwell SH, Oelsner DH, Iezzoni JC, et al. Cryptogenic cirrhosis: clinical characterization and risk factors for underlying disease. *Hepatology* 1999; **29**: 664–669.

70 Poonawala A, Nair SP, Thuluvath PJ. Prevalence of obesity and diabetes in patients with cryptogenic cirrhosis: a case–control study. *Hepatology* 2000; **32**: 689–692.

71 Bugianesi E, Leone N, Vanni E, et al. Expanding the natural history of nonalcoholic steatohepatitis: from cryptogenic cirrhosis to hepatocellular carcinoma. *Gastroenterology* 2002; **123**: 134–140.

72 Clark JM, Diehl AM. Nonalcoholic fatty liver disease: an underrecognized cause of cryptogenic cirrhosis. *JAMA* 2003; **289**: 3000–3004.

73 Brunt EM, Janney CG, Di Bisceglie AM, et al. Nonalcoholic steatohepatitis: a proposal for grading and staging the histological lesions. *Am J Gastroenterol* 1999; **94**: 2467–2474.

74 Yeh MM, Brunt EM. Pathology of nonalcoholic fatty liver disease. *Am J Clin Pathol* 2007; **128**: 837–847.

75 Brunt EM, Neuschwander-Tetri BA, Kent DO, et al. Nonalcoholic steatohepatitis: histologic features and clinical correlations with 30 blinded biopsy specimens. *Hum Pathol* 2004; **35**: 1070–1082.

76 Negro, F. Hepatitis C virus and liver steatosis: is it the virus? Yes it is, but not always. *Hepatology* 2002; **36**: 1050–1052.

77 Bedossa P, Moucari R, Chelbi E, et al. Evidence for a role of nonalcoholic steatohepatitis in hepatitis C: a prospective study. *Hepatology* 2007; **46**: 380–387.

78 Lewis JH, Mullick F, Ishak KG, et al. Histopathologic analysis of suspected amiodarone hepatotoxicity. *Hum Pathol* 1990; **21**: 59–67.

79 Brunt EM, Ramrakhiani S, Cordes BG, et al. Concurrence of histologic features of steatohepatitis with other forms of chronic liver disease. *Mod Pathol* 2003; **16**: 49–56.

80 Engler S, Elsing C, Flechtenmacher C, et al. Progressive sclerosing cholangitis after shock: a new variant of vanishing bile duct disorders. *Gut* 2003; **52**: 688–693.

81 Uchida T, Kao H, Quispe-Sjogren M, et al. Alcoholic foamy degeneration – a pattern of acute alcoholic injury of the liver. *Gastroenterology* 1983; **84**: 683–692.

82 Suri S, Mitros FA, Ahluwalia JP. Alcoholic foamy degeneration and a markedly elevated GGT. A case report and literature review. *Dig Dis Sci* 2003; **48**: 1142–1146.

83 Lefkowitch JH, Rushton AR, Feng-Chen KC. Hepatic fibrosis in fetal alcohol syndrome. Pathologic similarities to adult alcoholic liver disease. *Gastroenterology* 1983; **85**: 951–957.

84 Goodman ZD, Ishak KG. Occlusive venous lesions in alcoholic liver disease. A study of 200 cases. *Gastroenterology* 1982; **83**: 786–796.

85 Burt AD, MacSween RN. Hepatic vein lesions in alcoholic liver disease: retrospective biopsy and necropsy study. *J Clin Pathol* 1986; **39**: 63–67.

86 Morgan MY, Sherlock S, Scheuer PJ. Portal fibrosis in the livers of alcoholic patients. *Gut* 1978; **19**: 1015–1021.

87 Siu L, Foont J, Wands JR. Hepatitis C virus and alcohol. *Semin Liver Dis* 2009; **29**: 188–199.

General reading

Browning JD, Horton JD. Molecular mediators of hepatic steatosis and liver injury. *J Clin Invest* 2004; **114**: 147–152.

Ekstedt M, Franzén LE, Mathiesen UL, et al. Long-term follow-up of patients with NAFLD and elevated liver enzymes. *Hepatology* 2006; **44**: 865–873.

Farrell GC, George J, Hall P de la M, McCullough AJ, eds. Fatty Liver Disease: NASH and Related Disorders. Oxford: Blackwell Publishing, 2005.

Lucey MR, Mathurin P, Morgan TR. Medical progress: alcoholic hepatitis. *N Engl J Med* 2009; **360**: 2758–2769.

Mofrad P, Contos MJ, Haque M, et al. Clinical and histologic spectrum of nonalcoholic fatty liver disease associated with normal ALT values. *Hepatology* 2003; **37**: 1286–1292.

Reuben A. Pearls of pathology. *Hepatology* 2003; **37**: 715–718.

Yeh MM, Brunt EM. Pathology of nonalcoholic fatty liver disease. *Am J Clin Pathol* 2007; **128**: 837–847.

Zafrani ES. Non-alcoholic fatty liver disease: an emerging pathological spectrum. *Virchows Arch* 2004; **444**: 3–12.

Zatloukal K, French SW, Stumptner C, et al. From Mallory to Mallory–Denk bodies: what, how and why? *Exp Cell Res* 2007; **313**: 2033–2049.

Drugs and Toxins

Introduction

This chapter deals with the pathology of the important liver lesions attributed to drugs and toxins, with their recognition, and with their differential diagnosis. There are many hundreds of hepatotoxic drugs and other chemicals, and new reports of adverse drug reactions appear regularly in the literature under the acronym 'DILI' (drug-induced liver injury). Details of the lesions attributed to each of the many individual drugs are not considered appropriate for a bench book of this kind. If required, the information can be found in one of several comprehensive reviews.[1-5] There is also a regularly updated bibliography in the French literature.[6] The pathologist reporting a liver biopsy should, however, bear in mind that a drug cannot be exonerated simply because an adverse reaction has not been reported; there is always a first time.

Chemical injury is not confined to drugs listed in pharmacopoeias. Herbal medicines,[7,8] illicit drugs,[9-17] criminally administered poisons,[18] industrial chemicals,[19-22] vitamins[23,24] and foods[25,26] have all been held responsible for liver disease. Drugs used for the treatment of liver disease have themselves been suspected of causing liver damage.[27]

In his foreword to the second edition of Stricker's *Drug-Induced Hepatic Injury*[2] Zimmerman wrote: '... virtually all known acute and chronic hepatic lesions can result from drug injury.' This important observation implies that drugs should be considered as a possible cause of any liver lesion found on biopsy, but some lesions are more often produced by drugs than others. Hepatocellular necrosis, hepatitis and cholestasis in particular should arouse a greater degree of suspicion, especially if no other cause has been found. Also, some groups of drugs are associated with particular kinds of injury; non-steroidal anti-inflammatory drugs (NSAIDs), for example, are often associated with hepatocellular injury, while neuroleptic drugs mostly cause cholestasis. However, these are generalisations and a drug which causes a dose-related hepatocellular necrosis in one patient may cause non-dose-related hepatitis, cholestasis or granulomas in another.[28,29]

The diagnostic pathologist should be aware of the potential of drugs and other substances to cause this wide variety of acute and chronic liver lesions and to know which lesions are most likely to be drug induced. He or she should be familiar with their likely course and outcome, and the main points of similarity and difference from other, non-drug-related liver diseases. Finally, the pathologist should know where to look up the effects of individual drugs.

DOI: 10.1016/B978-0-7020-3410-7.00014-9

Table 8.1 Examples of liver lesions due to drugs and toxins

Lesion	Example of substance
Intrinsic hepatotoxicity	
Microvesicular steatosis	Valproate
Phospholipidosis	Amiodarone
Hepatocellular necrosis	Paracetamol (acetaminophen)
Fibrosis	Vitamin A
Cholestasis	Contraceptive steroids
Venous occlusion	Pyrrolizidine alkaloids
Angiosarcoma	Vinyl chloride
Idiosyncratic hepatotoxicity	
Hepatitis	Isoniazid
Cholestasis	Amoxicillin–clavulanic acid
Granuloma formation	Allopurinol

Classification and mechanisms

Drugs may be regarded as producing liver injury in two main ways (**Table 8.1**). **Intrinsic (predictable) hepatotoxins** are those which predictably produce liver damage when taken in sufficient quantities. The type of damage is often characteristic of a particular drug; for example, the typical result of paracetamol (acetaminophen) overdose is hepatocellular necrosis and steatosis. Intrinsic hepatotoxicity can often be studied in laboratory animals. This type of hepatotoxicity is also frequently **zonal** in distribution; examples of this are the perivenular lesions of paracetamol and carbon tetrachloride and the periportal necrosis seen in phosphorus toxicity. The mechanism of intrinsic hepatotoxicity can be **direct** or **indirect**; in the former, the chemical or its metabolites causes structural damage to cells and organelles, while in indirect intrinsic hepatotoxicity the chemical interferes with a specific metabolic pathway or cell component.

The commoner kind of drug-related liver damage is **idiosyncratic (unpredictable)**. Only a small proportion of patients on a particular drug is affected, so that the adverse reaction is not detected in initial human trials. Many different mechanisms for idiosyncratic hepatotoxicity have now been elucidated. They include individual genetic variation in the metabolism of drugs, and the development of immune reactions to a drug or its metabolites.[30] The immune reactions may be directed to neoantigens produced by the binding of reactive metabolites to hepatic drug metabolising enzymes of the P450 system.[31,32] In some instances the distinction between an idiosyncratic and intrinsic drug reaction is difficult to make. Typical idiosyncratic damage may follow a small dose of the offending drug, and cannot easily be studied in the laboratory. With the exception of a few drugs shown to cause liver damage in patients using a particular metabolic pathway, idiosyncratic drug injury is unpredictable in the sense that the susceptibility of individual patients cannot be tested before the drug is given.

Most intrinsic hepatotoxins produce liver damage within a few hours or days, whereas in the idiosyncratic type of injury there is often a latent period of many days, weeks or months[33] before liver disease becomes apparent. The latent period tends to shorten with repeated adminstration of the drug. Because of the latent period and the tendency for idiosyncratic injury to mimic non-drug-related liver diseases, clinicians and pathologists need to be alert to the possibility of idiosyncratic drug injury if diagnostic errors are to be avoided. The clinician may be helped by a clinical scale or scoring system,[34] and the pathologist by a suspicious or characteristic pattern of injury. Conclusive proof that a particular drug or combination of drugs is responsible is often impossible to obtain, although re-challenge (usually inadvertent) can provide strong circumstantial evidence. Liver injury may follow inadvertent re-challenge many years after a first episode.[35] Biochemical evidence of improvement after drug withdrawal is occasionally supported by a return to normal histology.[33]

Morphological categories

The categories described below represent the main changes attributed to drugs and toxins, apart from alcohol-related liver damage (**Ch 7**), neoplasms (**Ch 11**) and vascular lesions (**Ch 12**). A mixture of lesions may be found in the same liver; amiodarone, for example, produces both phospholipidosis and steatohepatitis, but by different mechanisms.[36] As already indicated, a single drug may give rise to different forms of hepatotoxicity in different patients. Phenylbutazone, for example, can cause necrosis, cholestasis, granuloma formation or combinations of these,[37] while the NSAIDs nimesulide and diclofenac can cause either severe hepatitis or cholestasis.[38,39]

Adaptation

Not all changes seen under the microscope necessarily represent liver damage. The increase in endoplasmic reticulum produced by long-term treatment with anticonvulsant drugs is commonly regarded as an adaptive phenomenon.[40,41] By light microscopy, this increase is seen as an abundance of pale-staining cytoplasm in hepatocytes (**see Figs 4.8 and 8.1**), which is difficult to distinguish from simple abundance of glycogen on a haematoxylin–eosin (H&E)-stained section.

Figure 8.1 Adaptation. Hepatocytes in this biopsy from a patient on anti-epileptic drugs are enlarged and have abundant pale-staining cytoplasm. (Needle biopsy, H&E.)

**Figure 8.2
Microvesicular
steatosis.**
In this example of
valproate toxicity the
hepatocytes are
swollen and finely
vacuolated.
(Recipient liver at
transplantation,
H&E.) (The section
was kindly provided
by Professor B. C.
Portmann, London,
UK.)

Non-hepatitic liver-cell damage

One of the commonest manifestations of intrinsic hepatotoxicity is **steatosis**. As discussed
in **Chapter 7**, this may be macrovesicular or microvesicular. Macrovesicular steatosis, in
which the nucleus of the hepatocyte is displaced by one or more fat vacuoles easily visible
by light microscopy, is produced by chlorinated hydrocarbons and methotrexate, for
example. It is common in patients on total parenteral nutrition,[42,43] although underlying
disease may also contribute to the liver changes.[44] In patients treated with gold compounds
for rheumatoid arthritis, intralobular lipogranulomas (focal accumulations of lipid-
containing macrophages) have been found to contain gold pigment in the form of fine
black or brown granules. These were also seen within portal lipid droplets.[45]

Causes of the more serious microvesicular steatosis[46] (**Fig. 8.2**) include treatment with
the anticonvulsant drug valproate[47] and with the nucleoside analogue fialuridine.[48] This
leads to the combination of microvesicular steatosis with mitochondrial abnormalities,
found also in Reye's syndrome (**see Ch. 13**). Similar changes are reported after zidovudine,[49] didanosine (**see Fig. 8.3**) and other nucleoside reverse transcriptase inhibitors in
highly active antiretroviral therapy (HAART) for AIDS.[50–52] In the microvesicular form of
steatosis the fat within the hepatocytes is finely divided and is not always obvious with
conventional stains. The hepatocyte nuclei remain in their normal central location, in
contrast to macrovesicular steatosis. There is a variable degree of associated hepatocellular
necrosis.

Several drugs, among them amiodarone[36] and trimethoprim-sulphamethoxazole (co-
trimoxazole),[53] are causes of acquired **phospholipidosis**. Similar changes have been
reported in patients receiving total parenteral nutrition.[54] Lamellar inclusions are seen
within hepatocytes and other cells by electron microscopy (**see Fig. 17.3**). Light microscopy of conventionally stained sections is not diagnostic.

Figure 8.3
Didanosine-induced microvesicular steatosis.
Small-droplet fat vacuoles are prominent in hepatocytes, most of which show nuclei maintained in a central position. (Needle biopsy, H&E.)

In acute arsenic intoxication, a striking increase in hepatocyte mitoses has been reported, accompanied by ballooning, cholestasis and mild inflammation.[18] Markers of cell proliferation were also markedly increased.

An unusual form of cell injury is produced by cyanamide, used in alcohol aversion therapy.[55-57] Periportal hepatocytes contain large, pale-staining **cytoplasmic inclusion bodies**, giving the cells a superficial resemblance to the ground-glass cells of chronic type B hepatitis (**see Figs 4.8 and 9.13**). The inclusions are, however, orcein-negative and diastase–periodic acid–Schiff positive.

Hepatocellular necrosis

Hepatocellular necrosis without the diffuse inflammatory lesion of hepatitis is usually a consequence of the intrinsic type of hepatotoxicity. A common example is suicidal or accidental overdose with the analgesic paracetamol (acetaminophen).[58] Jaundice develops after an interval of days, during which available glutathione, which reacts with a toxic metabolite, is used up. The necrosis – like that of shock or heatstroke (**see Fig. 12.2**) – is most severe in perivenular regions (acinar zones 3) and is accompanied by little or no inflammation (**Fig. 8.4**). Kupffer cells contain brown ceroid pigment. Portal tracts usually remain normal. Complete recovery is possible. While most paracetamol-induced necrosis follows suicidal overdose, it is occasionally found in habitual drinkers taking large doses in the high therapeutic range.[59]

Hepatocellular necrosis, sometimes accompanied by steatosis, is also a feature of cocaine intoxication,[9,11,13] of glue sniffing and of solvent abuse.[14,60] In most instances the necrosis is perivenular and mid-zonal (in acinar zones 3 and 2), but periportal (zone 1) necrosis has been reported in a cocaine user.[61] 'Ecstasy' (3,4-methylenedioxymethamphetamine, MDMA) can cause a hepatitic lesion of the kind described in the next section,[15,16,62] but there may also be confluent hepatocellular necrosis as a result of concurrent hyperthermia.[17] Other agents capable of causing confluent necrosis include industrial hydrochlorofluorocarbons.[19]

Figure 8.4
Hepatocellular
necrosis due to
paracetamol
(acetaminophen).
Confluent necrosis
with little
inflammation is seen
in a perivenular area.
(Needle biopsy,
H&E.)

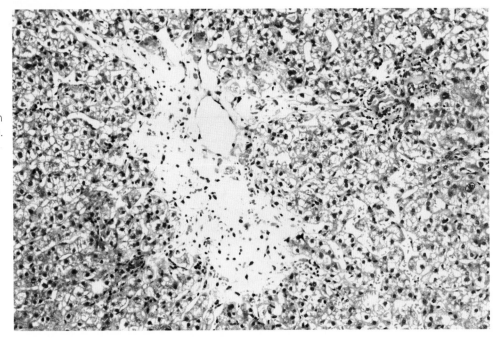

Acute drug-induced hepatitis

A large number of drugs of different chemical structure and with widely differing pharmacological actions occasionally give rise to acute hepatitis, and any drug should be regarded as a potential offender. Acute drug-induced hepatotoxicity is of the idiosyncratic type. The histological lesion is very like that of acute viral hepatitis, and often indistinguishable from it (**Figs 8.5, 8.6**). Incriminated substances include antituberculous drugs,[63] NSAIDs, anaesthetics,[64,65] herbal remedies[8] and many others.

In the idiosyncratic injury of hepatitic type the latent period between exposure to the drug and clinically evident liver disease ranges from a few days to several months, a long latent period sometimes making diagnosis difficult. However, correct diagnosis of idiosyncratic drug-induced hepatitis is most important, because inadvertent re-challenge may have serious consequences.

The hepatitis ranges in severity from a mild inflammatory lesion, sometimes combined with a cholestatic reaction (see under Cholestasis, below), to severe and even fatal disease.[66] In milder cases, removal of the drug usually leads to rapid improvement. Later uncommon outcomes also include cirrhosis and the development of autoimmune hepatitis.[67]

Differential diagnosis

The possibility of drug idiosyncrasy should be considered in all patients with acute hepatitis, because in many cases the histological appearances are identical to those of viral hepatitis. A higher than usual degree of suspicion should be aroused when the hepatitis is histologically unusual (**Table 8.2**). Well-demarcated centrilobular confluent necrosis (**Fig. 8.5**) is common.

Table 8.2 Features sometimes associated with drug-induced hepatitis

Demarcated perivenular (acinar zone 3) necrosis
Minimal hepatitis with canalicular cholestasis
Poorly developed portal inflammatory reaction
Abundant neutrophils
Abundant eosinophils
Epithelioid-cell granulomas

Figure 8.5 Drug-induced liver injury: hepatitic type.
In this acute hepatitis attributed to indometacin, necrosis in acinar zone 3 is well demarcated from the remaining parenchyma. The latter shows steatosis. Note the very mild portal inflammation (below right). (Needle biopsy, H&E.)

Figure 8.6 Drug-induced liver injury: hepatitic type.
There is a severe lobular hepatitis with disruption of liver-cell plates and apoptosis, attributed to ecstasy (3,4-methylenedi-oxymethampheta-mine). The patient is the second of the two reported by Fidler and colleagues.[16] (Needle biopsy, H&E.)

There may be a very mild lobular hepatitis together with canalicular cholestasis. The portal inflammatory reaction may be poorly developed or even absent. Conversely, the portal infiltrate may be unusually rich in neutrophils or eosinophils, although the latter are neither proof of drug aetiology nor necessary for its diagnosis. The presence of epithelioid-cell granulomas increases the likelihood that drug idiosyncrasy is the correct diagnosis.

Figure 8.7 Drug-induced chronic hepatitis. Liver damage, here attributed to methyldopa, has taken the form of extensive interface hepatitis. There is a heavy lymphoplasmacytic infiltrate. (Needle biopsy, H&E.)

Chronic drug-induced hepatitis

In some patients drug-induced hepatitis becomes chronic after prolonged or repeated exposure. A chronic course proved to be unexpectedly common in a recent follow-up study.[68] A high degree of suspicion of possible drug aetiology is particularly important because of the possibility of improvement after withdrawal of the drug. The histological pattern is that of chronic hepatitis with or without cirrhosis (**Fig. 8.7**). In patients still taking the offending drug there is usually substantial necrosis and inflammation; inflammation confined to portal tracts is not a common pattern of drug injury. Drugs considered to be responsible for chronic hepatitis include such widely used agents as nitrofurantoin[69,70] and phenytoin.[71] Among other incriminated substances is the Chinese herbal product Jin Bu Huan[7,72] as well as products with combinations of herbal agents.[73] Autoantibodies may be present in the serum of patients with drug-induced chronic hepatitis, leading to potential confusion with non-drug-related autoimmune hepatitis.[74] Drugs have indeed been cited as a possible trigger of autoimmune hepatitis.[75,76] The tetracycline derivative minocycline can itself give rise to a chronic hepatitis closely resembling autoimmune hepatitis clinically, immunologically and histologically.[77,78]

Differential diagnosis

The appearances of drug-induced chronic hepatitis are indistinguishable from those of chronic hepatitis of viral or autoimmune aetiology.

Steatohepatitis

Steatohepatitis refers to a specific form of hepatic injury characterised by steatosis, hepatocellular ballooning, Mallory body formation, inflammation and pericellular fibrosis, sometimes progressing to cirrhosis. The commonest cause is alcohol abuse (**see Ch. 7**).

**Figure 8.8
Steatohepatitis
attributed to
tamoxifen toxicity.**
Hepatocytes in the
lower part of the
field are swollen and
surrounded by
collagen, stained
blue. There is also
steatosis and nuclear
vacuolation. (Needle
biopsy, trichrome).
The patient is the
third of the three
reported by Pinto
and colleagues.[83]
(The biopsy was
kindly provided by
Professor Amelia
Baptista, Lisbon,
Portugal.)

Drugs are among the causes of non-alcoholic steatohepatitis (NASH). Incriminated agents include synthetic oestrogens,[79] amiodarone[36,80] and tamoxifen[81–83] (**Fig. 8.8**). Similar changes are sometimes seen in patients on parenteral nutrition[42] and in industrial workers exposed to volatile petrochemical products.[20] In the case of amiodarone, steatosis itself may be mild or absent,[84] but otherwise there is a close resemblance to other forms of NASH and to alcoholic steatohepatitis, including the potential for cirrhosis. However, amiodarone-related steatohepatitis has a periportal predilection in contrast to the perivenular distribution seen with other causes of steatohepatitis. It is interesting to note that some patients with reported drug-related steatohepatitis were also obese,[83] which raises the possibility of an interaction between drug and other factors.

Fibrosis and cirrhosis

As already stated, cirrhosis may result from chronic drug-induced hepatitis. Progressive fibrosis and portal hypertension in a non-hepatitic setting are known complications of long-term exposure to arsenic or vinyl chloride. Excess intake of vitamin A (hypervitaminosis A) affects hepatic stellate cells which may appear unusually prominent[85] (**Fig. 8.9**). Perisinusoidal fibrosis, veno-occlusive disease and cirrhosis[24] are other consequences.

Pathologists are sometimes asked to report on liver biopsies from patients given or about to receive long-term methotrexate for psoriasis or rheumatoid arthritis. Although methotrexate was initially considered to be a potent hepatotoxin, doubt has more recently been thrown on its potential to cause serious liver disease in the absence of additional risk factors.[86] These include regular or heavy alcohol intake[87] and obesity.[88] Significant liver injury is reputedly less common in patients with rheumatoid arthritis than in those with psoriasis. Histological abnormalities attributed to methotrexate include steatosis, hepatocyte pleomorphism, portal fibrosis and inflammation, formation of fibrous septa extending from the portal tracts (**Fig. 8.10**) and cirrhosis. A grading system for methotrexate liver injury was developed by Roenigk and colleagues which scores the degree of fat, inflam-

**Figure 8.9
Hypervitaminosis
A.**

Prominent, hypertrophied stellate cells with lipid vacuoles and peripheral dark, compressed nuclei are seen between hepatocytes, in perisinusoidal spaces (arrows). Some of the stellate cells are multivesicular (arrowheads). (Needle biopsy, H&E.)

**Figure 8.10
Liver damage
attributed to
methotrexate.**

Two portal tracts in this field show chronic inflammation and fibrosis extending outwards. The parenchyma shows steatosis. (Needle biopsy, H&E.)

mation and fibrosis.[89] Minor changes such as focal necrosis and steatosis are common in baseline pretreatment biopsies, and are presumably related to the underlying disease (e.g. psoriasis) or to additional risk factors. Periportal septum formation is more likely to be due to methotrexate, whereas fibrosis mainly in perivenular regions should lead to suspicion of alcohol abuse or non-alcoholic steatohepatitis.

Steroid-induced cholestasis

Steroid-induced cholestasis[90,91] lies on the borderline between intrinsic and idiosyncratic hepatotoxicity. On the one hand, it is reproducible in laboratory animals and some steroids cause biochemical abnormalities in humans in a predictable and dose-dependent manner. On the other hand, clinical liver disease cannot be predicted in the individual patient and is seen in only a small proportion of patients receiving anabolic or contraceptive steroids. Patients susceptible to contraceptive steroid-induced jaundice are also prone to develop cholestasis in late pregnancy.

The histological picture is one of canalicular cholestasis in perivenular areas, with little or no necrosis or inflammation beyond that attributable to the cholestasis itself. Isolated hepatocytes may undergo feathery degeneration, and in prolonged cholestasis liver-cell rosettes are a common finding (**see Fig. 4.4**). Portal tracts usually remain normal but may be minimally inflamed. Because of the lack of necrosis and inflammation, this type of lesion is sometimes known as pure or bland cholestasis.

Differential diagnosis

The differential diagnosis is from other causes of bland cholestasis such as benign recurrent intrahepatic cholestasis, which is discussed in detail in **Chapter 5**.

Idiosyncratic drug-induced cholestasis

Idiosyncratic drug-induced cholestasis, typified by chlorpromazine jaundice[92] but also caused by many other drugs, differs from bland cholestasis in that some degree of portal inflammation is usually present (**Fig. 8.11**). There is sometimes inflammatory infiltration of the lobules and evidence of hepatocellular damage. Zimmerman and Ishak[5] therefore refer to this type of lesion as 'hepatocanalicular'. The portal infiltrate often includes eosinophils and these are occasionally abundant, but their absence does not exclude a

Figure 8.11 Drug-induced liver injury: hepatocanalicular type.
In this patient with jaundice following chlorpromazine therapy there is mild inflammation of the portal tract (lower left) and swelling of hepatocytes, especially in the perivenular area (above, centre and right). (Needle biopsy, H&E.)

Figure 8.12 Drug-induced liver injury: hepatocanalicular type.

An inflamed portal tract from a patient with jaundice attributed to Augmentin (amoxicillin and clavulanic acid). The epithelium of an interlobular bile duct is irregular, vacuolated and infiltrated by lymphocytes. (Needle biopsy, H&E.) (Biopsy kindly provided by Dr Karin Oien, Glasgow, UK.)

diagnosis of drug-induced hepatocanalicular cholestasis. Small interlobular ducts often show abnormalities such as irregular distribution of epithelial cell nuclei, cytoplasmic vacuolation, variation in nuclear size and infiltration by lymphocytes. These changes are usually mild, but occasionally more severe (**Fig. 8.12**), even leading to ductopenia (see **vanishing bile duct syndrome**, below). The lobular changes (**Fig. 8.11**) are as in bland cholestasis, except for the additional element of inflammation and necrosis which is sometimes found, as mentioned above. There is therefore a spectrum of appearances in this type of cholestasis, from an almost bland cholestatic lesion to one resembling mild acute viral hepatitis. Even in the absence of necrosis and inflammation, hepatocellular changes are seen which possibly result from prolonged cholestasis itself, but which may also include an element of adaptive proliferation of the smooth endoplasmic reticulum. These changes include prominent hepatocellular swelling, abundant pale-staining cytoplasm and, commonly, multinucleation. Mitotic figures may be evident.[92]

Differential diagnosis

The differential diagnosis of idiosyncratic drug-induced cholestasis is from bile-duct obstruction, acute viral- or drug-induced hepatitis, and cholestasis of the bland type. Portal oedema, prominent neutrophils, marked ductular reaction and absence of lobular inflammation favour the first. In the absence of substantial portal inflammation the distinction between idiosyncratic drug jaundice and bland steroid-induced cholestasis becomes difficult to make and requires clinical information. In such circumstances bile-duct obstruction cannot be completely ruled out. The differential diagnosis also includes other causes of bland cholestasis, such as benign recurrent cholestasis (**see Ch. 4**). Severe liver-cell damage and inflammation favour viral hepatitis or the drug injury of hepatitic type already discussed.

The clinical course of idiosyncratic drug jaundice varies. In most patients removal of the offending drug leads to rapid improvement. Occasionally the cholestasis is slow to improve but liver biopsy shows cholestasis only, with no fibrosis or other evidence of progressive disease. In rare instances true chronic disease develops on the basis of severe bile-duct damage and duct loss, with consequent fibrosis and other features of chronic biliary disease. The clinical picture resembles primary biliary cirrhosis. This **vanishing bile duct syndrome** has been reported after a number of drugs[93,94] including chlorpromazine,[92] a combination of chlorpropamide with erythromycin ethylsuccinate,[95] prochlorperazine,[96] gold salts,[97] ciprofloxacin,[98] haloperidol,[99] ajmaline,[100] glycyrrhizin,[101] and amoxycillin and flucloxacillin[102] among others. Augmentin (amoxycillin and clavulanic acid; **Fig. 8.10**) is a well-documented cause of cholestasis, with striking focal destruction of bile ducts in some biopsies.[103–106] This is occasionally associated with granuloma formation. Prolonged cholestasis may be the result of the duct damage and, in some patients, of duct loss.

More acute bile-duct injury is seen in poisoning with the herbicide paraquat.[107] Zimmerman and Ishak[5] designate this type of injury as ductal or cholangiodestructive, in contrast to canalicular and hepatocanalicular cholestasis.

Long-term parenteral nutrition, already noted in relation to steatosis and steatohepatitis in adults, may be associated in infants and children with a progressive form of liver injury, typified by cholestasis, hepatocellular damage, ductular reaction, fibrosis and even cirrhosis.[42,43,108] Whether the parenteral nutrition itself is responsible for all these changes is not proven.[43,44] The lesion may mimic bile-duct obstruction[109] (**Fig. 13.18**).

Granulomas

Drugs are an important cause of otherwise unexplained granulomas. They are sometimes the only or main manifestation of a drug reaction, but can also form part of a cholestatic or hepatitic picture.[80] The granulomas may be portal (**Fig. 8.13**), parenchymal, or both. They usually show little or no necrosis, and are infiltrated by a variety of inflammatory cells including plasma cells and eosinophils. Allopurinol has been reported to cause granulomas of the fibrin-ring type.[110] The list of drugs associated with hepatic granulomas is small compared with the list of those causing hepatitis or cholestasis, but it is nevertheless substantial.[5,111,112]

Figure 8.13 Drug-induced granuloma formation.
A portal tract contains a granuloma with many multinucleated giant cells. The patient became jaundiced after taking phenylbutazone. (Needle biopsy, H&E.)

Other lesions

Drugs may produce other hepatic lesions such as **nodular regenerative hyperplasia**[113] as described with the combined chemotherapy agents 5-fluorouracil and oxaliplatin.[114]

Veno-occlusive disease, sinusoidal obstruction syndrome and obliterative venopathy are other consequences of chemotherapy[115] (**see Fig. 16.21**).

References

1 Navarro VJ, Senior JR. Drug-related hepatotoxicity. *N Engl J Med* 2006; **354**: 731–739.

2 Stricker BHC. Drug-Induced Hepatic Injury. Amsterdam: Elsevier, 1992.

3 Farrell GC. Drug-Induced Liver Disease. Edinburgh: Churchill Livingstone, 1994.

4 Pessayre D, Larrey D, Biour M. Drug-induced liver injury. In: Bircher J, Benhamou J-P, McIntyre N, Rizzetto M, Rodés J, eds. Oxford Textbook of Clinical Hepatology, 2nd edn. Oxford: Oxford University Press, 1999: Ch. 17, p. 1261.

5 Zimmerman HJ, Ishak KG. Hepatic injury due to drugs and toxins. In: MacSween RNM, Burt AD, Portmann BC, Ishak KG, Scheuer PJ, Anthony PP, eds. Pathology of the Liver, 4th edn. Edinburgh: Churchill Livingstone, 2002: Ch. 14, p. 621.

6 Biour M, Poupon R, Grange JD, et al. Drug-induced hepatotoxicity. The 13th updated edition of the bibliographic database of drug-related liver injuries and responsible drugs. *Gastroenterol Clin Biol* 2000; **24**: 1052–1091.

7 Stickel F, Patsenker E, Schuppan D. Herbal hepatotoxicity. *J Hepatol* 2005; **43**: 901–910.

8 Fogden E, Neuberger J. Alternative medicines and the liver. *Liver Int* 2003; **23**: 213–220.

9 Kanel GC, Cassidy W, Shuster L, et al. Cocaine-induced liver cell injury: comparison of morphological features in man and in experimental models. *Hepatology* 1990; **11**: 646–651.

10 Trigueiro de Araújo MS, Gerard F, Chossegros P, et al. Vascular hepatotoxicity related to heroin addiction. *Virchows Arch [A]* 1990; **417**: 497–503.

11 Wanless IR, Dore S, Gopinath N, et al. Histopathology of cocaine hepatotoxicity. Report of four patients. *Gastroenterology* 1990; **98**: 497–501.

12 Mallat A, Dhumeaux D. Cocaine and the liver. *J Hepatol* 1991; **12**: 275–278.

13 Silva MO, Roth D, Reddy KR, et al. Hepatic dysfunction accompanying acute cocaine intoxication. *J Hepatol* 1991; **12**: 312–315.

14 McIntyre AS, Long RG. Fatal fulminant hepatic failure in a 'solvent abuser'. *Postgrad Med J* 1992; **68**: 29–30.

15 Ellis AJ, Wendon JA, Portmann B, et al. Acute liver damage and ecstasy ingestion. *Gut* 1996; **38**: 454–458.

16 Fidler H, Dhillon A, Gertner D, et al. Chronic ecstasy (3,4-methylenedioxymethamphetamine) abuse: a recurrent and unpredictable cause of severe acute hepatitis. *J Hepatol* 1996; **25**: 563–566.

17 Milroy CM, Clark JC, Forrest ARW. Pathology of deaths associated with 'ecstasy' and 'eve' misuse. *J Clin Pathol* 1996; **49**: 149–153.

18 Brenard R, Laterre P-F, Reynaert M et al. Increased hepatocyte mitotic activity as a diagnostic marker of acute arsenic intoxication. A report of two cases. *J Hepatol* 1996; **25**: 218–220.

19 Hoet P, Graf MLM, Bourdi M, et al. Epidemic of liver disease caused by hydrochlorofluorocarbons used as ozone-sparing substitutes of chlorofluorocarbons. *Lancet* 1997; **350**: 556–559.

20 Cotrim HP, Andrade ZA, Parana R, et al. Nonalcoholic steatohepatitis: a toxic liver disease in industrial workers. *Liver* 1999; **19**: 299–304.

21 Kahl R. Toxic liver injury. In: Bircher J, Benhamou J-P, McIntyre N, Rizzetto M, Rodés J, eds. Oxford Textbook of Clinical Hepatology, 2nd edn. Oxford: Oxford University Press, 1999: Ch. 18. p. 1319.

22. Cave M, Falkner KC, Ray M, et al. Toxicant-associated steatohepatitis in vinyl chloride workers. *Hepatology* 2010; **51**: 474–481.

23 Bioulac-Sage P, Quinton A, Saric J, et al. Chance discovery of hepatic fibrosis in patient with asymptomatic hypervitaminosis A. *Arch Pathol Lab Med* 1988; **112**: 505–509.

24 Jorens PG, Michielsen PP, Pelckmans PA, et al. Vitamin A abuse: development of cirrhosis despite cessation of vitamin A. A six-year clinical and histopathologic follow-up. *Liver* 1992; **12**: 381–386.

25 Galler GW, Weisenberg E, Brasitus TA. Mushroom poisoning: the role of orthotopic liver transplantation. *J Clin Gastroenterol* 1992; **15**: 229–232.

26 Nagai K, Hosaka H, Kubo S, et al. Vitamin A toxicity secondary to excessive intake of yellow-green vegetables, liver and laver. *J Hepatol* 1999; **31**: 142–148.

27 Silva MO, Reddy KR, Jeffers LJ, et al. Interferon-induced chronic active hepatitis? *Gastroenterology* 1991; **101**: 840–842.

28 Lindgren A, Aldenborg F, Norkrans G, et al. Paracetamol-induced cholestatic and granulomatous liver injuries. *J Int Med* 1997; **241**: 435–439.

29 Andrade RJ, Lucena MI, Garcia-Escaño MD, et al. Severe idiosyncratic acute hepatic injury caused by paracetamol (Letter). *J Hepatol* 1998; **28**: 1078.

30 Kenna JG. Immunoallergic drug-induced hepatitis: lessons from halothane. *J Hepatol* 1997; **26**(Suppl. 1): 5–12.

31 Robin M-A, Le Roy M, Descatoire V, et al. Plasma membrane cytochromes P450 as neoantigens and autoimmune targets in drug-induced hepatitis. *J Hepatol* 1997; **26**(Suppl. 1): 23–30.

32 Eliasson E, Stål POA, Lytton S. Expression of autoantibodies to specific cytochromes P450 in a case of disulfiram hepatitis. *J Hepatol* 1998; **29**: 819–825.

33 Grieco A, Vecchio FM, Greco AV, et al. Cholestatic hepatitis due to ticlopidine: clinical and histological recovery after drug withdrawal. Case report and review of the literature. *J Hepatol* 1998; **10**: 713–715.

34 Aithal GP, Rawlins MD, Day CP. Clinical diagnostic scale: a useful tool in the evaluation of suspected hepatotoxic adverse drug reactions. *J Hepatol* 2000; **33**: 949–952.

35 Paiva LA, Wright PJ, Koff RS. Long-term hepatic memory for hypersensitivity to nitrofurantoin. *Am J Gastroenterol* 1992; **87**: 891–893.

36 Lewis JH, Mullick F, Ishak KG, et al. Histopathologic analysis of suspected amiodarone hepatotoxicity. *Hum Pathol* 1990; **21**: 59–67.

37 Benjamin SB, Ishak KG, Zimmerman HJ, et al. Phenylbutzone liver injury: a clinical-pathologic survey of 23 cases and review of the literature. *Hepatology* 1981; **1**: 255–263.

38 Banks AT, Zimmerman HJ, Ishak KG, et al. Diclofenac-associated hepatotoxicity: analysis of 180 cases reported to the Food and Drug Administration as adverse reactions. *Hepatology* 1995; **22**: 820–827.

39 Van Steenbergen W, Peeters P, De Bondt J, et al. Nimesulide-induced acute hepatitis: evidence from six cases. *J Hepatol* 1998; **29**: 135–141.

40 Jezequel AM, Librari ML, Mosca P, et al. Changes induced in human liver by long-term anticonvulsant therapy. Functional and ultrastructural data. *Liver* 1984; **4**: 307–317.

41 Pamperl H, Gradner W, Fridrich L, et al. Influence of long-term anticonvulsant treatment on liver ultrastructure in man. *Liver* 1984; **4**: 294–300.

42 Klein S, Nealon WH. Hepatobiliary abnormalities associated with total parenteral nutrition. *Semin Liver Dis* 1988; **8**: 237–246.

43 Quigley EM, Marsh MN, Shaffer JL, et al. Hepatobiliary complications of total parenteral nutrition. *Gastroenterology* 1993; **104**: 286–301.

44 Wolfe BM, Walker BK, Shaul DB, et al. Effect of total parenteral nutrition on hepatic histology. *Arch Surg* 1988; **123**: 1084–1090.

45 Landas SK, Mitros FA, Furst DE, et al. Lipogranulomas and gold in the liver in rheumatoid arthritis. *Am J Surg Pathol* 1992; **16**: 171–174.

46 Fromenty B, Berson A, Pessayre D. Microvesicular steatosis and steatohepatitis: role of mitochondrial dysfunction and lipid peroxidation. *J Hepatol* 1997; **26**(Suppl. 1): 13–22.

47 Zimmerman HJ, Ishak KG. Valproate-induced hepatic injury: analyses of 23 fatal cases. *Hepatology* 1982; **2**: 591–597.

48 Kleiner DE, Gaffey MJ, Sallie R, et al. Histopathologic changes associated with fialuridine hepatotoxicity. *Mod Pathol* 1997; **10**: 192–199.

49 Chariot P, Drogou I, de Lacroix-Szmania I, et al. Zidovudine-induced mitochondrial disorder with massive liver steatosis, myopathy, lactic acidosis, and mitochondrial DNA depletion. *J Hepatol* 1999; **30**: 156–160.

50 Van Huyen J-PD, Batisse D, Heudes D, et al. Alteration of cytochrome oxidase subunit I labeling is associated with severe mitochondriopathy in NRTI-related hepatotoxicity in HIV patients. *Mod Pathol* 2006; **19**: 1277–1288.

51 Spengler U, Lichterfeld M, Rockstroh JK. Antiretroviral drug toxicity – a challenge for the hepatologist? *J Hepatol* 2002; **36**: 283–294.

52 Clark SJ, Creighton S, Portmann B et al. Acute liver failure associated with antiretroviral treatment for HIV: a report of six cases. *J Hepatol* 2002; **36**: 295–301.

53 Muñoz SJ, Martinez-Hernandez A, Maddrey WC. Intrahepatic cholestasis and phospholipidosis associated with the use of trimethoprim–sulfamethoxazole. *Hepatology* 1990; **12**: 342–347.

54 Degott C, Messing B, Moreau D, et al. Liver phospholipidosis induced by parenteral nutrition: histologic, biochemical, and ultrastructural investigations. *Gastroenterology* 1988; **95**: 183–191.

55 Vazquez JJ, Guillen FJ, Zozaya J, et al. Cyanamide-induced liver injury. A predictable lesion. *Liver* 1983; **3**: 225–230.

56 Bruguera M, Lamar C, Bernet M, et al. Hepatic disease associated with ground-glass inclusions in hepatocytes after cyanamide therapy. *Arch Pathol Lab Med* 1986; **110**: 906–910.

57 Yokoyama A, Sato S, Maruyama K, et al. Cyanamide-associated alcoholic liver disease: a sequential histological evaluation. *Alcohol Clin Exp Res* 1995; **19**: 1307–1311.

58 Portmann B, Talbot IC, Day DW, et al. Histopathological changes in the liver following a paracetamol overdose: correlation with clinical and biochemical parameters. *J Pathol* 1975; **117**: 169–181.

59 Maddrey WC. Hepatic effects of acetaminophen. Enhanced toxicity in alcoholics. *J Clin Gastroenterol* 1987; **9**: 180–185.

60 Baerg RD, Kimberg DV. Centrilobular hepatic necrosis and acute renal failure in 'solvent sniffers'. *Ann Intern Med* 1970; **73**: 713–720.

61 Perino LE, Warren GH, Levine JS. Cocaine-induced hepatotoxicity in humans. *Gastroenterology* 1987; **93**: 176–180.

62 Andreu V, Mas A, Bruguera M, et al. Ecstasy: a common cause of severe acute hepatotoxicity. *J Hepatol* 1998; **29**: 394–397.

63 Mitchell I, Wendon J, Fitt S, et al. Antituberculous therapy and acute liver failure. *Lancet* 1995; **345**: 555–556.

64 Neuberger J. Halothane hepatitis. *Eur J Gastroentrol Hepatol* 1998; **10**: 631–633.

65 Lo SK, Wendon J, Mieli-Vergani G, et al. Halothane-induced acute liver failure: continuing occurrence and use of liver transplantation. *Eur J Gastroenterol Hepatol* 1998; **10**: 635–639.

66 Paterson D, Kerlin P, Walker N, et al. Piroxicam induced submassive necrosis of the liver. *Gut* 1992; **33**: 1436–1438.

67 Björnsson E, Davidsdottir L. The long-term follow-up after idiosyncratic drug-induced liver injury with jaundice. *J Hepatol* 2009; **50**: 511–517.

68 Aithal PG, Day CP. The natural history of histologically proved drug induced liver disease. *Gut* 1999; **44**: 731–735.

69 Sharp JR, Ishak KG, Zimmerman HJ. Chronic active hepatitis and severe hepatic necrosis associated with nitrofurantoin. *Ann Intern Med* 1980; **92**: 14–19.

70 Stricker BH, Blok AP, Claas FH, et al. Hepatic injury associated with the use of nitrofurans: a clinicopathological study of 52 reported cases. *Hepatology* 1988; **8**: 599–606.

71 Roy AK, Mahoney HC, Levine RA. Phenytoin-induced chronic hepatitis. *Dig Dis Sci* 1993; **38**: 740–743.

72 Picciotto A, Campo N, Brizzolara R, et al. Chronic hepatitis induced by Jin Bu Huan. *J Hepatol* 1998; **28**: 165–167.

73 Stickel F. Slimming at all costs: Herbalife-induced liver injury. *J Hepatol* 2007; **47**: 444–446.

74 Scully LJ, Clarke D, Barr RJ. Diclofenac induced hepatitis. Three cases with features of autoimmune chronic active hepatitis. *Dig Dis Sci* 1993; **38**: 744–751.

75 Kamiyama T, Nouchi T, Kojima S, et al. Autoimmune hepatitis triggered by administration of an herbal medicine. *Am J Gastroenterol* 1997; **92**: 703–704.

76 Sterling MJ, Kane M, Grace ND. Pemoline-induced autoimmune hepatitis. *Am J Gastroenterol* 1996; **91**: 2233–2234.

77 Gough A, Chapman S, Wagstaff K, et al. Minocycline induced autoimmune heapitis and systemic lupus erythematosus-like syndrome. *BMJ* 1996; **312**: 169–172.

78 Malcolm A, Heap TR, Eckstein RP, et al. Minocycline-induced liver injury. *Am J Gastroenterol* 1996; **91**: 1641–1643.

79 Seki K, Minami Y, Nishikawa M, et al. 'Nonalcoholic steatohepatitis' induced by massive doses of synthetic estrogen. *Gastroenterol Japon* 1983; **18**: 197–203.

80 Harrison RF, Elias E. Amiodarone-associated cirrhosis with hepatic and lymph node granulomas. *Histopathology* 1993; **22**: 80–82.

81 Van Hoof M, Rahier J, Horsmans Y. Tamoxifen-induced steatohepatitis [letter]. *Ann Intern Med* 1996; **124**: 855–856.

82 Cai Q, Bensen M, Greene R, et al. Tamoxifen-induced transient multifocal hepatic fatty infiltration. *Am J Gastroenterol* 2000; **95**: 277–279.

83 Pinto HC, Baptista A, Camilo ME, et al. Tamoxifen-associated steatohepatitis – report of three cases. *J Hepatol* 1995; **23**: 95–97.

84 Chang C-C, Petrelli M, Tomashefski JFJ, et al. Severe intrahepatic cholestasis caused by amiodarone toxicity after withdrawal of the drug. A case report and review of the literature. *Arch Pathol Lab Med* 1999; **123**: 251–256.

85 Nollevaux M-C, Guiot J, Horsmans Y, et al. Hypervitaminosis A-induced liver fibrosis: stellate cell activation and daily dose consumption. *Liver Int* 2006; **26**: 182–186.

86 Tang H, Neuberger J. Review article: methotrexate in gastroenterology – dangerous villain or simply misunderstood? *Aliment Pharmacol Ther* 1996; **10**: 851–858.

87 Whiting OK, Fye KH, Sack KD. Methotrexate and histologic hepatic abnormalities: a meta-analysis. *Am J Med* 1991; **90**: 711–716.

88 Newman M, Auerbach R, Feiner H, et al. The role of liver biopsies in psoriatic patients receiving long-term methotrexate treatment. Improvement in liver abnormalities after cessation of treatment. *Arch Dermatol* 1989; **125**: 1218–1224.

89 Roenigk HH Jr, Auerbach R, Maibach HI, et al. Methotrexate guidelines – revised. *J Am Acad Dermatol* 1982; **6**: 145–155.

90 Sánchez-Osorio M, Duarte-Rojo A, Martinez-Benitez B, et al. Anabolic–androgenic steroids and liver injury. *Liver International* 2008; **28**: 278–282.

91 Ishak KG. Hepatic lesions caused by anabolic and contraceptive steroids. *Semin Liver Dis* 1981; **1**: 116–128.

92 Ishak KG, Irey NS. Hepatic injury associated with phenothiazines. Clinicopathologic and follow-up study of 36 patients. *Arch Pathol* 1972; **93**: 283–304.

93 Degott C, Feldmann G, Larrey D, et al. Drug-induced prolonged cholestasis in adults: a histological semi-quantitative study demonstrating progressive ductopenia. *Hepatology* 1992; **15**: 244–251.

94 Desmet VJ. Vanishing bile duct syndrome in drug-induced liver disease. *J Hepatol* 1997; **26**(Suppl. 1): 31–35.

95 Geubel AP, Nakad A, Rahier J, et al. Prolonged cholestasis and disappearance of interlobular bile ducts following chlorpropamide and erythromycin ethylsuccinate. Case of drug interaction? *Liver* 1988; **8**: 350–353.

96 Lok ASF, Ng IOL. Prochlorperazine-induced chronic cholestasis. *J Hepatol* 1988; **6**: 369–373.

97 Basset C, Vadrot J, Denis J, et al. Prolonged cholestasis and ductopenia following gold salt therapy. *Liver Int* 2003; **23**: 89–93.

98 Bataille L, Rahier J, Geubel A. Delayed and prolonged cholestatic hepatitis with ductopenia after long-term ciprofloxacin therapy for Crohn's disease. *J Hepatol* 2002; **37**: 696–699.

99 Dincsoy HP, Saelinger DA. Haloperidol-induced chronic cholestatic liver disease. *Gastroenterology* 1982; **83**: 694–700.

100 Larrey D, Pessayre D, Duhamel G, et al. Prolonged cholestasis after ajmaline-induced acute hepatitis. *J Hepatol* 1986; **2**: 81–87.

101 Ishii M, Miyazaki M, Yamamoto T, et al. A case of drug-induced ductopenia resulting in fatal biliary cirrhosis. *Liver* 1993; **13**: 227–231.

102 Davies MH, Harrison RF, Elias E, et al. Antibiotic-associated acute vanishing bile duct syndrome: a pattern associated with severe, prolonged, intrahepatic cholestasis. *J Hepatol* 1994; **20**: 112–116.

103 Richardet J-P, Mallat A, Zafrani ES, et al. Prolonged cholestasis with ductopenia after administration of amoxicillin/clavulanic acid. *Dig Dis Sci* 1999; **44**: 1997–2000.

104 O'Donohue J, Oien KA, Donaldson P, et al. Co-amoxiclav jaundice: clinical and histological features and HLA class II association. *Gut* 2000; **47**: 717–720.

105 Hautekeete ML, Horsmans Y, Van Waeyenberge C, et al. HLA association of amoxicillin–clavulanate-induced hepatitis. *Gastroenterology* 1999; **117**: 1181–1186.

106 Ryley NG, Fleming KA, Chapman RWG. Focal destructive cholangiopathy associated with amoxycillin/clavulinic acid (Augmentin). *J Hepatol* 1995; **23**: 278–282.

107 Mullick FG, Ishak KG, Mahabir R, et al. Hepatic injury associated with paraquat toxicity in humans. *Liver* 1981; **1**: 209–221.

108 Baker AL, Rosenberg IH. Hepatic complications of total parenteral nutrition. *Am J Med* 1987; **82**: 489–497.

109 Body JJ, Bleiberg H, Bron D, et al. Total parenteral nutrition-induced cholestasis mimicking large bile duct obstruction. *Histopathology* 1982; **6**: 787–792.

110 Vanderstigel M, Zafrani ES, Lejonc JL, et al. Allopurinol hypersensitivity syndrome as a cause of hepatic fibrin-ring granulomas. *Gastroenterology* 1986; **90**: 188–190.

111 Ishak KG, Zimmerman HJ. Drug-induced and toxic granulomatous hepatitis. *Baillières Clin Gastroenterol* 1988; **2**: 463–480.

112 Lewis JH, Kleiner DE. Hepatic injury due to drugs, chemicals and toxins. In: MacSween's Pathology of the Liver, 5th edn. Burt AD, Portmann BC, Ferrell LD, eds.

Edinburgh: Churchill Livingstone/Elsevier, 2007: 649–760.

113 Reshamwala PA, Kleiner DE, Heller T. Nodular regenerative hyperplasia: not all nodules are created equal. *Hepatology* 2006; **44**: 7–14.

114 Hubert C, Sempoux C, Horsmans Y, et al. Nodular regenerative hyperplasia: a deleterious consequence of chemotherapy for colorectal liver metastases? *Liver Int* 2007; **27**: 938–943.

115 De Bruyne R, Portmann B, Samyn M, et al. Chronic liver disease related to 6-thioguanine in children with acute lymphoblastic leukaemia. *J Hepatol* 2006; **44**: 407–410.

General reading

Aithal PG, Day CP. The natural history of histologically proved drug induced liver disease. *Gut* 1999; **44**: 731–735.

Biour M, Poupon R, Grange JD, Chazouilleres O. Drug-induced hepatotoxicity. The 13th updated edition of the bibliographic database of drug-related liver injuries and responsible drugs. *Gastroenterol Clin Biol* 2000; **24**: 1052–1091.

Goodman ZD. Drug hepatotoxicity. *Clin Liver Dis* 2002; **6**: 381–398.

Larrey D. Drug-induced liver diseases. *J Hepatol* 2000; **32** (Suppl. 1): 77–88.

Lewis JH, Kleiner DE. Hepatic injury due to drugs, chemicals and toxins. In: Burt AD, Portmann BC, Ferrell LD, eds. MacSween's Pathology of the Liver, 5th edn. Edinburgh: Churchill Livingstone/Elsevier, 2007: 649–760.

Navarro VJ, Senior JR. Drug-related hepatotoxicity. *N Engl J Med* 2006; **354**: 731–739.

Ramachandran R, Kakar S. Histological patterns in drug-induced liver disease. *J Clin Pathol* 2009; **62**: 481–492.

Watkins PB, Seeff LB. Drug-induced liver injury: summary of a single topic clinical research conference. *Hepatology* 2006; **43**: 618–631.

Chronic Hepatitis

Definition and causes

Chronic hepatitis is a common reason for persistently abnormal liver function tests[1] and forms the background for the development of much cirrhosis[2] and hepatocellular carcinoma. It is defined as persistence of liver injury with raised aminotransferase levels or viral markers for more than 6 months.[3] This definition, though artificial, helps to establish a borderline in studies of acute and chronic hepatitis. In practice, however, this borderline is not always easy to draw, because acute self-limiting hepatitis is sometimes prolonged beyond 6 months and chronic hepatitis may have an acute or indefinable onset. Many chronic liver diseases have an inflammatory component, but the term chronic hepatitis is often restricted to a limited number of causes (**Table 9.1**). Some of the histological features of this group, such as interface hepatitis and lymphocytic infiltration, are also found in other conditions (**Table 9.2**) not included in this chapter. For the sake of clarity, a diagnosis of chronic hepatitis should therefore include the probable cause whenever possible.

Table 9.1 Classic causes of chronic hepatitis
Hepatitis B, with or without HDV infection
Hepatitis C
Autoimmune hepatitis
Drug-induced hepatitis
Chronic hepatitis of unknown cause

Table 9.2 Conditions sharing pathological features with classic forms of chronic hepatitis
Wilson's disease
α_1-Antitrypsin deficiency
Primary biliary cirrhosis
Primary sclerosing cholangitis

Classification and nomenclature

In 1994, two international working parties recommended the replacement of the old histological classification into chronic active, chronic persistent and chronic lobular hepatitis by a predominantly aetiological classification supplemented by semi-quantitative scoring.[4,5] This reflected the fact that the cause of a chronic hepatitis could, by 1994, be determined

©2010 Elsevier Ltd
DOI: 10.1016/B978-0-7020-3410-7.00015-0

in most patients and appropriate treatment given. Also, it had become apparent that the future course of a chronic hepatitis could not after all be accurately predicted from the histological appearances. The several systems available for semi-quantitative scoring are discussed in detail at the end of the chapter.

Use of liver biopsy in chronic hepatitis

Opinion is divided on the need for biopsy in the diagnosis and management of patients with chronic hepatitis.[6,7] Histology continues to play a central role in the assessment of new treatment regimens, however, and is used by many physicians to establish a diagnosis and to guide management.[8,9] Criteria used by physicians for the latter include the severity of the hepatitis (grading), the extent of progression towards cirrhosis (staging) and individual features such as steatosis and iron deposition. In the case of auto-immune hepatitis, liver biopsy plays an important part in the decision to stop treatment.[10] In patients with multiple aetiological agents, biopsy may help to establish their relative importance; an example of this is the patient with thalassaemia and viral hepatitis. Large-cell and small-cell change (dysplasia), possible predictors of hepatocellular carcinoma, are sometimes found before cirrhosis develops but will be discussed with the latter, in **Chapter 10**.

Table 9.3 lists the possible reasons for liver biopsy in chronic hepatitis.

Table 9.3 Uses of liver biopsy in chronic hepatitis

Establishment of the diagnosis

Diagnosis of incidental lesions

Assessment of histological activity (grading)

Evaluation of types of necrosis

Evaluation of structural changes (staging)

Clues to aetiology and possible superinfection

Immunohistochemical assessment of viral antigens

Monitoring of therapy

Histological features of chronic hepatitis

Portal changes

Most small portal tracts are infiltrated to a variable extent by lymphocytes together with smaller numbers of plasma cells and occasional segmented leucocytes. A few eosinophils are often present. Lymphoid aggregates and lymphoid follicles with germinal centres are common in, but not exclusive to, hepatitis C. Larger conducting tracts are less affected than small terminal tracts and this has to be taken into account in assessing the severity of a hepatitis.

In the mildest forms of chronic hepatitis, the infiltrate is confined to portal tracts (**Fig. 9.1**) and the margins of the tracts remain regular. In the more severe forms, infiltration extends into the adjacent parenchyma, as described below. In mild chronic hepatitis, the tracts are often enlarged and short fibrous spurs may be seen extending from them (**Fig. 9.2**). These and other structural changes are most easily evaluated in reticulin or collagen stains. Interlobular bile ducts may be damaged, as shown by irregularity of the epithelial wall, vacuolation and infiltration by lymphocytes.

Parenchymal changes

The periportal lesion: interface hepatitis

In all but the mildest forms of chronic hepatitis, the inflammatory infiltrate extends from the portal tracts into the adjacent parenchyma and there is destruction of hepatocytes (**Figs 9.3, 9.4**). This process of interface hepatitis or piecemeal necrosis is most easily identified

Figure 9.1 Chronic hepatitis B, mild. The portal tract is heavily infiltrated with lymphocytes. These do not extend beyond the margins of the tract, the limiting plate of hepatocytes is intact and interface hepatitis is absent. Some hepatocytes have a ground-glass appearance. (Needle biopsy, H&E.)

Figure 9.2 Chronic hepatitis. Short septa extend from the slightly enlarged portal tract (P) but normal architectural relationships are preserved. (Needle biopsy, reticulin.)

by the irregularity of the limiting plates of hepatocytes around the portal tracts. The term 'interface hepatitis' is now often preferred to the older term 'piecemeal necrosis' because there is evidence to suggest that apoptosis rather than necrosis may be involved.[11,12] However, the relative roles played by apoptosis and necrosis in viral hepatitis are not yet entirely clear, because the two processes share several characteristics.[13]

Figure 9.3
Interface hepatitis.
In contrast to the upper margin of this portal tract, the edges of the lower margin are blurred by inflammatory infiltration and hepatocyte loss. (Needle biopsy, H&E.)

Figure 9.4
Interface hepatitis.
At a higher magnification than **Fig. 9.3**, lymphocytes are seen infiltrating between surviving hepatocytes. The interface between inflamed portal tract and parenchyma is irregular. (Needle biopsy, H&E.)

Interface hepatitis at its mildest is recognised by lymphocytes in the periportal parenchyma, in association with hepatocellular damage. In more severe examples, trapped surviving hepatocytes may be seen within the inflammatory infiltrate (**Fig. 9.5**) and fibrous septa extend from the portal tract (**Fig. 9.6**). In cirrhotic livers the process is seen at the edges of nodules and septa rather than immediately around portal tracts (**see Fig. 10.19**);

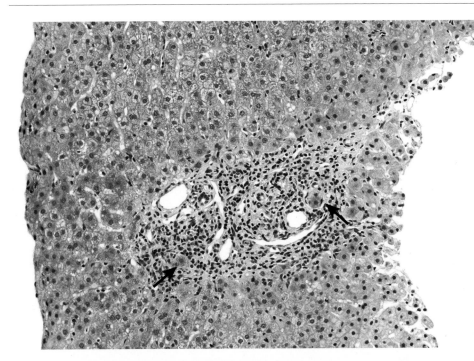

Figure 9.5 Chronic hepatitis, mild to moderate.
The lower edge of the portal tract shows interface hepatitis, with trapping of hepatocytes in the infiltrate (arrows). (Needle biopsy, H&E.)

Figure 9.6 Chronic hepatitis with fibrosis.
Fibrosis extends from the portal tract above into the parenchyma. (Needle biopsy, reticulin.)

Figure 9.7 Ductular reaction in chronic hepatitis with marked activity.
The margins of the portal tract (P) above and below are expanded and effaced by marked interface hepatitis. The white arrow marks the native bile duct. Within the irregular border of interface hepatitis at bottom are bile ductular structures (ductular reaction), one of which (arrow) is enlarged in the inset. *Inset*: Scattered neutrophils surround and partially infiltrate the flattened ductule (arrow) in this area of lymphoplasmacytic interface hepatitis. (Needle biopsy, H&E.)

in either case, however, the hepatitic process involves the interface between connective tissue and parenchyma.

Interface hepatitis varies not only in severity, but also in the extent of involvement of the interface, whatever its exact location. This is taken into consideration in some grading systems. With more severe interface hepatitis and liver-cell damage, periportal progenitor cells may become activated to produce a ductular reaction (proliferated bile ductules).[14] The blurring of the margins of the portal tracts in such instances then results from the combination of periportal chronic inflammatory cells and the ductular structures (**Fig. 9.7**). The presence of scattered neutrophils near the ductules should not be confused with biliary obstruction, cholangitis or a presumed drug reaction; they are normal constituents of the ductular reaction, mediated by cytokines expressed by the ductular cells.[15]

The lobular lesion

Deeper within the parenchyma there are varying degrees of hepatocellular damage and inflammation, sometimes called the lobular component or lobular hepatitis. Most commonly, this takes the form of focal necrosis, but confluent and bridging necrosis may also be seen. Panlobular necrosis is rare in chronic hepatitis. Also uncommon is the finding of severe lobular hepatitis in the absence of substantial portal and periportal inflammation.[16] The severity of lobular hepatitis correlates with the accumulation of progenitor cells.[17]

Figure 9.8 Chronic hepatitis with lobular activity. Clumps of inflammatory cells, some of them associated with hepatocyte loss, extend through the parenchyma. The portal tract above is inflamed. (Needle biopsy, H&E.)

Focal (spotty) necrosis is seen as areas of hepatocyte loss with infiltration by lymphocytes, macrophages and other cells. Each area covers the space normally occupied by up to about four or five hepatocytes (**Fig. 9.8**). Larger areas of hepatocyte loss are referred to as confluent necrosis (**see Ch. 4**). As in acute hepatitis, bridging necrosis refers to confluent necrosis and collapse linking vascular structures and is usually restricted to bridges linking portal tracts to terminal hepatic venules.

Severe lobular hepatitis is often accompanied by the formation of small rounded or ovoid gland-like clusters of surviving hepatocytes, so-called hepatitic rosettes (**Fig. 9.9**). Unlike cholestatic rosettes (**Ch. 4**), these are embedded in connective tissue and probably form as a result of hyperplasia of hepatocytes trapped in a collapsed and inflamed area of parenchyma.

In a minority of patients with chronic hepatitis some of the hepatocytes fuse to form multinucleated giant cells like those of neonatal hepatitis (**Fig. 9.10**). In adults this is termed *postinfantile giant-cell transformation*; it is an occasional feature of autoimmune hepatitis and of chronic hepatitis C (with or without human immunodeficiency virus (HIV) co-infection),[18,19] typically present only in perivenular regions.

Other hepatocyte changes seen in chronic hepatitis include steatosis, iron deposition and oncocytic change. Steatosis is commonest in chronic hepatitis C and is further discussed under that heading below, as is siderosis. Iron deposits are sometimes focal.[20] Substantial hepatocellular siderosis should always lead to consideration of possible hereditary haemochromatosis, but siderosis is not necessarily related to an *HFE* gene mutation.[21] Oncocytic change results from the accumulation of large numbers of closely packed mitochondria in hepatocytes, giving them a granular, densely eosinophilic appearance[22,23] (**Fig. 9.11**). These cells are most common within hepatitic rosettes. Mitochondrial hyperplasia in these cells appears to be a compensatory response to mitochondrial DNA dysfunction.[24] Finally, the appearance of bile thrombi in dilated canaliculi is most unusual in chronic hepatitis. While this type of cholestasis could result from an acute

Figure 9.9 Chronic hepatitis, severe, with rosette formation.
Parenchymal architecture has been completely disrupted. Surviving hepatocytes have formed gland-like rosettes, which are separated by bridges of collapse and inflammation. (Needle biopsy, H&E.)

Figure 9.10 Post-infantile giant-cell transformation in chronic hepatitis.
The affected perivenular hepatocytes are enlarged and pale with multiple nuclei (arrows). In adults this may be seen in autoimmune hepatitis or in chronic hepatitis C with or without HIV co-infection. (Needle biopsy, H&E.)

exacerbation of chronic disease, alternative explanations such as drug hepatotoxicity should be considered.

In some patients with chronic viral or autoimmune hepatitis, distinctive eosinophilic and diastase periodic acid–Schiff (PAS)-positive inclusions are seen in sinusoidal endothelial cells[25] (**Fig. 9.12**). The inclusions have been shown to contain immunoglobulins.[26]

Figure 9.11 Oncocyte formation in chronic hepatitis. Some of the hepatocytes in this severe chronic hepatitis have intensely eosinophilic granular cytoplasm. Others have a ground-glass appearance. (Needle biopsy, H&E.)

Figure 9.12 Sinusoidal inclusion-containing endothelial cells. In this example of chronic hepatitis C, multiple small granular inclusions are seen in the endothelium. (Needle biopsy, diastase–PAS.)

Individual causes of chronic hepatitis

Chronic hepatitis B and D

Chronic hepatitis B infection in both adults and children[27,28] goes through a series of phases marked by different serological, histological and immunocytochemical findings.[29] It begins with a period of immune tolerance, in which there are high levels of hepatitis B

Figure 9.13 Chronic hepatitis B with ground-glass hepatocytes.
In many hepatocytes the central part of the cytoplasm has a homogeneous ground-glass appearance. A paler-staining halo is seen around the ground-glass areas in some cells. (Needle biopsy, H&E.)

virus (HBV)-DNA in serum. Hepatitis B e antigen (HbeAg) is positive and anti-HBe negative. Histological activity varies, and both interface hepatitis and lobular hepatitis may be seen on liver biopsy. However, low levels of activity are more common. The surface antigen, HbsAg, is most abundant in the characteristic **ground-glass hepatocytes** (**Fig. 9.13**). The ground-glass cells are typically scattered singly throughout the parenchyma at this stage of infection. Their name derives from the finely granular appearance of the central part of the cytoplasm, which is rich in endoplasmic reticulum and hepatitis B surface material. Other organelles are located at the cell periphery and often appear to be separated from the ground-glass area by a pale halo. HBsAg can be demonstrated immunohistochemically (**Fig. 9.14**) and with orcein or Victoria blue methods. It is most abundant in the ground-glass hepatocytes, but can also be seen in a membranous or submembranous location in hepatocytes without a ground-glass pattern. The differential diagnosis of ground-glass hepatocytes is from the oncocytic cells described in the previous section, from drug-induced hypertrophy of the endoplasmic reticulum (**Fig. 8.1**) and from inclusion-containing hepatocytes in cyanamide toxicity (**Ch. 8**), Lafora's disease, immunosuppressed transplant patients (**Ch. 16**) and fibrinogen storage disease.[30] Clinical circumstances together with immunostaining for HBsAg make confusion unlikely.

The core antigen, HBcAg, is also demonstrable by immunostaining (**Fig. 9.14**). It is mainly located in hepatocyte nuclei, but also in cytoplasm when necroinflammatory activity is high. Positive nuclear staining correlates with viral load.[31] Nuclei which contain large amounts of core protein sometimes have a pale, homogeneous appearance on haematoxylin and eosin (H&E)-stained sections and have been described as 'sanded'[32] (**Fig. 9.15**).

The immunotolerant phase of chronic HBV infection is followed by immune clearance and seroconversion to a non-replicative phase in which HBeAg disappears from serum to be replaced by anti-HBe. During the phase of immune clearance, of very variable length, histological activity is typically high.

In the third, non-replicative phase, histological activity is usually considered to be low, as are markers of viral replication. However, in a large study of liver biopsies from patients in this phase, about one-third showed varying degrees of interface hepatitis, sometimes in

Figure 9.14 Hepatitis B surface and core antigens with immunohistochemistry.
A: Characteristic cytoplasmic inclusions of HBsAg are present. *Inset*: HBsAg staining is sometimes membranous or submembranous. **B:** Nuclear as well as cytoplasmic staining of HBcAg is present in this case, consistent with active viral replication. (Explant liver, specific immunoperoxidase stains.)

**Figure 9.15
'Sanded' nuclei
with hepatitis B
core antigen.**
In this case of
chronic hepatitis
B the pale
homogeneous
appearance of the
affected hepatocyte
nuclei (long arrows)
reflects the presence
of many intra-
nuclear core
particles. Several
normal-appearing
nuclei are in the field
(short arrows). Many
hepatocytes have
ground-glass
inclusions. (Needle
biopsy, H&E.)

the presence of normal aminotransferase levels.[33] Lobular activity was not necessarily accompanied by portal and periportal inflammation. Ground-glass hepatocytes may be aggregated in focal accumulations in the non-replicative phase.

Reactivation of virus replication and histological activity are common and are some-times associated with the emergence of viral mutants. In some of these mutants, expression of HBeAg is defective and histological activity is unexpectedly high, in spite of the negative HBeAg and presence of anti-HBe.

Finally, in a minority of patients with chronic HBV infection, HBsAg becomes negative and anti-HBs appears in the serum. HBV-DNA may still be detectable in small amounts in serum and liver.

This complex evolution, not always as orderly as the above simplified description might suggest, is marked by a very variable degree of fibrosis, depending on the severity and timing of the hepatic process. Cirrhosis may develop at any stage, especially in patients whose HBV infection is complicated by infection with other viruses such as HCV and HDV.[34]

Apart from the presence of ground-glass hepatocytes and HBV antigens, there are other features which characterise chronic hepatitis B. Marked variation in the size and appear-ance of hepatocyte nuclei has been described,[35] as has close contact between hepatocytes and lymphocytes,[36] in keeping with the immunological nature of the hepatitis. The lym-phocytes are usually of CD8+ type, in contrast to the portal infiltrate, which is rich in CD4+ lymphocytes, B lymphocytes and dendritic cells.[37] Lymphoid follicles are occasion-ally found in portal tracts but are less common and less prominent than in hepatitis C.[38]

Infection with the delta virus (HDV) modifies infection with HBV, as already noted in **Chapter 6**. Its presence is associated with relatively high histological activity except after liver transplantation. Inflammation is rarely restricted to portal tracts, and there is likely to be substantial inflammation in periportal areas as well as deeper within the lobules.

Positive immunostaining for HDV (**see Fig. 6.16**) denotes active infection. A 'sanded' appearance similar to that produced by hepatitis core protein may be seen when there is abundant HDV in hepatocyte nuclei.[39] In the presence of HDV infection there is a greater risk of chronicity than with HBV alone, and liver-associated mortality is increased.[40] Once cirrhosis has developed in patients with hepatitis B, HDV infection confers a greater risk of developing hepatocellular carcinoma and a higher mortality.[41] The prevalence of HDV infection has declined since the 1970s and 1980s as a result of measures to eradicate HBV infection.[42]

Chronic hepatitis C

Chronic hepatitis C affects more than 170 million persons worldwide.[43] It is not usually life-threatening until cirrhosis develops, typically several decades after onset of the hepatitis. Factors associated with faster progression to cirrhosis include older age,[44] male sex, fibrosis on initial biopsy,[45] high necroinflammatory activity on initial biopsy,[46] iron deposition (see Pathological features, below), alcohol consumption, previous HBV infection[47] and HIV infection.[48] There are six different genotypes of the virus[49] affecting disease severity and response to specific treatment;[50] patients with genotypes 2 and 3 respond best to specific therapy.

The use of liver biopsy in the management of patients with HCV infection has been the subject of extensive discussion. There are serious efforts to replace biopsy to some extent with formulae based on biochemical findings,[51,52] but these fail to predict histological findings accurately.[8,9] Repeatedly normal or near-normal serum aminotransferases suggest mild histological changes,[53] yet a substantial proportion of such patients has been found to have serious liver damage and even cirrhosis.[54,55] The consensus view appears to be that liver biopsy currently continues to provide useful information not obtainable in other ways.[7,56,57]

Pathological features

The histological features of chronic hepatitis C, although not completely diagnostic in themselves, are very characteristic[38,58] (**Table 9.4**). The portal infiltrate is rich in lymphocytes which often form aggregates or follicles, some of them with prominent germinal centres (**Fig. 9.16**). These follicles are easily identified in reticulin preparations (**Fig. 9.17**). Follicles are not restricted to hepatitis C and can also be found in hepatitis B, autoimmune hepatitis and primary biliary cirrhosis, but in hepatitis C they are particularly common and prominent. Within, or to one side of the lymphoid infiltrates, damaged interlobular bile ducts may be seen, as in acute hepatitis. The damage takes the form of vacuolation, stratification and crowding of epithelial cells, and infiltration by lymphocytes.[59] The virus has been demonstrated in bile-duct epithelium and in bile.[60] Bile-duct damage is occasionally, but by no means always, associated with a clinically cholestatic course, and rare ductopenia has been reported.[61,62]

The intralobular changes typically include acidophilic degeneration of hepatocytes and formation of acidophil bodies, already described in **Chapter 6**. Confluent necrosis is uncommon. Sinusoids are focally or diffusely infiltrated by lymphocytes, giving rise in some biopsies to a striking beaded appearance reminiscent of infectious mononucleosis. Epithelioid-cell granulomas are occasionally found in lobules or portal tracts[63,64] and clumped material somewhat like Mallory bodies has been reported in periportal hepatocytes.[65] The presence

Table 9.4 Histological features of chronic type C hepatitis
Difficult to distinguish from acute hepatitis C
Often mild, but cirrhosis commonly develops
Lymphoid follicles in portal tracts
Damaged interlobular bile ducts
Lobular activity including acidophil bodies
Large-droplet steatosis
Lymphocytes in sinusoids
Granulomas

Figure 9.16
Chronic hepatitis C.
The portal tract (top left) is heavily infiltrated by lymphocytes, which extend irregularly into the adjacent tissue. A lymphoid follicle with germinal centre has formed. (Needle biopsy, H&E.) (Colour version of a half-tone figure in Scheuer et al.,[38] reproduced with permission from the publishers.)

Figure 9.17
Chronic hepatitis C.
The prominent pale area in the portal tract is the site of a lymphoid follicle. (Needle biopsy, reticulin.)

of talc crystals in liver tissue, seen by polarised light microscopy, is a specific but insensitive marker of intravenous drug abuse.[66]

Iron deposition is common even in the absence of the frequently found *HFE* mutations of hereditary haemochromatosis and may influence progression of the disease.[67,68] Iron is seen not only in hepatocytes, but also in macrophages, endothelial cells and portal tracts.[69,70]

There is an extensive recent literature on the significance of steatosis in chronic hepatitis C. As already noted, steatosis is more common in hepatitis C than in other forms of chronic hepatitis and may be quite severe. It is a risk factor for progression,[71,72] and can interfere with therapy. The steatosis is often associated with obesity, diabetes or alcohol consumption.[63-76] However, in infection with HCV genotype 3[77,78] and very occasionally other genotypes,[79] the virus appears to have a direct effect and the steatosis improves after successful treatment.[80,81] The mechanism for the steatosis may be interference by the viral core protein with lipoprotein assembly and secretion.[82] In addition to steatosis, features of steatohepatitis such as pericellular fibrosis have been reported.[83]

The development of reliable and clinically useful methods for detecting viral proteins by immunohistochemistry has been hampered by the small amounts of virus present in each cell, at least in immunocompetent patients. Although results using a monoclonal antibody against HCV envelope protein have been reported,[84] an immunostain for the identification of HCV in routine practice currently remains unavailable.

In biopsies taken early in the course of the disease, the hepatitis is often mild, with little interface hepatitis or fibrosis. With time, fibrous septa extend from expanded portal tracts and link vascular structures. Fibrosis linking portal tracts has the appearance of web-like membranes on three-dimensional reconstruction.[85] A pericellular pattern of fibrosis in perivenular areas has been reported in children.[86] Spontaneous clearance of virus[87] or specific treatment of the infection[88] may bring about dramatic improvement of the fibrosis and structural changes.

Autoimmune hepatitis

Autoimmune hepatitis (AIH) is diagnosed mainly on the basis of serum autoantibodies and absence of evidence for other causes of chronic hepatitis. The autoantibody profile is the basis for subclassification into different types.[89] The commonly assayed autoantibodies include anti-nuclear and anti-smooth muscle antibodies (ANA, ASMA) and liver–kidney microsomal (LKM) antibodies. Other non-standard antibodies which may be present include soluble liver antigen (SLA), atypical peripheral anti-neutrophil cytoplasmic antibodies (atypical pANCA) and anti-liver cytosol antibodies.[90-92] Anti-mitochondrial antibodies (AMAs) may be present in up to 35% of patients with otherwise typical AIH; they may persist for many years without clinical impact or evidence of primary biliary cirrhosis.[93] Histological evidence is important not only for confirming the diagnosis, but also as a means of detecting other conditions with which AIH may be confused. Histology is therefore one component of scoring systems which can be utilised in clinical practice.[94,95]

While there are no pathognomonic histological features of AIH, there is a characteristic picture in many patients before treatment. Biopsy shows active disease, with much hepatocellular damage and a heavy infiltrate of lymphocytes and plasma cells in portal tracts, at the interface and deep within the parenchyma (**Figs 9.18, 9.19**). Plasma cells in clusters in interface regions are often striking. Eosinophils may also be present.[96] Lymphoid follicles are less prominent than in hepatitis C. Bridging necrosis is common and surviving hepatocytes often form hepatitic rosettes (**Fig. 9.14**). Prominent syncytial giant hepatocytes in an adult hepatitis (**Fig. 9.10**), while not diagnostic, should always raise the possibility of AIH.[97,98]

This classic histological picture is not, however, the only one seen in AIH, and communication between pathologist and clinician is important to ensure a correct diagnosis.[99] Plasma cells are not always present in large numbers. In some patients the hepatitis is much milder, and in some there may be cholestasis, bile-duct damage or even ductopenia.[100,101] In adults, this has to be distinguished from the bile-duct lesions of primary biliary cirrhosis and the relatively uncommon overlap syndromes (**Ch. 5**). In children, AIH is often associated with an autoimmune form of sclerosing cholangitis.[102,103]

Figure 9.18 Autoimmune hepatitis with rosette formation. Rounded hepatitic rosettes, some with a visible lumen (arrow), are surrounded by compressed sinusoids, fibrous tissue and inflammatory cells. (Needle biopsy, H&E.)

Figure 9.19 Autoimmune hepatitis. Inflammatory cells including plasma cells extend from the portal tract (left) into the parenchyma as part of the process of interface hepatitis. (Needle biopsy, H&E.)

Autoimmune hepatitis is regarded as a chronic disease in all patients, but the clinical onset is sometimes acute. In a study of 26 patients biopsied within 6 months of onset,[104] most showed evidence of chronicity and a few had cirrhosis. However, careful analysis of connective tissue septa with the help of several connective tissue stains (**Ch. 6**) sometimes suggests recent onset with rapid development of nodules. Furthermore there are a few

Figure 9.20 Autoimmune hepatitis with confluent perivenular necrosis. The parenchyma around an efferent venule (top centre) has been almost completely replaced by necrotic debris and inflammatory cells. (Needle biopsy, H&E.)

patients with AIH in whom the principal features on presentation are confluent necrosis and inflammation in perivenular areas, as in an acute hepatitis[105-108] (**Fig. 9.20**). This lesion may also be accompanied by the portal and periportal lymphoplasmacytic inflammation more typical of AIH. Exacerbation of disease severity may favour the development of confluence of the two patterns, resulting in central-to-portal bridging necrosis or even multilobular and massive necrosis.

Patients with AIH usually respond rapidly to corticosteroid therapy. Biopsy following treatment shows varying degrees of resolution of the necroinflammatory process and sometimes dramatic improvement in fibrosis and structural changes.[109,110] Liver biopsy helps to determine when corticosteroid treatment can safely be withdrawn.[10] The degree of plasma-cell infiltration is a predictor of relapse,[111] and worsening histological activity appears to correlate with progression of fibrosis.[112] Biopsy therefore continues to play an important role in patient management.

Other conditions with features of autoimmune hepatitis

Histological changes closely resembling AIH may occur in other settings (**Table 9.5**), sometimes accompanied by positive serum autoantibodies and elevated γ-globulin levels. The microscopic changes and generation of autoantibodies may be triggered by viral infection (chronic hepatitis C with autoimmune features[113]), drugs with idiosyncratic effects (minocycline,[114] statins,[115] black cohosh[116]) or medication-related immunomodulatory changes in an immunosuppressed individual (immune reconstitution after antiretroviral therapy in HIV disease;[117] after liver transplantation –

Table 9.5 Conditions sometimes associated with features of autoimmune hepatitis

Drug hepatotoxicity (e.g. minocycline, statins)
Chronic hepatitis C
HIV disease with immune reconstitution
Transition from other autoimmune diseases (e.g. primary biliary cirrhosis)
Overlap syndromes (autoimmune hepatitis/PBC; autoimmune hepatitis/PSC)
After liver transplantation
Recurrent chronic hepatitis C
Recurrent chronic hepatitis C treated with interferon
De novo autoimmune hepatitis
Alloimmune late rejection

see Ch. 16). In such cases, the interpretation of AIH-like features merits clinical discussion along with review of current or recently changed medications. The type and titre of auto-antibodies, γ-globulin level and the biopsy findings need to be factored into specific changes in management.

The potential for AIH to 'overlap' with other liver diseases of autoimmune nature, such as primary biliary cirrhosis and primary sclerosing cholangitis, was discussed in **Chapter 5**. Infrequently, one autoimmune disease may transition over time to another, such as primary biliary cirrhosis evolving to AIH. The transition may be evident as heightened necroinflammation, including interface hepatitis and bridging necrosis.[118,119]

Differential diagnosis of chronic hepatitis

In biopsies with inflammation confined to portal tracts, other possibilities to be considered include **resolving acute hepatitis, non-specific inflammation near a focal lesion, primary biliary cirrhosis** and **lymphoma**. The nature of the infiltrate and involvement of most or all portal tracts in chronic hepatitis should resolve the issue in most cases, but clinical information is also needed.

More severe chronic hepatitis needs to be distinguished from **acute hepatitis**, which is sometimes difficult. As discussed in **Chapter 6**, staining for elastic fibres may enable recently formed bridges to be distinguished from old fibrous septa. Canalicular cholestasis, common in acute hepatitis, is not often found in chronic hepatitis. In HBV infection in an immunocompetent patient the presence of HBsAg-containing ground-glass hepatocytes indicates chronic disease.

Other diseases to be considered in the more severe forms include **chronic biliary diseases**, especially primary biliary cirrhosis and primary sclerosing cholangitis, α_1-**antitrypsin deficiency**, **Wilson's disease**, **lymphoma** and **drug injury**. Loss of bile ducts and periportal accumulation of copper-associated protein suggest biliary disease rather than chronic hepatitis. α_1-Antitrypsin deficiency can be diagnosed by appropriate staining (**Ch. 13**), while Wilson's disease (**Ch. 14**) should be established principally by clinical features and biochemical findings. The infiltrates of various lymphomas are usually extensive and irregular and may undergo necrosis. Drugs sometimes cause a liver disease closely resembling AIH, or may act as a trigger, unmasking latent autoimmunity, as discussed above. As in all liver diseases, correlation of clinical and histological findings reduces the risk of diagnostic error.

Semi-quantitative scoring: grading and staging

Scoring is now widely used to evaluate liver biopsies before treatment, to monitor the effects of treatment and to assess the effects of new therapies in clinical trials. It consists of two components, their names borrowed from oncology: **grading** and **staging**. Grading refers to the scoring of the necroinflammatory lesion of a hepatitis, including the various types and degrees of hepatocellular damage and the location and extent of the inflammatory process. Staging records the extent of fibrosis and of changes in structure, including the development of cirrhosis. In many scoring systems, grading is subdivided into categories such as portal inflammation, interface hepatitis and lobular hepatitis, whereas staging is expressed as a single scale.

Assessment of fibrosis can also be carried out using morphometric measurement of collagen.[120,121] This gives an accurate measurement of the amount of fibrous tissue per unit area, but does not take structural changes such as nodule formation into account. Staging and morphometry should therefore be viewed as complementary to each other and not as alternatives.

Table 9.6 A simple scoring system for chronic hepatitis

1.	**Grade**
A.	**Portal inflammation and interface hepatitis**
	0 Absent or minimal
	1 Portal inflammation only
	2 Mild or localised interface hepatitis
	3 Moderate or more extensive interface hepatitis
	4 Severe and widespread interface hepatitis
B.	**Lobular activity**
	0 None
	1 Inflammatory cells but no hepatocellular damage
	2 Focal necrosis or apoptosis
	3 Severe hepatocellular damage
	4 Damage includes bridging confluent necrosis
2.	**Stage**
	0 No fibrosis
	1 Fibrosis confined to portal tracts
	2 Periportal or portal–portal septa but intact vascular relationships
	3 Fibrosis with distorted structure but no obvious cirrhosis
	4 Probable or definite cirrhosis

Modified by permission from Elsevier from Scheuer.[122]

Scoring is semi-quantitative rather than quantitative, in the sense that, while scores are usually expressed as numbers, they do not represent measurements. Scoring involves subjective assessment of the various relevant histological features in a biopsy, and the scores allotted will inevitably vary somewhat from observer to observer depending on experience and personal bias. For this reason, scores allotted at different times or by different observers cannot be directly compared. This limits the usefulness of scoring as a routine reporting procedure.

Before embarking on scoring, the pathologist should consider carefully why the scores are required. This will help to determine the most suitable system for the particular purpose or project. For example, if what is needed is a decision as to whether the chronic hepatitis in a particular patient is mild, moderate or severe, a simple system will suffice, and will usually have the advantage over more complex systems in so far as the latter tend to be associated with greater intra- and inter-observer variation and are also more time-consuming. If, on the other hand, the purpose is to evaluate a group of biopsies in a clinical trial of a new treatment regime, then a complex system is more appropriate. A complex system would allow analysis not only of the overall severity of the changes, but also of individual features such as interface hepatitis and lobular activity. Examples of two simple systems are given in **Table 9.6**[122] and **Table 9.8**.[123] The simple staging system proposed by the METAVIR group[124] is given in **Table 9.7**, and the more complex and widely

Table 9.7 The METAVIR staging system

F0 No fibrosis

F1 Stellate enlargement of portal tracts but without septum formation

F2 Enlargement of portal tracts with rare septum formation

F3 Numerous septa without cirrhosis

F4 Cirrhosis

Modified by permission of Wiley-Liss, Inc., from Bedossa et al.[124]

Table 9.8 The METAVIR algorithm

Interface hepatitis[a] (piecemeal necrosis)		Lobular necrosis[b]		Overall histological activity[c]
0	+	0	=	0
0	+	1	=	1
0	+	2	=	2
1	+	0	=	1
1	+	1	=	1
1	+	2	=	2
2	+	0	=	2
2	+	1	=	2
2	+	2	=	3
3	+	0	=	3
3	+	1	=	3
3	+	2	=	3

[a]Interface hepatitis scored 0 (none), 1 (mild), 2 (moderate), 3 (severe).
[b]Lobular necrosis scored 0 (none or mild), 1 (moderate), 2 (severe).
[c]Histological activity scored 0 (none), 1 (mild), 2 (moderate), 3 (severe).
Modified by permission of Wiley-Liss, Inc., from Bedossa et al.[123]

used Ishak system,[124] derived from the earlier Knodell Histology Activity Index,[125] in **Table 9.9**. Examples of grading and staging are shown in **Figs 9.21 and 9.22**.

The results of a particular study can be compared in a general way with those of another, but, because of the subjective nature of scoring, the numbers themselves cannot be directly compared or combined. Each study therefore stands on its own to some extent and the observers are free to modify a published scoring system to suit a particular purpose. For instance, a scoring range for steatosis, siderosis or bile-duct damage could be devised and added if required.

Reproducibility of scoring is improved when it is performed by more than one observer.[126] There should then be an initial discussion using a multi-headed microscope in order to ensure that all observers agree on the criteria used to score each feature. At the end of a study, discrepancies between observers can be resolved by joint discussion at the microscope. In a clinical trial, it may be helpful to re-assess a proportion of biopsies in order to test intra-observer variation. The scoring should be performed by the same observer or observers throughout, and is usually done without knowledge of clinical data.

Interpretation of the results of scoring

When the scores from a group of biopsies are assessed, the statistical methods used to evaluate the results must be appropriate for categorical data. An example of a suitable method is that used by Lagging et al.[127] Some grading systems are divided into several categories. In the case of the Ishak score, these are interface hepatitis, confluent necrosis, lobular activity and portal inflammation. For each of these four categories the scale from 0 to 4 or 0 to 6 is not exactly linear, and it is therefore not acceptable to add the four scores together and then to manipulate the result as if it were a true mathematical sum. To put the matter another way, a score of 2 for any particular feature does not denote exactly twice 1 or precisely half of 4, but simply a score somewhere between 1 and 3.

Table 9.9 The Ishak scoring system

Category	Score
Grading	
A. Periportal or periseptal interface hepatitis	
Absent	0
Mild (focal, few portal areas)	1
Mild/moderate (focal, most portal areas)	2
Moderate (continuous around <50% of tracts or septa)	3
Severe (continuous around >50% of tracts or septa)	4
B. Confluent necrosis	
Absent	0
Focal	1
Zone 3 necrosis in some areas	2
Zone 3 necrosis in most areas	3
Zone 3 necrosis + occasional portal–central bridging	4
Zone 3 necrosis + multiple portal–central bridging	5
Panacinar or multiacinar necrosis	6
C. Focal (spotty) lytic necrosis, apoptosis and focal inflammation[a]	
Absent	0
<2 foci per 10 × objective	1
2–4 foci per 10 × objective	2
5–10 foci per 10 × objective	3
>10 foci per 10 × objective	4
D. Portal inflammation	
None	0
Mild, some or all portal areas	1
Moderate, some or all portal areas	2
Moderate/marked, all portal areas	3
Marked, all portal areas	4
Staging	
No fibrosis	0
Fibrous expansion of some portal areas, with or without short fibrous septa	1
Fibrous expansion of most portal areas, with or without short fibrous septa	2
Fibrous expansion of most portal areas with occasional portal–portal bridging	3
Fibrous expansion of portal areas with marked bridging (portal–portal and portal–central)	4
Marked bridging (portal–portal and/or portal–central) with occasional nodules (incomplete cirrhosis)	5
Cirrhosis, probable or definite	6

[a]Does not include diffuse sinusoidal infiltration by inflammatory cells.
Adapted by permission from Elsevier from Ishak et al.[125]

Figure 9.21 Grading of chronic hepatitis.
The examples of grading shown in these four panels emphasise the portal/periportal necroinflammatory component of chronic hepatitis; lobular activity also should be taken into account, but
is frequently less prominent. **A:** *Minimal activity (grade 1)*. Inflammation is confined to the portal tracts
and there is no interface hepatitis. The lobular parenchyma is quiescent. **B:** *Mild activity (grade 2)*.
Focal interface hepatitis is now present (right periportal region) in addition to portal tract
inflammation. A few lobular necroinflammatory foci are also seen at right. **C:** *Moderate activity (grade
3)*. More extensive interface hepatitis is present than in grade 2, but involving <50% of the
circumference of most portal tracts. In this example, the portal tract edges above and to the right
show relative sparing. **D:** *Marked activity (grade 4)*. The portal tract is diffusely inflamed and shows
extensive circumferential interface hepatitis. Similar changes affect virtually all portal tracts with this
grade of activity, often with considerable lobular activity. (Needle biopsies, H&E.)

Nevertheless, total grading scores are often used and published. In routine practice a total
grading score gives an approximate indication of the severity of a patient's hepatitis, but
no information on the relative contribution of each category. In clinical trials of new
therapies, total grading scores are potentially misleading and the effect of the therapy on
each individual grading category should be examined.

The possibility or indeed likelihood of sampling variation must also be kept in mind.[128]
In chronic hepatitis C, there are differences between the findings in the left and the right
lobe of the liver.[129] More important, small needle biopsy samples may be misleading.
Recent studies have thrown light on this particular issue. In one study using image analysis
to assess fibrosis, the ability of the image analysis to predict a METAVIR fibrosis score
diminished progressively in specimens less than 25 mm long.[120] In another study, reducing
the sample size optically led to underestimation of disease severity in samples less than
20 mm long and 1.4 mm wide.[130] According to this study, samples obtained with fine
needles were considered unsatisfactory for scoring. Another group recommended that the

Figure 9.22 Staging of chronic hepatitis.
A: *Minimal fibrosis (stage 1)*. This type of modest fibrosis sometimes takes the form of rounded fibrous expansion of some portal tracts (shown at left). In other cases, minimal fibrosis consists of occasional short fibrous scars at the edges of some, but not all, portal tracts (shown at arrows in right panel). **B:** *Mild fibrosis (stage 2)*. Most portal tracts have a stellate contour due to periportal fibrosis as shown here.

Figure 9.22, cont'd
C: *Extensive bridging fibrosis with nodularity, but without cirrhosis (stage 3).* This biopsy specimen consisted of several cores of liver tissue. Portal-to-portal bridging fibrosis is prominent in the left-hand portions of both cores, while more architecturally preserved parenchyma with stellate scarring of portal tracts is evident at right. Developing parenchymal nodules are also seen at left. Fully established cirrhosis is not demonstrated.
D: *Cirrhosis (stage 4).* Architecturally abnormal regenerative nodules are evident and are circumscribed by diffuse fibrosis. Needle biopsy samples sometimes contain fragments of cirrhotic nodules (at arrow) which have been shelled out and separated from the adjacent fibrous septa. Such regenerative fragments frequently have a 'squared-off' or 'flat-top' appearance at their edges. (A&B, needle biopsies: trichrome stain; C&D, needle biopsies: reticulin stain.)

use of fine needles in diffuse HCV-related liver disease should be restricted to early non-fibrotic lesions.[131] While not all investigators agree that fine-needle specimens are inadequate for grading and staging,[132] specimen size is clearly a critical issue.

In conclusion, many factors limit the accuracy of semi-quantitative scoring in chronic hepatitis.[133] Awareness of these factors, careful attempts to minimise observer variation and appropriate interpretation of the results should ensure the continued usefulness of grading and staging in clinical practice and research.

References

1 Berasain C, Betes M, Panizo A, et al. Pathological and virological findings in patients with persistent hypertransaminasaemia of unknown aetiology. *Gut* 2000; 47: 429–435.

2 Hano H, Takasaki S. Three-dimensional observations on the alterations of lobular architecture in chronic hepatitis with special reference to its angioarchitecture for a better understanding of the formal pathogenesis of liver cirrhosis. *Virchows Arch* 2003; 443: 655–663.

3 Diseases of the Liver and Biliary Tract. Standardization of Nomenclature, Diagnostic Criteria, and Prognosis. New York: Raven Press, 1994.

4 Desmet VJ, Gerber M, Hoofnagle JH, et al. Classification of chronic hepatitis: diagnosis, grading and staging. *Hepatology* 1994; 19: 1513–1520.

5 International Working Party. Terminology of chronic hepatitis, hepatic allograft rejection, and nodular lesions of the liver: summary of recommendations developed by an international working party, supported by the World Congresses of Gastroenterology, Los Angeles 1994. *Am J Gastroenterol* 1994; 89: S177–S181.

6 Andriulli A, Festa V, Leandro G, et al. Usefulness of a liver biopsy in the evaluation of patients with elevated ALT values and serological markers of hepatitis viral infection: an AIGO study. *Dig Dis Sci* 2001; 46: 1409–1415.

7 Saadeh S, Cammell G, Carey WD, et al. The role of liver biopsy in chronic hepatitis C. *Hepatology* 2001; 33: 196–200.

8 Ghany MG, Strader DB, Thomas DL, Seeff LB. Diagnosis, management, and treatment of hepatitis C: an update. *Hepatology* 2009; 49: 1335–1374.

9 Bain VG, Bonacini M, Govindarajan S, et al. A multicentre study of the usefulness of liver biopsy in hepatitis C. *J Viral Hepat* 2004; 11: 375–382.

10 Czaja AJ, Carpenter HA. Histological features associated with relapse after corticosteroid withdrawal in type 1 autoimmune hepatitis. *Liver Int* 2003; 23: 116–123.

11 Lau JYN, Xie X, Lai MMC, et al. Apoptosis and viral hepatitis. *Semin Liver Dis* 1998; 18: 169–176.

12 Oksuz M, Akkiz H, Isiksal F, et al. Expression of Fas antigen in liver tissue of patients with chronic hepatitis B and C. *Eur J Gastroenterol Hepatol* 2004; 16: 341–345.

13 Jaeschke H, Gujral J, Bajt M. Apoptosis and necrosis in liver disease. *Liver Int* 2004; 24: 85–89.

14 Eleazar JA, Memeo L, Jhang JS, et al. Progenitor cell expansion: an important source of hepatocyte regeneration in chronic hepatitis. *J Hepatol* 2004; 39: 552–556.

15 Isse K, Harada K, Nakanuma Y. IL-8 expressed by biliary epithelial cells is associated with neutrophilic infiltration and reactive bile ductules. *Liver Int* 2007; 27: 672–680.

16 Liaw YF, Chu CM, Chen TJ, et al. Chronic lobular hepatitis: a clinicopathological and prognostic study. *Hepatology* 1982; 2: 258–262.

17 Libbrecht L, Desmet V, Van Damme B, et al. Deep intralobular extension of human hepatic 'progenitor cells' correlates with parenchymal inflammation in chronic viral hepatitis: can 'progenitor cells' migrate? *J Pathol* 2000; 192: 373–378.

18 Protzer U, Dienes HP, Bianchi L, et al. Post-infantile giant cell hepatitis in patients with primary sclerosing cholangitis and autoimmune hepatitis. *Liver* 1996; 16: 274–282.

19 Micchelli STL, Thomas D, Boitnott JK, et al. Hepatic giant cells in hepatitis C virus (HCV) mono-infection and HCV/HIV co-infection. *J Clin Pathol* 2008; 61: 1058–1061.

20 Lefkowitch JH, Yee HT, Sweeting J, et al. Iron-rich foci in chronic viral hepatitis. *Hum Pathol* 1998; 29: 116–118.

21 Martinelli AL, Filho AB, Franco RF, et al. Liver iron deposits in hepatitis B patients: association with severity of liver disease but not with hemochromatosis gene mutations. *Gastroenterol Hepatol* 2004; 19: 1036–1041.

22 Lefkowitch JH, Arborgh BA, Scheuer PJ. Oxyphilic granular hepatocytes. Mitochondrion-rich liver cells in hepatic disease. *Am J Clin Pathol* 1980; 74: 432–441.

23 Gerber MA, Thung SN. Hepatic oncocytes. Incidence, staining characteristics, and ultrastructural features. *Am J Clin Pathol* 1981; 75: 498–503.

24 Tanji K, Bhagat G, Vu TH, et al. Mitochondrial DNA dysfunction in oncocytic hepatocytes. *Liver Int* 2003; 23: 397–403.

25 Iwamura S, Enzan H, Saibara T, et al. Appearance of sinusoidal inclusion-containing endothelial cells in liver disease. *Hepatology* 1994; 20: 604–610.

26 Iwamura S, Enzan H, Saibara T, et al. Hepatic sinusoidal endothelial cells can store and metabolize serum immunoglobulin. *Hepatology* 1995; 22: 1456–1461.

27 Broderick AL, Jonas MM. Hepatitis B in children. *Semin Liver Dis* 2003; 23: 59–68.

28 Boxall E, Sira J, Standish RA, et al. The natural history of hepatitis B in perinatally infected carriers. *Arch Dis Child – Fetal Neonatal Edn* 2004; 89: F456–F460.

29 Fattovich G. Natural history and prognosis of hepatitis B. *Semin Liver Dis* 2003; 23: 47–58.

30 Callea F, De Vos R, Togni R, et al. Fibrinogen inclusions in liver cells: a new type of ground-glass hepatocyte. Immune light and electron microscopic characterization. *Histopathology* 1986; 10: 65–73.

31 Serinoz E, Varli M, Erden E, et al. Nuclear localization of hepatitis B core antigen and its relations to liver injury, hepatocyte proliferation, and viral load. *J Clin Gastroenterol* 2003; 36: 269–272.

32 Bianchi L, Gudat F. Sanded nuclei in hepatitis B: eosinophilic inclusions in liver cell nuclei due to excess in hepatitis B core antigen formation. *Lab Invest* 1976; **35**: 1–5.

33 Ter Borg F, ten Kate FJ, Cuypers HT, et al. A survey of liver pathology in needle biopsies from HBsAg and anti-HBe positive individuals. *J Clin Pathol* 2000; **53**: 541–548.

34 Mathurin P, Thibault V, Kadidja K, et al. Replication status and histological features of patients with triple (B, C, D) and dual (B, C) hepatic infections. *J Viral Hepat* 2000; **7**: 15–22.

35 Bianchi L, Gudat F. Chronic hepatitis. In: MacSween RNM, Anthony PP, Scheuer PJ, et al, eds. Pathology of the Liver, 3rd edn. Edinburgh: Churchill Livingstone, 1994: 349–396.

36 Dienes HP, Popper H, Arnold W, et al. Histologic observations in human hepatitis non-A, non-B. *Hepatology* 1982; **2**: 562–571.

37 van den Oord JJ, De Vos R, Facchetti F, et al. Distribution of non-lymphoid, inflammatory cells in chronic HBV infection. *J Pathol* 1990; **160**: 223–230.

38 Scheuer PJ, Ashrafzadeh P, Sherlock S, et al. The pathology of hepatitis C. *Hepatology* 1992; **15**: 567–571.

39 Moreno A, Ramón y Cahal S, Marazuela M, et al. Sanded nuclei in delta patients. *Liver* 1989; **9**: 367–371.

40 Abiad H, Ramani R, Currie JB, et al. The natural history of hepatitis D virus infection in Illinois state facilities for the developmentally disabled. *Am J Gastroenterol* 2001; **96**: 534–540.

41 Fattovich G, Giustina G, Christensen E, et al. Influence of hepatitis delta virus infection on morbidity and mortality in compensated cirrhosis type B. The European Concerted Action on Viral Hepatitis (Eurohep). *Gut* 2000; **46**: 420–426.

42 Rizzetto M. Hepatitis D: thirty years after. *J Hepatol* 2009; **50**: 1043–1050.

43 Poynard T, Ratziu V, Benhamou Y, et al. Natural history of HCV infection. *Best Pract Res Clin Gastroenterol* 2000; **14**: 211–228.

44 Ghany MG, Kleiner DE, Alter H, et al. Progression of fibrosis in chronic hepatitis C. *Gastroenterology* 2003; **124**: 97–104.

45 Ryder SD. Progression of hepatic fibrosis in patients with hepatitis C: a prospective repeat liver biopsy study. *Gut* 2004; **53**: 451–455.

46 Fontaine H, Nalpas B, Poulet B, et al. Hepatitis activity index is a key factor in determining the natural history of chronic hepatitis C. *Hum Pathol* 2001; **32**: 904–909.

47 Giannini E, Ceppa P, Botta F, et al. Previous hepatitis B virus infection is associated with worse disease stage and occult hepatitis B virus infection has low prevalence and pathogenicity in hepatitis C virus-positive patients. *Liver Int* 2003; **23**: 12–18.

48 Poynard T, Mathurin P, Lai CL, et al. A comparison of fibrosis progression in chronic liver diseases. *J Hepatol* 2003; **38**: 257–265.

49 Webster G, Barnes E, Brown D, et al. HCV genotypes – role in pathogenesis of disease and response to therapy. *Best Pract Res Clin Gastroenterol* 2000; **14**: 229–240.

50 Roffi L, Redaelli A, Colloredo G, et al. Outcome of liver disease in a large cohort of histologically proven chronic hepatitis C: influence of HCV genotype. *Eur J Gastroenterol Hepatol* 2001; **13**: 501–506.

51 Imbert-Bismut F, Ratziu V, Pieroni L, et al. Biochemical markers of liver fibrosis in patients with hepatitis C virus infection: a prospective study. *Lancet* 2001; **357**: 1069–1075.

52 Afdhal NH. Diagnosing fibrosis in hepatitis C: is the pendulum swinging from biopsy to blood tests? *Hepatology* 2003; **37**: 972–974.

53 Persico M, Persico E, Suozzo R, et al. Natural history of hepatitis C virus carriers with persistently normal aminotransferase levels. *Gastroenterology* 2000; **118**: 760–764.

54 Nutt AK, Hassan HA, Lindsey J, et al. Liver biopsy in the evaluation of patients with chronic hepatitis C who have repeatedly normal or near-normal serum alanine aminotransferase levels. *Am J Med* 2000; **109**: 62–64.

55 Kyrlagkitsis I, Portmann B, Smith H, et al. Liver histology and progression of fibrosis in individuals with chronic hepatitis C and persistently normal ALT. *Am J Gastroenterol* 2003; **98**: 1588–1593.

56 Dienstag JL. The role of liver biopsy in chronic hepatitis C. *Hepatology* 2002; **36**: S152–S160.

57 Rockey DC, Caldwell SH, Goodman ZD, Nelson RC, Smith AD. Liver biopsy. *Hepatology* 2009; **49**: 1017–1044.

58 Bach N, Thung SN, Schaffner F. The histological features of chronic hepatitis C and autoimmune chronic hepatitis: a comparative analysis. *Hepatology* 1992; **15**: 572–577.

59 Kaji K, Nakanuma Y, Sasaki M, et al. Hepatitic bile duct injuries in chronic hepatitis C: histopathologic and immunohistochemical studies. *Mod Pathol* 1994; **7**: 937–945.

60 Haruna Y, Kanda T, Honda M, et al. Detection of hepatitis C virus in the bile and bile duct epithelial cells of hepatitis C virus-infected patients. *Hepatology* 2001; **33**: 977–980.

61 Delladetsima JK, Makris F, Psichogiou M, et al. Cholestatic syndrome with bile duct damage and loss in renal transplant recipients with HCV infection. *Liver* 2001; **21**: 81–88.

62 Kumar KS, Saboorian MH, Lee WM. Cholestatic presentation of chronic hepatitis C: a clinical and histological study with a review of the literature. *Dig Dis Sci* 2001; **46**: 2066–2073.

63 Gaya DR, Thorburn D, Oien KA, et al. Hepatic granulomas: a 10 year single centre experience. *J Clin Pathol* 2003; **56**: 850–853.

64 Ozaras R, Tahan V, Mert A, et al. The prevalence of hepatic granulomas in chronic hepatitis C. *J Clin Gastroenterol* 2004; **38**: 449–452.

65 Lefkowitch JH, Schiff ER, Davis GL, et al. Pathological diagnosis of chronic hepatitis C: a multicenter comparative study with chronic hepatitis B. *Gastroenterology* 1993; **104**: 595–603.

66 Sherman KE, Lewey SM, Goodman ZD. Talc in the liver of patients with chronic hepatitis C infection. *Am J Gastroenterol* 1995; **90**: 2164–2166.

67 Bonkovsky HL, Troy N, McNeal K, et al. Iron and HFE or TfR1 mutations as comorbid factors for development and progression of chronic hepatitis C. *J Hepatol* 2002; **37**: 848–854.

68 Martinelli AL, Ramalho LN, Zucoloto S. Hepatic stellate cells in hepatitis C patients: relationship with liver iron deposits and severity of liver disease. *J Gastroenterol Hepatol* 2004; **19**: 91–98.

69 Pirisi M, Scott CA, Avellini C, et al. Iron deposition and progression of disease in chronic hepatitis C. Role of interface hepatitis, portal inflammation, and HFE missense mutations. *Am J Clin Pathol* 2000; **113**: 546–554.

70 Metwally MA, Zein CO, Zein NN. Clinical significance of hepatic iron deposition and serum iron values in patients with chronic hepatitis C infection. *Am J Gastroenterol* 2004; **99**: 286–291.

71 Wyatt J, Baker H, Prasad P, et al. Steatosis and fibrosis in patients with chronic hepatitis C. *J Clin Pathol* 2004; **57**: 402–406.

72 Fartoux L, Chazoullières O, Wendum D, Poupon R, Serfaty L. Impact of steatosis on progression of fibrosis in patients with mild hepatitis C. *Hepatology* 2005; **41**: 82–87.

73 Adinolfi LE, Gambardella M, Andreana A, et al. Steatosis accelerates the progression of liver damage of chronic hepatitis C patients and correlates with specific HCV genotype and visceral obesity. *Hepatology* 2001; **33**: 1358–1364.

74 Monto A, Alonzo J, Watson JJ, et al. Steatosis in chronic hepatitis C: relative contributions of obesity, diabetes mellitus, and alcohol. *Hepatology* 2002; **36**: 729–736.

75 Sheikh MY, Choi J, Qadri I, et al. Hepatitis C virus infection: molecular pathways to metabolic syndrome. *Hepatology* 2008; **47**: 2127–2133.

76 Hu KQ, Kyulo NL, Esrailian E, et al. Overweight and obesity, hepatic steatosis, and progression of chronic hepatitis C: a retrospective study on a large cohort of patients in the United States. *J Hepatol* 2004; **40**: 147–154.

77 Rubbia-Brandt L, Quadri R, Abid K, et al. Hepatocyte steatosis is a cytopathic effect of hepatitis C virus genotype 3. *J Hepatol* 2000; **33**: 106–115.

78 Serfaty L, Andreani T, Giral P, et al. Hepatitis C virus induced hypobetalipoproteinemia: a possible mechanism for steatosis in chronic hepatitis C. *J Hepatol* 2001; **34**: 428–434.

79 Colloredo G, Sonzogni A, Rubbia-Brandt L, et al. Hepatitis C virus genotype 1 associated with massive steatosis of the liver and hypo-β-lipoproteinemia. *J Hepatol* 2004; **40**: 562–563.

80 Hofer H, Bankl HC, Wrba F, et al. Hepatocellular fat accumulation and low serum cholesterol in patients infected with HCV-3a. *Am J Gastroenterol* 2002; **97**: 2880–2885.

81 Kumar D, Farrell GC, Fung C, et al. Hepatitis C virus genotype 3 is cytopathic to hepatocytes: reversal of hepatic steatosis after sustained therapeutic response. *Hepatology* 2002; **36**: 1266–1272.

82 Lonardo A, Adinolfi LE, Loria P, et al. Steatosis and hepatitis C virus: mechanisms and significance for hepatic and extrahepatic disease. *Gastroenterology* 2004; **126**: 586–597.

83 Clouston AD, Jonsson JR, Purdie DM, et al. Steatosis and chronic hepatitis C: analysis of fibrosis and stellate cell activation. *J Hepatol* 2001; **34**: 314–320.

84 Verslype C, Nevens F, Sinelli N, et al. Hepatic immunohistochemical staining with a monoclonal antibody against HCV-E2 to evaluate antiviral therapy and reinfection of liver grafts in hepatitis C viral infection. *J Hepatol* 2003; **38**: 208–214.

85 Hoofring A, Boitnott J, Torbenson M. Three-dimensional reconstruction of hepatic bridging fibrosis in chronic hepatitis C viral infection. *J Hepatol* 2003; **39**: 738–741.

86 Badizadegan K, Jonas MM, Ott MJ, et al. Histopathology of the liver in children with chronic hepatitis C infection. *Hepatology* 1998; **28**: 1416–1423.

87 Sugiyasu Y, Yuki N, Nagaoka T, et al. Histological improvement of chronic liver disease after spontaneous serum hepatitis C virus clearance. *J Med Virol* 2003; **69**: 41–49.

88 Pol S, Carnot F, Nalpas B, et al. Reversibility of hepatitis C virus-related cirrhosis. *Hum Pathol* 2004; **35**: 107–112.

89 Al Khalidi JA, Czaja AJ. Current concepts in the diagnosis, pathogenesis, and treatment of autoimmune hepatitis. *Mayo Clin Proc* 2001; **76**: 1237–1252.

90 Krawitt EL. Autoimmune hepatitis. *N Engl J Med* 2006; **354**: 54–66.

91 Heneghan MA, McFarlane IG. Of mice and women: toward a mouse model of autoimmune hepatitis. *Hepatology* 2005; **42**: 17–20.

92 Czaja AJ, Bayraktar Y. Non-classical phenotypes of autoimmune hepatitis and advances in diagnosis and treatment. *World J Gastroenterol* 2009; **15**: 2314–2328.

93 O'Brien C, Joshi S, Feld JJ, Guindi M, Dienes HP, Heathcote EJ. Long-term follow-up of antimitochondrial antibody-positive autoimmune hepatitis. *Hepatology* 2008; **48**: 550–556.

94 Alvarez F, Berg PA, Biandin FB, et al. International Autoimmune Hepatitis Group report: review of criteria for diagnosis of autoimmune hepatitis. *J Hepatol* 1999; **31**: 929–938.

95 Hennes EM, Zeniya M, Czaja AJ, et al. Simplified criteria for the diagnosis of autoimmune hepatitis. *Hepatology* 2008; **48**: 169–176.

96 Goldstein NS, Soman A, Gordon SC. Portal tract eosinophils and hepatocyte cytokeratin 7 immunoreactivity helps distinguish early-stage, mildly active primary biliary cirrhosis and autoimmune hepatitis. *Am J Clin Pathol* 2001; **116**: 846–853.

97 Devaney K, Goodman ZD, Ishak KG. Postinfantile giant-cell transformation in hepatitis. *Hepatology* 1992; **16**: 327–333.

98 Lau JYN, Koukoulis G, Mieli-Vergani G, et al. Syncytial giant-cell hepatitis – a specific disease entity? *J Hepatol* 1992; **15**: 216–219.

99 Carpenter HA, Czaja AJ. The role of histologic evaluation in the diagnosis and management of autoimmune hepatitis and its variants. *Clin Liver Dis* 2002; **6**: 397–417.

100 Czaja AJ, Carpenter HA. Autoimmune hepatitis with incidental histologic features of bile duct injury. *Hepatology* 2001; **34**: 659–665.

101 Zolfino T, Heneghan MA, Norris S, et al. Characteristics of autoimmune hepatitis in patients who are not of European Caucasoid ethnic origin. *Gut* 2002; **50**: 713–717.

102 Gregorio GV, Portmann B, Karani J, et al. Autoimmune hepatitis/sclerosing cholangitis overlap syndrome in childhood: a 16-year prospective study. *Hepatology* 2001; **33**: 544–553.

103 Mieli-Vergani G, Vergani D. Autoimmune hepatitis in children. *Clin Liver Dis* 2002; **6**: 335–346.

104 Burgart LJ, Batts KP, Ludwig J, et al. Recent-onset autoimmune hepatitis. Biopsy findings and clinical correlations. *Am J Surg Pathol* 1995; **19**: 699–708.

105 Pratt DS, Fawaz KA, Rabson A, et al. A novel histological lesion in glucocorticoid-responsive chronic hepatitis. *Gastroenterology* 1997; **113**: 664–668.

106 Te HS, Koukoulis G, Ganger DR. Autoimmune hepatitis: a histological variant associated with prominent centrilobular necrosis. *Gut* 1997; **41**: 269–271.

107 Singh R, Nair S, Farr G, et al. Acute autoimmune hepatitis presenting with centrizonal liver disease: case report and review of the literature. *Am J Gastroenterol* 2002; **97**: 2670–2673.

108 Misdraji J, Thiim M, Graeme-Cook FM. Autoimmune hepatitis with centrilobular necrosis. *Am J Surg Pathol* 2004; **28**: 471–478.

109 Cotler SJ, Jakate S, Jensen DM. Resolution of cirrhosis in autoimmune hepatitis with corticosteroid therapy. *J Clin Gastroenterol* 2001; **32**: 428–430.

110 Czaja AJ, Carpenter HA. Decreased fibrosis during corticosteroid therapy of autoimmune hepatitis. *J Hepatol* 2004; **40**: 646–652.

111 Verma S, Gunuwan B, Mendler M, et al. Factors predicting relapse and poor outcome in type I autoimmune hepatitis: role of cirrhosis development, patterns of transaminases during remission and plasma cell activity in the liver biopsy. *Am J Gastroenterol* 2004; **99**: 1510–1516.

112 Czaja AJ, Carpenter HA. Progressive fibrosis during corticosteroid therapy of autoimmune hepatitis. *Hepatology* 2004; **39**: 1631–1638.

113 Czaja AJ, Carpenter HA. Histological findings in chronic hepatitis C with autoimmune features. *Hepatology* 1997; **26**: 459–466.

114 Goldstein NS, Bayati N, Silverman AL, Gordon SC. Minocycline as a cause of drug-induced autoimmune hepatitis. Report of four cases and comparison with autoimmune hepatitis. *Am J Clin Pathol* 2000; **114**: 591–598.

115 Alla V, Abraham J, Siddiqui J, et al. Autoimmune hepatitis triggered by statins. *J Clin Gastroenterol* 2006; **40**: 757–761.

116 Lynch CR, Folkers ME, Hutson WR. Fulminant hepatic failure associated with the use of black cohosh: a case report. *Liver Transplant* 2006; **12**: 989–992.

117 O'Leary JG, Zachary K, Misdraji J, Chung RT. De novo autoimmune hepatitis during immune reconstitution in an HIV-infected patient receiving highly active antiretroviral therapy. *Clin Infect Dis* 2008; **46**: e12–e14.

118 Poupon R, Chazouillieres O, Corpechot C, Chrétien,Y. Development of autoimmune hepatitis in patients with typical primary biliary cirrhosis. *Hepatology* 2006; **44**: 85–90.

119 Twaddell WS, Lefkowitch J, Berk PD. Evolution from primary biliary cirrhosis to primary biliary cirrhosis/ autoimmune hepatitis overlap syndrome. *Semin Liver Dis* 2008; **28**: 128–134.

120 Bedossa P, Dargere D, Paradis V. Sampling variability of liver fibrosis in chronic hepatitis C. *Hepatology* 2003; **38**: 1449–1457.

121 Wright M, Thursz M, Pullen R, et al. Quantitative versus morphological assessment of liver fibrosis: semi-quantitative scores are more robust than digital image fibrosis area estimation. *Liver Int* 2003; **23**: 28–34.

122 Scheuer PJ. Classification of chronic viral hepatitis: a need for reassessment. *J Hepatol* 1991; **13**: 372–374.

123 Bedossa P, Poynard T, the METAVIR cooperative study group. An algorithm for the grading of activity in chronic hepatitis C. *Hepatology* 1996; **24**: 289–293.

124 Bedossa P, Bioulac-Sage P, Callard P, et al. Intraobserver and interobserver variations in liver biopsy interpretation in patients with chronic hepatitis C. *Hepatology* 1994; **20**: 15–20.

125 Ishak K, Baptista A, Bianchi L, et al. Histological grading and staging of chronic hepatitis. *J Hepatol* 1995; **22**: 696–699.

126 Knodell RG, Ishak KG, Black WC, et al. Formulation and application of a numerical scoring system for assessing histological activity in asymptomatic chronic active hepatitis. *Hepatology* 1981; **1**: 431–435.

127 Lagging LM, Westin J, Svensson E, et al. Progression of fibrosis in untreated patients with hepatitis C virus infection. *Liver* 2002; **22**: 136–144.

128 Guido M, Rugge M. Liver biopsy sampling in chronic viral hepatitis. *Semin Liver Dis* 2004; **24**: 89–97.

129 Regev A, Berho M, Jeffers LJ, et al. Sampling error and intraobserver variation in liver biopsy in patients with chronic HCV infection. *Am J Gastroenterol* 2002; **97**: 2614–2618.

130 Colloredo G, Guido M, Sonzogni A, et al. Impact of liver biopsy size on histological evaluation of chronic viral hepatitis: the smaller the sample, the milder the disease. *J Hepatol* 2003; **39**: 239–244.

131 Brunetti E, Silini E, Pistorio A, et al. Coarse vs. fine needle aspiration biopsy for the assessment of diffuse liver disease from hepatitis C virus-related chronic hepatitis. *J Hepatol* 2004; **40**: 501–506.

132 Petz D, Klauck S, Rohl FW, et al. Feasibility of histological grading and staging of chronic viral hepatitis using specimens obtained by thin-needle biopsy. *Virchows Arch* 2003; **442**: 238–244.

133 Rousselet M-C, Michalak S, Dupré F, et al. Sources of variability in histological scoring of chronic hepatitis. *Hepatology* 2005; **41**: 257–264.

General reading

Carpenter HA, Czaja AJ. The role of histologic evaluation in the diagnosis and management of autoimmune hepatitis and its variants. *Clin Liver Dis* 2002; **6**: 397–417.

Czaja AJ. Autoimmune liver disease. *Curr Opin Gastroenterol* 2003; **19**: 232–242.

De Vos R, Verslype C, Depla E, et al. Ultrastructural visualization of hepatitis C virus components in human and primate liver biopsies. *J Hepatol* 2002; **37**: 370–379.

Fattovich G, Bortolotti F, Donato F. Natural history of chronic hepatitis B: special emphasis on disease progression and prognostic factors. *J Hepatol* 2008; **48**: 335–352.

Ganem D, Prince AM. Hepatitis B virus infection – natural history and clinical consequences. *N Engl J Med* 2004; **350**: 1118–1129.

Goodman ZD. Grading and staging systems for inflammation and fibrosis in chronic liver diseases. *J Hepatol* 2007; **47**: 598–607.

Ishak KG. Pathologic features of chronic hepatitis. A review and update. *Am J Clin Pathol* 2000; **113**: 40–55.

Lai CL, Ratziu V, Yuen MF, et al. Viral hepatitis B. *Lancet* 2003; **362**: 2089–2094.

Mani H, Kleiner DE. Liver biopsy findings in chronic hepatitis B. *Hepatology* 2009; **49**: S61–S71.

McFarlane IG. Definition and classification of autoimmune hepatitis. *Semin Liver Dis* 2002; **22**: 317–324.

Penin F, Dubuisson J, Rey FA, et al. Structural biology of hepatitis C virus. *Hepatology* 2004; **39**: 5–19.

Ramadori G, Saile B. Portal tract fibrogenesis in the liver. *Lab Invest* 2004; **84**: 153–159.

Scheuer PJ, Standish RA, Dhillon AP. Scoring of chronic hepatitis. *Clin Liver Dis* 2002; **6**: 335–347.

Seeff LB. Natural history of chronic hepatitis C. *Hepatology* 2004; **36**: S35–S46.

Washington MK. Autoimmune liver disease: overlap and outliers. *Mod Pathol* 2007; **20**: S15–S30.

Cirrhosis

Introduction

Cirrhosis is a diffuse process in which the normal lobules are replaced by architecturally abnormal nodules separated by fibrous tissue.[1,2] The nodules, which are most commonly the result of regenerative hyperplasia following hepatocellular injury, are functionally less efficient than normal hepatic parenchyma and there is a profound disturbance of vascular relationships.

Several different kinds of information can be obtained about the cirrhotic liver by means of liver biopsy (**Table 10.1**). The most important functions of biopsy are to establish a diagnosis, to assess the cause of the cirrhosis as far as possible and to detect hepatocellular carcinoma.

Table 10.1 Main information from liver biopsy in cirrhosis
Diagnosis of cirrhosis
Assessment of cause
Stage of development
Histological activity
Detection of hepatocellular carcinoma

Diagnosis of cirrhosis by liver biopsy

The ease with which the pathologist can diagnose cirrhosis from a biopsy specimen depends on the sample as well as on the criteria used. The sample may be sufficiently big, and the nodules sufficiently small, to make the diagnosis obvious. On the other hand a slender core from within a large cirrhotic nodule can be difficult to identify as such (**Fig. 1.4**). There are occasions when the pathologist can do no more than hint at the possible diagnosis.

The type of biopsy needle used also influences the ease of diagnosis. Very narrow needles may be adequate to obtain tumour samples, but may be inadequate for the accurate diagnosis of medical conditions. For example, in staging chronic hepatitis thin-needle biopsies obtained under computed tomographic guidance may underdiagnose cirrhosis for advanced bridging fibrosis.[3] Some clinicians prefer to use the Trucut type of needle when cirrhosis is suspected in order to lessen the risk of fragmentation,[4,5] but suitable samples can usually be obtained with needles of the aspiration type.[6,7] Transjugular biopsy is used when there is a risk of haemorrhage by other routes. The combination of biopsy with laparoscopy has been advocated.[8,9] Operative wedge biopsies of cirrhotic liver give

DOI: 10.1016/B978-0-7020-3410-7.00016-2

Table 10.2 Cirrhosis: diagnostic criteria

A.	**Fundamental**
Nodularity	
Fibrosis	
B.	**Relative**
Fragmentation	
Abnormal structure	
Hepatocellular changes	
Regenerative hyperplasia	
Pleomorphism	
Large-cell dysplasia (large-cell change)	
Small-cell dysplasia (small-cell change)	
Excess copper-associated protein	

an accurate idea of the relative proportions of parenchyma and stroma in the liver as a whole.[10]

The histological criteria for a diagnosis of cirrhosis are outlined in **Table 10.2**. The two fundamental criteria, nodularity and fibrosis, reflect the definition of cirrhosis. When there are well-defined, rounded nodules surrounded by fibrous septa the diagnosis is easily established. Underestimating the stage of fibrosis because of specimen fragmentation (see below) is a concern, particularly when scoring biopsies in chronic hepatitis.[10a] Correlation with clinical and laboratory data help surmount this problem. Occasionally, a nodular appearance just deep to the liver capsule is not representative of the whole liver but has resulted from transection of a tongue or peninsula extending from the main bulk of the parenchyma.

In many patients the relative criteria listed in **Table 10.2** are equally important. They allow a tentative diagnosis of cirrhosis to be reached, readily converted to a firm diagnosis when correlated with other data. A diagnosis of cirrhosis therefore requires communication between pathologist and clinician, and cannot be exactly equated with a histological stage.[11]

Fragmentation

Fragmentation of the specimen, either at the time of biopsy or during processing in the laboratory, should itself suggest the possibility of cirrhosis (**Fig. 10.1**). The specimen is more likely to break into fragments when needles of the aspiration type (e.g. Menghini) are used. Other biopsy specimens that are likely to fragment are metastatic tumours surrounded by reactive fibrous tissue, and hepatocellular carcinoma.

Figure 10.1 Cirrhosis: fragmented sample.

A specimen obtained by the aspiration biopsy method has broken into rounded fragments peripherally circumscribed by fibrosis. (Needle biopsy, reticulin.)

Abnormal structure

Structural changes should be assessed by means of a reticulin preparation, preferably not counterstained. This may show two features not readily seen with other stains. First, although nodules are readily cored out of the dense fibrous stroma of a cirrhotic liver during aspiration biopsy, a thin layer of connective tissue tends to adhere to the nodules over much of their surface (**Fig. 10.2**). This layer may be difficult to see even with the help of collagen stains, and is easily missed in haematoxylin and eosin (H&E)-stained sections (**Fig. 10.3**). Second, minor alterations of structure become apparent even in those nodules which closely mimic normal liver. Such alterations include abnormal orientation of reticulin fibres resulting from different patterns and rates of growth in different areas (**Fig. 10.4**) and approximation of portal tracts and terminal venules. The number of venules may be abnormally large in relation to the number of portal tracts (**Fig. 10.5**), and the latter are sometimes abnormally small and poorly formed (**see Fig. 1.4**). A more obvious structural abnormality in cirrhosis is the presence of septa linking central veins (terminal hepatic venules) to portal tracts. These septa must be distinguished from recently formed necrotic bridges.

In wedge biopsies, excess fibrous tissue in and near the capsule and crowding of vessels must be distinguished from the changes of cirrhosis. The latter extend through the specimen, whereas the former is confined to the capsular and immediately subcapsular area.[12] Very occasionally a wedge biopsy of part of a large, well-differentiated regeneration nodule fails to show the histological features of cirrhosis.

Hepatocellular changes

In some biopsies from cirrhotic livers the hepatocytes are normal in appearance and arrangement, so that diagnosis rests on the structural changes discussed above. In others there are more or less obvious abnormalities of growth.

Regeneration is suggested by thickening of the liver-cell plates (**Fig. 10.6**). In any liver an oblique plane of sectioning will cause a few plates to appear more than one cell thick,

Figure 10.2 Cirrhosis: selective sampling.
A nodule has been cored out of the connective tissue by the biopsy procedure, but a thin layer of connective tissue (arrow) has adhered to the nodule margin. (Needle biopsy, reticulin.)

Figure 10.3
Cirrhosis: selective sampling.
Same field as in **Fig. 10.2**. In a haematoxylin and eosin preparation the thin layer of connective tissue is not easily seen. (Needle biopsy, H&E.)

Figure 10.4
Cirrhosis: distorted reticulin pattern.
The distortion has resulted from abnormal and irregular hepatocyte growth patterns. (Needle biopsy, reticulin.)

but widespread double-cell plates are seen when there is active growth. Hepatocytes in hyperplastic areas contain little or no lipofuscin pigment, even near terminal venules. Regeneration is not always evident in cirrhosis because it is not a continuous process. Its absence does not therefore exclude the diagnosis. Conversely, its presence does not prove cirrhosis, because it is found also in other circumstances, for example after an acute hepatitis and in the precirrhotic stages of chronic biliary diseases.

A very characteristic feature of cirrhosis is the presence of adjacent populations of hepatocytes growing at different rates and having different cell and nuclear characteristics

Figure 10.5 Cirrhosis: abnormal vascular relationships. Several venous channels are seen near to each other. (Wedge biopsy, H&E.)

Figure 10.6 Cirrhosis: hepatocellular regeneration. Liver-cell plates are two or more cells thick, indicating active growth. (Needle biopsy, H&E.)

(**Fig. 10.7**). This **pleomorphism** gives rise to the abnormalities of reticulin pattern already mentioned, notably a tendency for reticulin fibres in the different growth areas to lie in different directions.

In a minority of cirrhotic livers the hepatocytes show structural atypia of a degree sufficient to warrant a label of **dysplasia**, an appearance further discussed in **Chapter 11**. Two

Figure 10.7
Cirrhosis: different cell populations.
The parenchymal cells in area A are smaller than those in area B which also show a rounded and nodular growth pattern. (Wedge biopsy, H&E.)

Figure 10.8
Cirrhosis: large-cell dysplasia (large-cell change).
The nuclei of the enlarged hepatocytes at centre and left are irregular in shape and vary greatly in size and staining intensity. Several of these cells are multinucleated. Compare with the normal hepatocytes at right and in the upper left-hand corner. (Wedge biopsy, H&E.)

types have been described, large-cell dysplasia[13] and small-cell dysplasia.[14] Because of the controversial status of either type as a precursor of malignant change,[15] some authors prefer to call them large-cell change and small-cell change.[15,16] In the large-cell form, the cells are enlarged and their nuclei are hyperchromatic and irregular in shape, with prominent nucleoli (**Fig. 10.8**). Nuclear–cytoplasmic ratio is normal or only moderately increased.[17] This type of dysplasia was first described in an African population with a high incidence

Figure 10.9
Cirrhosis: small-cell dysplasia (small-cell change).
The hepatocytes below and to the right have normal-sized nuclei, but their overall size is reduced. Nuclear–cytoplasmic ratios are therefore increased. (Needle biopsy, H&E.)

of hepatocellular carcinoma (HCC) and hepatitis B virus (HBV) infection.[13] It is most often seen in patients with HBV and HCV infection but may also be evident in other chronic liver diseases.[18] There is evidence of an association of large-cell dysplasia with an increased risk of development of HCC independently of other risk factors.[19,20] Decreased expression of cell cycle checkpoint markers, presence of cytoplasmic DNA micronuclei and shortened telomeres in large-cell change are evidence favouring a disposition to HCC.[21] Demonstration of an increased hepatocyte proliferation rate as a risk for carcinoma is also important.[22] Care should be taken not to interpret the nuclear atypia which may be associated with cholestasis as large-cell dysplasia.[16]

In small-cell dysplasia the nuclear–cytoplasmic ratio is increased but the overall size of the affected cells is less than normal (**Fig. 10.9**). Zones of dysplastic hepatocytes of either type support a diagnosis of cirrhosis, and are regarded by some clinicians as an indication for increased monitoring for HCC. A finding of dysplasia of either type should therefore be specifically mentioned in liver biopsy reports.

Differential diagnosis

When there is nodularity and evidence of regeneration but little or no fibrosis, **nodular regenerative hyperplasia** should be considered. In **congenital hepatic fibrosis** the acinar architecture remains intact and the ductal plate malformation is seen. In **chronic hepatitis** with fibrosis and structural abnormalities, the differential diagnosis is between active cirrhosis and chronic hepatitis that has not yet reached the stage of cirrhosis. This problem cannot always be resolved on the basis of a liver biopsy. Similar doubt may arise in steatohepatitis. The presence of substantial quantities of copper and copper-associated protein in non-cholestatic chronic liver disease supports a diagnosis of cirrhosis.[23] Cirrhotic nodules can usually be distinguished from well-differentiated **hepatocellular carcinoma** (HCC). In the latter the cell plate architecture is more abnormal, reticulin may be scanty or absent and the cells have malignant cytological characteristics. Also, hepatocellular siderosis is often present secondarily in cirrhosis of varied aetiology (**see Ch. 14**) but is typically absent in tumour cells of HCC.

Assessment of cause

Biopsy may help to establish the cause of a cirrhosis. In some of the categories listed in **Table 10.3** the histological appearances are diagnostic. The term 'cryptogenic' should only be applied when full clinical and laboratory investigations have been completed and the features listed in **Table 10.4** have been assessed. This can be achieved by means of a small range of routine stains. There is evidence to suggest that many examples of cryptogenic cirrhosis result from non-alcoholic steatohepatitis (NASH), not evident histologically at the time of diagnosis.[24] Some cases of cirrhosis are due to mutations in genes for specific cellular keratins[25] or for bile canalicular transporter proteins.[26]

Table 10.3 Main causes of cirrhosis
Viral hepatitis (B, C, D)
Alcohol abuse
Obesity, insulin resistance/metabolic syndrome
Biliary disease
Metabolic disorders
Haemochromatosis
Wilson's disease
α_1-Antitrypsin deficiency, etc.
Venous outflow obstruction
Drugs and toxins
Autoimmune disease

Table 10.4 Cirrhosis: assessment of cause
Pattern of nodules and fibrosis
Bile ducts
Blood vessels
Steatohepatitis
Evidence of viral infection
Abnormal deposits
Iron
Copper, copper-associated protein
α_1-Antitrypsin globules

Pattern of nodules and fibrosis

Irregularly shaped nodules suggest the possibility of a biliary cause, especially if there is perinodular oedema, ductular reaction and chronic cholestasis. In a pre-cirrhotic stage of venous outflow obstruction there is regular fibrosis in perivenular regions (acinar zones 3). Sinusoids are dilated. Portal tracts show little or no abnormality or sometimes have changes mimicking biliary tract obstruction.[27] Certain features are indicative of earlier chronic hepatitis that evolved to cirrhosis. Irregular, slender fibrous septa emanating from portal tracts, lymphoplasmacytic infiltrates, lymphoid aggregates or follicles and foci of interface hepatitis should prompt consideration of the several causes of chronic hepatitis.

Confluent fibrosis which replaces multiple adjacent lobules is a common feature in several types of cirrhosis, particularly following steatohepatitis and chronic hepatitis of viral or autoimmune aetiology. It is also seen in the less common 'post-necrotic' cirrhosis which develops rapidly, within a few months of a severe viral or drug-induced acute hepatitis. Needle biopsy samples in such cases may show entire cores, portions of cores and especially the subcapsular region occupied by fibrous tissue, residual portal tracts and many ductular structures (**see Fig. 4.6c**), mild chronic inflammatory cell infiltrates, entrapped regenerative liver-cell rosettes and collections of small neo-vessels (see Blood vessels, below).

Bile ducts

Assessment of bile-duct numbers in cirrhosis is very important. The number of ducts should approximately equal the number of arteries of similar size and location, but the pathologist must bear in mind that not every portal tract will necessarily contain a bile duct in the plane of section. Definite duct loss should prompt consideration of primary biliary cirrhosis or primary sclerosing cholangitis. In some cases ductopenia is drug related or is associated with other conditions,[28] so the clinical history is important. In children or young adults, other ductopenic syndromes should also be considered. Typical bile-duct lesions of primary biliary cirrhosis, with or without granulomas, are still sometimes found at a stage of cirrhosis.

Periductal fibrosis may be very prominent in primary sclerosing cholangitis. Ductular reaction is a non-specific finding, but when severe and focal it often reflects biliary disease. Following extensive hepatocellular damage in cirrhosis – for example, after variceal haemorrhage – there is sometimes a very extensive ductular reaction which can be mistaken for cholangiocarcinoma.

Blood vessels

Occluded, narrowed or recanalised veins suggest that the cirrhosis may be the result of venous outflow block, but they are also found in cirrhosis from other causes.[29,30] Portal and hepatic venous thrombosis has indeed been implicated in the progression of cirrhosis in general.[31] Recognition of venous lesions is often difficult without the help of stains for collagen or elastic fibres. Neovascularisation of fibrotic portal tracts, areas of confluent fibrosis and bridging fibrous septa in cirrhosis produce numerous lymphatic and capillary channels, particularly in chronic hepatitis B and C.[32]

Steatohepatitis

This is found in alcohol abusers and in individuals at risk for non-alcoholic fatty liver disease, as a manifestation of drug toxicity, or for no obvious underlying reason (**see Ch. 7**). In amiodarone toxicity the fatty change is usually absent. Steatohepatitis must be distinguished from chronic cholestasis, in which there are also swollen hepatocytes containing Mallory bodies (**see Ch. 5**).

Evidence of viral infection

Features of chronic hepatitis, particularly interface hepatitis and lymphocytic infiltration, are often but by no means always due to infection with one of the hepatitis viruses. Liver-cell dysplasia also favours a viral cause. Ground-glass hepatocytes, Victoria blue or orcein stains (**Fig. 10.10**) and immunostains for viral antigens (**see Fig. 9.14**) help in the diagnosis of HBV infection, but tissue evidence of HBV antigens is not always present or detectable. Lymphoid aggregates or follicles should suggest the possibility of hepatitis C (**Fig. 10.11**). More than one virus or other causal agent may be responsible for a patient's cirrhosis. Abundant plasma cells raise the possibility of autoimmune hepatitis but are also sometimes found in viral hepatitis.

Abnormal deposits

Severe parenchymal siderosis should always raise the possibility of hereditary haemochromatosis, even when another cause is also evident. However, stainable iron often accumulates in cirrhosis from any cause.[33,34] Lack of significant haemosiderin in the connective tissue of portal tracts or fibrous septa in a cirrhosis points to a cause other than hereditary haemochromatosis (**see Fig. 14.12**). In hereditary haemochromatosis the nodules are sometimes irregular as in biliary cirrhosis.

Copper and copper-associated protein can often be detected in cirrhosis, whatever its cause.[23] Large amounts at the edges of the nodules suggest biliary disease. Staining of entire nodules is seen in Wilson's disease, but other nodules may be negative. In some stages of

Figure 10.10 Hepatitis B surface antigen in HBV-related cirrhosis. Many hepatocytes show positive cytoplasmic staining for HBV surface antigen. This staining method also demonstrates elastic tissue fibres in the fibrous tissue. (Recipient liver from transplantation, Victoria blue.)

Figure 10.11 Cirrhosis following hepatitis C virus infection. Lymphoid aggregates are still visible. The patient was also infected with GBV-C (the so-called hepatitis G virus). (Recipient liver from transplantation, H&E.)

the disease the copper is not histochemically demonstrable, so that negative staining does not exclude the diagnosis. Abundant copper and Mallory bodies are also features of Indian childhood cirrhosis and other forms of copper toxicosis.[35,36]

α_1-Antitrypsin bodies should always be looked for in cirrhosis. Immunocytochemical staining is more sensitive than diastase–PAS.

**Figure 10.12
Cirrhosis:
micronodular
pattern.**
Nodules are of
lobular size or
smaller. (Needle
biopsy, reticulin.)

Anatomical type

Because of possible sampling error, the pathologist cannot confidently assess nodule size in the rest of the liver on the basis of a biopsy specimen. This is usually of little consequence to the patient, though one biopsy study has suggested a significant correlation of the hepatic venous pressure gradient in portal hypertension with small nodule size.[37] Nevertheless, primary classification of cirrhosis by nodule size is no longer appropriate, because aetiology is clinically much more important.

However, nodule size does influence the ease of histological diagnosis. When nodules are of the size order of the lobules from which they are derived, several nodules are usually seen in one biopsy and diagnosis is easy (**Figs 10.12, 10.13**). When nodules are larger (**Fig. 10.14**), more subtle diagnostic criteria need to be considered. The most difficult anatomical type to recognise is **incomplete septal cirrhosis**. This is characterised by indistinct nodularity, slender septa, some of which end blindly, poorly formed small portal tracts and abnormal relationships between portal tracts and efferent venules[38] (**Fig. 10.15**). There is evidence of hepatocytic hyperplasia, giving rise to crowding of reticulin fibres in adjacent areas. Sinusoidal dilatation is common, while inflammation and necrosis are generally modest or absent. A reticulin preparation is important for diagnosis because the slender septa are easily missed (**Figs 10.15, 10.16**). The diagnosis is more easily made in wedge biopsies than in needle specimens. A relationship to various forms of non-cirrhotic portal hypertension has been demonstrated,[38–41] but it has also been postulated that incomplete septal cirrhosis can represent a burnt-out form of macronodular cirrhosis.[42] The incomplete septa could also reflect resorption of fibrous tissue, a type of 'regressed cirrhosis'.

**Figure 10.13
Cirrhosis:
micronodular
pattern.**
Similar field as in
Fig. 10.12. There is
steatosis. (Needle
biopsy, H&E.)

**Figure 10.14
Cirrhosis:
macronodular
pattern.**
Nodules are larger
than in **Figs 10.12
and 10.13**. The
magnification is
slightly smaller.
(Needle biopsy,
reticulin.)

**Figure 10.15
Cirrhosis:
incomplete septal
pattern.**
The parenchyma is
nodular but only
partially surrounded
by fibrous septa.
Note the
incompleted fibrous
septum emerging
vertically from the
portal tract at
bottom. (Wedge
biopsy, H&E.)

**Figure 10.16
Cirrhosis:
incomplete septal
pattern.**
Slender septa and
vessels are present.
There is a small
portal tract on the
right, towards the
top of the figure.
(Wedge biopsy,
reticulin.)

Figure 10.17 Early (developing) cirrhosis.
There is extensive fibrosis and architectural distortion in this biopsy from an alcohol abuser. Nodules are beginning to form but are not yet clearly defined. (Needle biopsy, reticulin.)

Stage of development

In some patients, cirrhosis is obvious and appears mature, in the sense that the well-demarcated nodules and dense fibrosis give an impression of long-standing disease. In others there is doubt as to whether there is cirrhosis or merely fibrosis. An impression may be gained that cirrhosis is incipient or at an early stage of development (**Fig. 10.17**). When doubt is unresolved, a report of 'developing cirrhosis' or 'incomplete cirrhosis' is sometimes appropriate. The concept of incomplete cirrhosis is recognised in the staging system of Ishak et al.[43] Once cirrhosis is fully established, reversion to a normal lobular pattern is unlikely. Indeed, reversibility of cirrhosis is a controversial subject[44] and the pathologist should consider this prospect cautiously, taking into account the type of biopsy sample, the underlying disease process and the possibility of sampling error. Diminished fibrosis following therapy does not automatically confer a return to normal liver-cell plate structure and vascular relationships.[2] Despite these caveats, reports of regression of cirrhosis of varied aetiologies[45] deserve attention.

Paradoxically, there may be confusion between mild chronic hepatitis and an inactive, well-established cirrhosis. This reflects difficulty in diagnosing some examples of late cirrhosis by needle biopsy, because of a tendency for nodule size to increase with time.

Histological activity

Activity is a convenient term to describe the rate of progression of the cirrhosis. It is usually taken to mean the various forms of liver-cell damage and inflammation typical of chronic viral hepatitis. In cirrhosis following steatohepatitis, however, the severity of the latter should also be taken into account.

In an inactive cirrhosis the interface between septa and nodules is sharply defined (**Fig. 10.18**). Cellular infiltration is mild and may be confined to the septa. There is little or no focal necrosis or intranodular inflammation. In an active, rapidly progressive cirrhosis on

Figure 10.18
Inactive cirrhosis.
Nodules are sharply outlined and inflammatory cells are scanty. (Wedge biopsy, H&E.)

Figure 10.19
Active cirrhosis.
The outline of the nodule is blurred by interface hepatitis and there is a heavy inflammatory infiltrate. (Wedge biopsy, H&E.)

the other hand the interface is blurred by hepatocellular damage and inflammation (**Fig. 10.19**). Isolated hepatocytes or groups of cells may be seen within the inflamed septa. There is hepatocellular damage and inflammation deep within the nodules.

Histological activity often varies in severity from one part of the liver to another. Comparison of activity in multiple biopsies from an individual patient should therefore be made with caution and with reference to clinical and biochemical data.

Complications

Hypoperfusion leads to coagulative necrosis involving whole nodules or their centres.[31] This is sometimes referred to as **nodular infarction**.

In recent years, advances in imaging and examination of explanted cirrhotic livers after transplantation have led to extensive discussion of the pathology and nomenclature of nodules different in appearance from the rest, and usually larger in diameter. The relationship of these nodules to hepatocellular carcinoma has been debated, and is further discussed in **Chapter 11**. An international working party[46] has recommended that the old term adenomatous hyperplasia should no longer be used, and that the nodules should be subdivided into **large regenerative nodules (macroregenerative nodules)** and **dysplastic nodules**. The latter are further subclassified as low grade and high grade. The dysplastic nodules differ from macroregenerative nodules in their content of dysplastic (atypical) hepatocytes and their more expansile growth pattern. However, the distinction between macroregenerative nodules and low-grade dysplastic nodules is often difficult, as is the distinction between high-grade dysplastic nodules and well-differentiated **hepatocellular carcinoma**, a very important complication of cirrhosis. In addition to the three large nodule types described by the working party, the group also defined **dysplastic foci**, clusters of dysplastic hepatocytes less than 1 mm in diameter.[47] In making a microscopic diagnosis and differentiating between these various possibly preneoplastic nodules, the pathologist must bear in mind that needle biopsy samples of a nodule may not be representative of the entire nodule, and that hepatocellular carcinoma may have arisen in a part not sampled by the needle.

References

1. Anthony PP, Ishak KG, Nayak NC, et al. The morphology of cirrhosis: definition, nomenclature, and classification. *Bull World Health Org* 1977; **55:** 521–540.

2. Desmet VJ, Roskams T. Cirrhosis reversal: a duel between dogma and myth. *J Hepatol* 2004; **40:** 860–867.

3. Petz D, Klauck S, Röhl, et al. Feasibility of histological grading and staging of chronic viral hepatitis using specimens obtained by thin-needle biopsy. *Virchows Arch* 2003; **442:** 238–244.

4. Rockey DC, Caldwell SH, Goodman ZD, et al. Liver biopsy. *Hepatology* 2009; **49:** 1017–1044.

5. Colombo M, Del Ninno E, de Francis R, et al. Ultrasound-assisted percutaneous liver biopsy: superiority of the Tru-Cut over the Menghini needle for diagnosis of cirrhosis. *Gastroenterology* 1988; **95:** 487–489.

6. Bateson MC, Hopwood D, Duguid HL, et al. A comparative trial of liver biopsy needles. *J Clin Pathol* 1980; **33:** 131–133.

7. Littlewood ER, Gilmore IT, Murray-Lyon IM, et al. Comparison of the Trucut and Surecut liver biopsy needles. *J Clin Pathol* 1982; **35:** 761–763.

8. Orlando R, Lirussi F, Okolicsanyi L. Laparoscopy and liver biopsy: further evidence that the two procedures improve the diagnosis of liver cirrhosis. A retrospective study of 1,003 consecutive examinations. *J Clin Gastroenterol* 1990; **12:** 47–52.

9. Jalan R, Harrison DJ, Dillon JF, et al. Laparoscopy and histology in the diagnosis of chronic liver disease. *Q J Med* 1995; **88:** 559–564.

10. Imamura H, Kawasaki S, Bandai, Y et al. Comparison between wedge and needle biopsies for evaluating the degree of cirrhosis. *J Hepatol* 1993; **17:** 215–219.

10a. Everhart JE, Wright EC, Goodman ZD, et al. Prognostic value of Ishak fibrosis stage: findings from the Hepatitis C Antiviral Long-Term Treatment Against Cirrhosis trial. *Hepatology* 2010; **51:** 585–594.

11. Desmet VJ, Roskams T. Reversal of cirrhosis: evidence-based medicine? *Gastroenterology* 2003; **125:** 629–630.

12. Petrelli M, Scheuer PJ. Variation in subcapsular liver structure and its significance in the interpretation of wedge biopsies. *J Clin Pathol* 1967; **20:** 743–748.

13. Anthony PP, Vogel CL, Barker LF. Liver cell dysplasia: a premalignant condition. *J Clin Pathol* 1973; **26:** 217–223.

14. Watanabe S, Okita K, Harada T, et al. Morphologic studies of the liver cell dysplasia. *Cancer* 1983; **51:** 2197–2205.

15. Lee RG, Tsamandas AC, Demetris AJ. Large cell change (liver cell dysplasia) and hepatocellular carcinoma in cirrhosis: matched case–control study, pathological analysis, and pathogenetic hypothesis. *Hepatology* 1997; **26:** 1415–1422.

16. Natarajan S, Theise ND, Thung SN, et al. Large-cell change of hepatocytes in cirrhosis may represent a reaction to prolonged cholestasis. *Am J Surg Pathol* 1997; **21:** 312–318.

17. Roncalli M, Borzio M, Tombesi MV, et al. A morphometric study of liver cell dysplasia. *Hum Pathol* 1988; **19:** 471–474.

18 Hodges TR, Millward-Sadler GH, Barbatis C, et al. Heterozygous MZ alpha-1-antitrypsin deficiency in adults with chronic active hepatitis and cryptogenic cirrhosis. *N Engl J Med* 1981; **304**: 557–560.

19 Libbrecht L, Craninx M, Nevens F, et al. Predictive value of liver cell dysplasia for development of hepatocellular carcinoma in patients with non-cirrhotic and cirrhotic chronic viral hepatitis. *Histopathology* 2001; **39**: 66–71.

20 Borzio M, Bruno S, Roncalli M, et al. Liver cell dysplasia is a major risk factor for hepatocellular carcinoma in cirrhosis: a prospective study. *Gastroenterology* 1995; **108**: 812–817.

21 Kim H, Oh B-K, Roncalli M, et al. Large liver cell change in hepatitis B virus-related liver cirrhosis. *Hepatology* 2009; **50**: 752–762.

22 Borzio M, Trerè D, Borzio F, et al. Hepatocyte proliferation rate is a powerful parameter for predicting hepatocellular carcinoma development in liver cirrhosis. *J Clin Pathol Mol Pathol* 1998; **51**: 96–101.

23 Guarascio P, Yentis F, Cevikbas U, et al. Value of copper-associated protein in diagnostic assessment of liver biopsy. *J Clin Pathol* 1983; **36**: 18–23.

24 Caldwell SH, Oelsner DH, Iezzoni JC, et al. Cryptogenic cirrhosis: clinical characterization and risk factors for underlying disease. *Hepatology* 1999; **29**: 664–669.

25 Ku N-O, Gish R, Wright TL, et al. Keratin 8 mutations in patients with cryptogenic liver disease. *N Engl J Med* 2001; **344**: 1580–1587.

26 Gotthardt D, Runz H, Keitel V, et al. A mutation in the canalicular phospholipid transporter gene, *ABCB4*, is associated with cholestasis, ductopenia, and cirrhosis in adults. *Hepatology* 2008; **48**: 1157–1166.

27 Kakar S, Batts KP, Poterucha JJ, et al. Histologic changes mimicking biliary disease in liver biopsies with venous outflow impairment. *Mod Pathol* 2004; **17**: 874–878.

28 Kim WR, Ludwig J, Lindor KD. Variant forms of cholestatic diseases involving small bile ducts in adults. *Am J Gastroenterol* 2000; **95**: 1130–1138.

29 Burt AD, MacSween RN. Hepatic vein lesions in alcoholic liver disease: retrospective biopsy and necropsy study. *J Clin Pathol* 1986; **39**: 63–67.

30 Nakanuma Y, Ohta G, Doishita K. Quantitation and serial section observations of focal venocclusive lesions of hepatic veins in liver cirrhosis. *Virchows Arch [A]* 1985; **405**: 429–438.

31 Wanless IR, Wong F, Blendis LM, et al. Hepatic and portal vein thrombosis in cirrhosis: possible role in development of parenchymal extinction and portal hypertension. *Hepatology* 1995; **21**: 1238–1247.

32 Yamauchi Y, Michitaka K, Onji M. Morphometric analysis of lymphatic and blood vessels in human chronic viral liver diseases. *Am J Pathol* 1998; **153**: 1131–1137.

33 Deugnier Y, Turlin B, Le Quilleuc D, et al. A reappraisal of hepatic siderosis in patients with end-stage cirrhosis: practical implications for the diagnosis of hemochromatosis. *Am J Surg Pathol* 1997; **21**: 669–675.

34 McGuinness PH, Bishop GA, Painter DM, et al. Intrahepatic hepatitis C RNA levels do not correlate with degree of liver injury in patients with chronic hepatitis C. *Hepatology* 1996; **23**: 676–687.

35 Mehrotra R, Pandey RK, Nath P. Hepatic copper in Indian childhood cirrhosis. *Histopathology* 1981; **5**: 659–665.

36 Müller T, Langner C, Fuchsbichler A, et al. Immunohistochemical analysis of Mallory bodies in Wilsonian and non-Wilsonian hepatic copper toxicosis. *Hepatology* 2004; **39**: 963–969.

37 Nagula S, Jain D, Groszmann RJ, et al. Histological–hemodynamic correlation in cirrhosis – a histological classification of the severity of cirrhosis. *J Hepatol* 2006; **44**: 111–117.

38 Sciot R, Staessen D, Van Damme B, et al. Incomplete septal cirrhosis: histopathologic aspects. *Histopathology* 1988; **13**: 593–603.

39 Lopez JI. Does incomplete septal cirrhosis link non-cirrhotic nodulations with cirrhosis? *Histopathology* 1989; **15**: 318–320.

40 Bernard P-H, Le Bail B, Cransac M, et al. Progression from idiopathic portal hypertension to incomplete septal cirrhosis with liver failure requiring liver transplantation. *J Hepatol* 2004; **22**: 495–499.

41 Nakanuma Y, Hoso M, Sasaki M, et al. Histopathology of the liver in non-cirrhotic portal hypertension of unknown etiology. *Histopathology* 1996; **28**: 195–204.

42 Nevens F, Staessen D, Sciot R, et al. Clinical aspects of incomplete septal cirrhosis in comparison with macronodular cirrhosis. *Gastroenterology* 1994; **106**: 459–463.

43 Ishak K, Baptista A, Bianchi L, et al. Histological grading and staging of chronic hepatitis. *J Hepatol* 1995; **22**: 696–699.

44 Friedman SL. Liver fibrosis – from bench to bedside. *J Hepatol* 2003; **38**: S38–S53.

45 Serpaggi J, Carnot F, Nalpas B, et al. Direct and indirect evidence for the reversibility of cirrhosis. *Hum Pathol* 2006; **37**: 1519–1526.

46 International Working Party. Terminology of nodular hepatocellular lesions. *Hepatology* 1995; **22**: 983–993.

47 International Consensus Group for Hepatocellular Neoplasia. Pathologic diagnosis of early hepatocellular carcinoma: a report of the international consensus group for hepatocellular neoplasia. *Hepatology* 2009; **49**: 658–664.

General reading

Crawford JM. Liver cirrhosis. In: MacSween RNM, Burt AD, Portmann BC, Ishak KG, Scheuer PJ, Anthony PP, eds. Pathology of the Liver, 4th edn. Edinburgh: Churchill Livingstone/Elsevier, 2002: 575–620.

Desmet VJ, Roskams T. Cirrhosis reversal: a duel between dogma and myth. *J Hepatol* 2004; **40**: 860–867.

International Consensus Group for Hepatocellular Neoplasia. Pathologic diagnosis of early hepatocellular carcinoma: a report of the International Consensus Group for Hepatocellular Neoplasia. *Hepatology* 2009; **49**: 658–664.

Neoplasms and Nodules

Introduction

This chapter is intended to provide a working overview of the tumours and tumour-like nodular lesions that the pathologist will encounter with some frequency in everyday practice. The majority of these can be classified according to the putative cells of origin (hepatocytes, bile-duct epithelium and endothelium) from which they arise (**Table 11.1**) and immunohistochemistry can often be used effectively to distinguish histogenesis. Neoplastic and nodular lesions of adults are covered first, followed by lesions in children and a section on cytopathological diagnosis. The reader is encouraged to consult the references and general reading list for additional details and coverage of some of the rarer tumours.

Neoplasms and nodules in adults

Benign lesions

Liver-cell adenoma

Liver-cell adenomas are solitary or occasionally multiple tumours composed of hepatocytes. Macroscopically they are well defined but often not encapsulated. The cells of the tumour closely resemble normal hepatocytes (**Fig. 11.1**). Nuclei are small and regular and mitoses are almost never seen. These features are evident in fine-needle aspiration biopsies.[1] The cells are arranged in normal or thickened trabeculae interspersed with prominent arteries and thin-walled blood vessels. In adenomas, reticulin is normal or reduced, but extensive loss is in most cases confined to areas of necrosis or haemorrhage. The latter are characteristically found in adenomas in oral contraceptive users, and are responsible for pain and for the serious complication of haemoperitoneum. They probably also explain the fibrous scars which are sometimes found in the lesions. Regular septa, portal tracts and bile ducts are, however, absent; this distinguishes liver-cell adenomas both from non-neoplastic liver and from macroregenerative nodules (large regenerative nodules) in cirrhosis as well as focal nodular hyperplasia. An exception to this rule may occur in patients with multiple adenomas (adenomatosis[2]) where bile ducts can become entrapped within the lesions.[3]

Adenomas may show small liver-cell rosettes (acini) with a central bile-filled or empty lumen, as in cholestatic liver. They may contain Dubin–Johnson-like pigment[4] or show

DOI: 10.1016/B978-0-7020-3410-7.00017-4

Table 11.1 Classification of liver tumours and nodular lesions

Putative cell of origin	Benign	Malignant
Hepatocyte	Liver-cell adenoma MRN FNH NRH PNT	Hepatocellular carcinoma Fibrolamellar carcinoma Hepatoblastoma
Bile-duct epithelium	Bile-duct adenoma Cystadenoma Adenofibroma	Cholangiocarcinoma Cystadenocarcinoma
Mixed liver-cell and bile-duct cell	Mesenchymal hamartoma	Combined hepatocellular cholangiocarcinoma
Endothelial cell	Haemangioma Infantile haemangioendothelioma*	Angiosarcoma Epithelioid haemangioendothelioma

MRN, macroregenerative nodule; FNH, focal nodular hyperplasia; NRH, nodular regenerative hyperplasia; PNT, partial nodular transformation.
*Some cases may behave more aggressively and are capable of metastasis.

Figure 11.1 Hepatocellular adenoma.
Liver cells appear normal or contain fat vacuoles. Blood vessels but no portal tracts are seen within the lesion. (Operative specimen, H&E.)

steatohepatitis with Mallory bodies.[5] Non-necrotising granulomas within adenomas are also described.[6] Genetic–histological correlations have allowed subclassification of adenomas into several types.[7] Approximately 30–50% of adenomas show *HNF-1α* mutations and these typically contain fat but show no cytological atypia.[8,9] Activating β-catenin gene mutations are seen in some 10–15% of adenomas with cytological atypia and acini[8] and these tumours are more likely to show transformation to hepatocellular carcinoma (HCC). A third type of adenoma ('inflammatory and/or telangiectatic adenoma') with chronic inflammatory cell infiltrates and/or sinusoidal dilatation has been linked to *IL6ST* gene mutations and increased interleukin-6 signalling[10] and represents some 35% of adenomas.

The distinction of adenoma from HCC is occasionally difficult. Loss of reticulin, nuclear atypia and mitotic activity and the presence of many acinar structures favour carcinoma. Immunohistochemical demonstration of nuclear and/or cytoplasmic β-catenin overexpression is often helpful evidence of transition to carcinoma, but is not invariably present.[11]

Most liver-cell adenomas arise in women of childbearing age, usually after prolonged use of oral contraceptives.[12] Use of anabolic/androgenic steroids is a risk factor for both adenoma and HCC,[13] particularly in Fanconi's anaemia.[14,15] **Adenomatosis**,[16,17] in which multiple tumours are seen throughout the liver, is much less common, is associated with *HNF-1α* mutations and shows female predominance.[2] A subgroup of these cases is familial and associated with diabetes.[2,17–19] Adenomatosis is also seen in patients taking anabolic/androgenic steroids[20] or in patients without risk factors.[21] Liver-cell adenomas may also arise in patients with diabetes[22] or type I glycogen storage disease,[23] and in children or young adults (see Neoplasms and nodules in children).

Macroregenerative nodules (large regenerative nodules)

The macroregenerative nodule (MRN) or large regenerative nodule is an unusually large regenerative nodule, which usually develops in cirrhotic liver. Because the MRN is one of several possible settings in which HCC may develop, it is covered in greater detail later in this chapter (see Precursors of hepatocellular carcinoma).

Focal nodular hyperplasia

Focal nodular hyperplasia (FNH) is a fairly common lesion, seen in either sex and at any age. FNH is a reactive, hyperplastic response of polyclonal[24] hepatocytes, fibrous stroma and bile ductules due to a putative pre-existing arterial malformation.[25–28] FNH, unlike liver-cell adenoma, does not appear to be caused by oral contraceptives. Although oral contraceptives may cause an increase in size and vascularity,[29] they do not appear to influence the number or size of these lesions.[30] Bleeding and rupture are rare, as is recurrence after resection.[31] Features of FNH and adenoma are only very occasionally seen in the same tumour, and the occurrence of the two lesions in the same liver may be coincidental.[32] There may be multiple FNHs in the same patient, and such individuals often have other lesions, including vascular anomalies (hepatic haemangioma, telangiectasis of the brain, berry aneurysm, dysplastic systemic arteries, portal-vein atresia), central nervous system neoplasms (meningioma, astrocytoma)[33,34] and hemihypertrophy.[35]

Macroscopically, the nodules are well demarcated from the normal hepatic parenchyma. They are usually pale, and are dissected by fibrous septa into nodules, giving them an appearance very like that of cirrhosis. There may be a prominent central fibrous scar **(Fig. 11.2)** with closely associated smooth muscle actin immunostain-positive activated stellate cells.[36] Histologically, the appearance is also very like that of inactive cirrhosis. The dense fibrous septa contain large thick-walled and sometimes narrowed arteries, as well as bile-duct-like structures probably derived from metaplastic liver-cell plates[37] or from progenitor cells.[27] Cytokeratin 7 immunostain is useful for demonstration of the bile ductular structures and helps distinguish FNH from adenoma.[38] The presence of bile-duct cells in fine-needle aspiration cytology of FNH is helpful in distinguishing this lesion from HCC.[39] In radiologically guided needle biopsies, the pathologist should be made aware that a mass lesion is being sampled, since the proliferated bile-duct-like structures and reactive stroma may otherwise suggest the diagnosis of mechanical bile-duct obstruction[40] **(Fig. 11.2)**.

**Figure 11.2.
Focal nodular
hyperplasia (FNH).
A:** Part of a central
scar with abnormal
arterioles has been
sampled. Radiating
fibrous septa show
small bile-duct-like
structures at their
edges (arrowheads).
The parenchyma is
nodular. (Operative
specimen, H&E.)
B: Needle core
biopsy from FNH has
sampled a portion of
the fibrous scar and
lesional parenchyma.
A portal tract-like
region (arrow) with
oedematous stroma
and bile ductular
structures shows
changes resembling
those of large
bile-duct
obstruction. *Inset
above*: Ductular
structures in
oedematous stroma.
(Needle biopsy,
H&E.) *Inset below*:
Cytokeratin 7
immunostaining
pattern of bile
ductular structures in
FNH. (Operative
specimen, specific
immunoperoxidase.)

**Figure 11.3
Nodular
regenerative
hyperplasia.**
This abnormal,
nodular growth
pattern is not
accompanied by
fibrosis and therefore
differs from cirrhosis.
The parenchymal
nodules (N) are often
adjacent to (nodule
at left) or surrounding
portal tracts. The
intervening liver
shows flattened and
compressed liver-cell
plates and/or
sinusoidal dilatation.
(Post-mortem liver,
H&E.)

Lesions that grossly resemble FNH are also occasionally seen in Budd–Chiari syndrome.[41] Microscopically, these masses show hyperplastic, regenerative nodules in combination with other features, including central scars and multiple arterial structures. Some vary histologically so as to suggest crossover lesions between large regenerative nodules, FNH and liver-cell adenoma.[42] They appear to result from hyperarterialisation of regions of decreased hepatic venous blood flow.[42,43] FNH is also seen after liver transplantation in allografts with vascular perfusion abnormalities.[43a]

Nodular regenerative hyperplasia

In nodular regenerative hyperplasia (NRH) multiple hyperplastic parenchymal nodules with thickened liver-cell plates are seen but fibrosis is absent or slight[44] (**Fig. 11.3**). This distinguishes the lesion from cirrhosis. In some cases perisinusoidal fibrosis is found in the compressed liver tissue between nodules. Portal tracts may be found at the centres of the nodules but this is not invariable. Diagnosis is often difficult in needle-biopsy specimens. The nodularity may be more clearly seen in reticulin preparations (**Fig. 11.4**). A wedge liver biopsy may be required to establish the diagnosis and to exclude an important differential: incomplete septal cirrhosis (**see Ch. 10**).

NRH is associated with a wide range of conditions, mainly rheumatic diseases, myeloproliferative disorders and chronic venous congestion.[45-47] Patients with NRH may have received therapeutic drugs, including corticosteroids, anabolic steroids, oral contraceptives, antineoplastics,[48] anticonvulsants and immunosuppressive agents.[45,49,50] NRH has also been associated with the toxic oil syndrome,[51] Behçet's disease,[52] early histological stages of primary biliary cirrhosis,[53] coeliac disease with anti-cardiolipin antibodies,[54] livers containing metastatic neuroendocrine tumours[55] and non-cirrhotic livers in which HCC has developed.[56] Some patients with NRH have portal hypertension. Serum alkaline phosphatase and γ-glutamyl transpeptidase levels may be elevated.[47,53]

Wanless and co-workers[57] have postulated that the basic lesion is portal venous thrombosis, leading to atrophy and compensatory hyperplasia. Arterial lesions, particularly arteriosclerosis of ageing, may also contribute to these changes.[47] Portal venous thrombosis

**Figure 11.4
Nodular
regenerative
hyperplasia.**
Reticulin stain of a
field similar to that
shown in **Fig. 11.3**
highlights the
regenerative nodules
and the absence of
fibrosis. (Post-
mortem liver,
reticulin.)

Table 11.2 Non-cirrhotic parenchymal nodules

Nodule type Number; *Involvement of liver*	Structure	Portal hypertension
Focal nodular hyperplasia		
Solitary or few; *Focal*	Mixed	No
Liver-cell adenoma		
Solitary or few; rarely many; *Focal*	Liver cells	No
Nodular regenerative hyperplasia		
Many; *Diffuse*	Liver cells	Sometimes
Partial nodular transformation		
Several; *Perihilar*	Liver cells, some fibrous tissue	Usually

has also been invoked in the pathogenesis of the rare **partial nodular transformation**, in which somewhat larger nodules are found, often localised to the perihilar region.[58,59] NRH, FNH and partial nodular transformation share the common feature of liver-cell hyperplastic growth in the form of nodules; they have accordingly been grouped under the umbrella heading of 'nodular transformation' by Wanless.[60] The main features of the various non-cirrhotic nodular conditions so far discussed are summarised in **Table 11.2**.

Bile-duct adenoma

Bile-duct adenomas are small, grey-white, usually subcapsular nodules measuring from 1 to 20 mm in diameter,[61] which may represent hamartomatous peribiliary glands rather

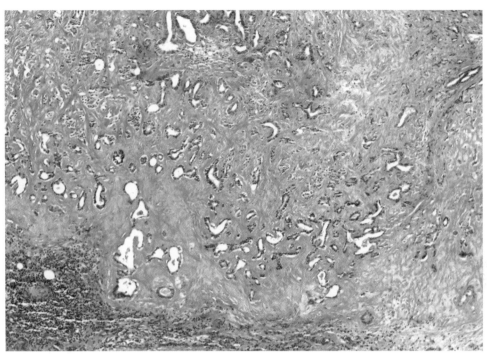

Figure 11.5
Bile-duct adenoma.
This subcapsular
tumour consists of
closely packed bile
ducts set in a dense
fibrous stroma. A
dense collection of
lymphocytes is seen
at the edge of the
lesion (bottom).
(Operative specimen,
H&E.)

than a neoplasm.[62] They are more often solitary than multiple. Histologically, they are composed of small, well-formed ducts embedded in a stroma of mature fibrous tissue which may contain chronic inflammatory cells, often densely aggregated at the periphery of the lesion[61,63,64] (**Fig. 11.5**). Their chief importance is that they may be mistaken for metastatic carcinoma, both macroscopically and microscopically. They differ from micro-hamartomas (von Meyenburg complexes) in that the ducts are smaller and more numerous, are usually not dilated and do not contain bile.[61,65] Periodic acid–Schiff (PAS)-positive, diastase-resistant globules of α_1-antitrypsin within the bile-duct epithelium of multiple adenomas were described in a patient with heterozygous α_1-antitrypsin deficiency.[66] The bile-duct adenoma should also be distinguished from the rare **biliary adenofibroma**, a much larger tumour composed of tubulocystic bile-duct structures with apocrine metaplasia and intraluminal bile embedded in fibrous stroma, resembling fibroadenoma of the breast.[67]

Biliary cystadenoma

Biliary cystadenoma is a multilocular tumour, the cystic spaces of which contain mucoid fluid and are lined by columnar, mucin-secreting epithelium which may form papillary projections. A variant with subepithelial **mesenchymal stroma** containing myofibroblasts occurs in women.[68,69] Malignant change is common.[70]

Haemangioma

The cavernous haemangioma is the most common benign tumour of the liver, found incidentally at autopsy or operation and occasionally seen in biopsy material.[71] A few reach a large and clinically significant size. As in other sites, the lesions are composed of endothelium-lined channels supported by a fibrous stroma (**Fig. 11.6**). Lesional tissue sometimes extends irregularly into adjacent liver.[72] Complications include thrombosis,

**Figure 11.6
Haemangioma.**
Blood-filled spaces
are separated by
fibrous septa. A thick
capsule is seen at
right. (Operative
specimen, H&E.)

sclerosis and calcification.[73] Spontaneous rupture is recorded but uncommon. A distinction should be made between cavernous haemangiomas and peliosis (**see Ch. 12**); the latter lacks the complete endothelial layer and fibrous trabeculae. **Lymphangioma** of the liver has been reported as part of multiorgan lymphangiomatosis or as a solitary hepatic lesion,[74] but is very rare. The endothelium-lined channels of this neoplasm are empty or contain lymph with occasional leucocytes. It should not be mistaken for mesenchymal hamartoma (see Neoplasms and nodules in children).

Mesenchymal and neural tumours

Connective-tissue elements, adipocytes and smooth muscle of the liver, nerve sheaths of intrahepatic nerves and other mesenchymal cells may give rise to rare tumours, including lipomas, myelolipomas, angiomyelolipomas,[75,76] schwannomas and neurofibromas,[77–79] solitary fibrous tumours[80] and chondromas.[81] **Angiomyolipomas** resemble their more common renal counterparts, and contain blood vessels, smooth muscle (myoid cells) and fat.[82] These components allow subcategorisation into mixed, lipomatous, myomatous and angiomatous types, in decreasing order of frequency.[83] Multiple tumours may be present.[84,85] Muscle cells may be partly of epithelioid type, with finely granular eosinophilic cytoplasm and pleomorphic nuclei[86–89] (**Fig. 11.7**). These may be mistaken for hepatocytes or malignant cells, particularly in cases where the component of fat is minimal. Megakaryocytes and other bone marrow elements are commonly present. Positive HMB-45 immunostaining of the myoid cells is a major diagnostic feature.[83,89] **Pseudolipomas**[90] probably represent separated nodules of peritoneal fat which become embedded in the liver capsule.

Inflammatory pseudotumour

Lesions of inflammatory pseudotumour may be solitary or multiple and usually occur in young, male patients with constitutional symptoms, fever and weight loss. They may sometimes involve structures near the porta hepatis with resultant biliary problems or portal hypertension. The microscopic hallmark of inflammatory pseudotumour is the

Figure 11.7
Angiomyolipoma.
The tumour shows myoid cells with ample granular cytoplasm resembling hepatocytes. Fat vacuoles, seen at right, were variably scattered through the tumour, as were small blood vessels. (Operative specimen, H&E.)

extensive polyclonal plasma-cell infiltrates which are intermixed with lymphocytes, eosinophils, foamy histiocytes and variable degrees of stromal proliferation, including spindle cells in bundles and whorls with associated fibrosis[91] (**Fig. 11.8**). Granulomas and partly obliterated blood vessels may be present. The lesion falls within a diagnostically controversial spectrum ranging from an inflammatory–reparative process (possibly infectious in aetiology) to a low-grade stromal malignancy termed inflammatory myofibroblastic tumour (IMT).[92,93] Some have been thought to be follicular dendritic cell tumours related to Epstein–Barr virus infection.[94] Immunostains are helpful to characterise individual cases. Among these, smooth muscle actin will highlight the extent of the myofibroblastic component and activin-like kinase 1 (ALK1) expression in the spindle cells favours a diagnosis of IMT.[92,93] Surgical resection is the treatment of choice, when possible.

Malignant lesions

Precursors of hepatocellular carcinoma

A number of hepatocellular changes and nodular lesions have been considered premalignant or precursors of hepatocellular carcinoma (HCC) and these are discussed below. Despite refinements in the terminology of these lesions (**Table 11.3**) provided by panels of hepatic pathologists,[95–97] the precise sequence of histological and molecular changes in the presumed multistep pathogenesis of HCC in humans has not been established. The importance of recognition of these worrisome lesions is based on the need for close patient surveillance and possible surgical resection (or liver transplantation) once they are identified pathologically. The presence of one or more of these lesions should be clearly stated in the pathologist's report.

Non-neoplastic liver tissue may show varying degrees of **liver-cell dysplasia (LCD)** of either large- or small-cell type (**see Figs 10.8, 10.9**). **Large-cell LCD (large-cell change)** is the type most often observed and features cell and nuclear enlargement, nuclear pleomorphism, multinucleation and multiple nucleoli and increased nuclear staining[98] (**see Figs 10.8 and 11.33**). Its distribution is random within lobules or cirrhotic nodules and

Figure 11.8 Inflammatory pseudotumour. Dense infiltrates of plasma cells, lymphocytes and histiocytes with interwoven bundles of collagen are seen. *Inset*: Plasma cells are unusually prominent. (Operative specimen, H&E.)

Table 11.3 Nomenclature of putative precursors of hepatocellular carcinoma

Current term	Synonym(s)
Large-cell liver-cell dysplasia	Large-cell change
Small-cell liver-cell dysplasia	Small-cell change
Macroregenerative nodule (MRN)	Adenomatous hyperplasia Large regenerative nodule Type I MRN

Dysplastic nodule
  Low grade
  High grade
	–
	Borderline lesion
	Type II MRN

Dysplastic foci (<1 mm diameter)	–

should be distinguished from the variations in nuclear morphology seen in perivenular hepatocytes with ageing, in the presence of cholestasis or in methotrexate therapy. This type of dysplasia was first associated with hepatitis B virus infection, cirrhosis and HCC[99,100] and subsequently with a four- to five-fold increased risk of HCC in several studies.[101,102] Affected cells are usually aneuploid[103] and may have attendant chromosomal abnormalities.[104] However, it has been considered merely an effect of cholestasis[105] or a derangement in normal liver-cell polyploidisation[106] and has not been proven to be a direct pathogenetic precursor lesion of HCC. Nevertheless, it is a strong independent risk factor for the development of HCC[107,108] and thereby identifies patients requiring more diligent surveillance.

Small-cell LCD (small-cell change) is characterised by enlarged, hyperchromatic nuclei within small hepatocytes (increased nuclear–cytoplasmic ratio) arranged in crowded

Figure 11.9
Macroregenerative nodule.
This low-magnification view demonstrates the increased size of the nodule at right compared with the cirrhotic nodules at left. (Operative specimen, H&E.) (Illustration kindly provided by Dr Kamal Ishak, Washington, DC, USA.)

clusters[109] (**see Figs 10.9 and 11.34**). These foci show high cellular proliferation rates[110] and an overall cytological resemblance to HCC, and may originate from progenitor cells.[107] These features have lent support to small-cell LCD as a true precursor lesion that is subject to the later cellular events leading to the development of HCC.[111]

Other cellular changes cited as indicators of pre-malignancy include intracytoplasmic Mallory bodies,[112] irregular areas of regeneration showing hepatocyte glycogenosis, oncocytic change (**see Ch. 9**) or bulging nodularity,[113] iron-negative foci in siderotic macroregenerative nodules[114] and 'iron-free foci' in livers of patients with hereditary haemochromatosis;[115] the last may show large-cell LCD.[115] Clusters of large-cell or small-cell dysplastic hepatocytes less than 1 mm in diameter have been termed **dysplastic foci** by an international working party.[96]

The **macroregenerative nodule (MRN)** is an unusually large regenerative nodule measuring 0.8 cm or more in diameter which develops in cirrhosis or other chronic liver disease[116] (**Fig. 11.9**). MRNs are particularly common in macronodular cirrhosis.[117] They may be paler or more bile-stained than the surrounding liver.[96] The cirrhotic liver may harbour several MRNs, which may coexist with HCC elsewhere in the liver or may contain foci of carcinoma. Cirrhotic explant livers should be carefully examined for these lesions[95,118] and for liver-cell dysplasia.[119]

The MRN histologically shows hyperplastic liver parenchyma arranged in plates two or three cells thick, which is typical of cirrhosis. The nodule contains portal tracts and fibrous septa with bile ducts, hepatic arteries and portal-vein branches, and shows no cellular atypia or disorder in the liver-cell plate arrangement. Steatosis, haemosiderin, bile plugs and Mallory bodies may be present.[116,120] The term 'adenomatous hyperplasia', a former synonym of MRN, as well as subdivisions into MRN types I and II[117] are not currently advocated for use.[96]

The **dysplastic nodule (borderline nodule)** shows atypical architectural and/or cytological features that are not acceptable for a benign macroregenerative nodule, but which fall diagnostically short of frank HCC.[96,121] Dysplastic nodules may show varying degrees

**Figure 11.10
Dysplastic nodule.**
The dysplastic nodule at right shows hepatocytes arranged in pseudoacini, with a less cohesive growth pattern centrally. A cirrhotic nodule is present at lower left. The patient had an inactive cirrhosis due to tyrosinaemia. (Explant liver, H&E.)

of large and small-cell LCD, increased cellularity and foci where the liver cords are less cohesive, focal loss of reticulin fibres or pseudoacini[95,96,118,121] (**Fig. 11.10**).

The major diagnostic concern is to distinguish MRNs and dysplastic nodules from HCC. Certain features seen in these nodules are associated with high risk of progression to carcinoma, including an increased ratio of nuclear density, clear-cell change, small-cell dysplasia and fatty change.[122] Increased mitotic activity, loss of reticulin fibres, formation of broad trabeculae and an infiltrative margin are helpful evidence of carcinoma.[95,118,123,124] Studies that have demonstrated clonality and loss of heterozygosity[125] and increased cell proliferative indices[126] combined with newer techniques such as spectral karyotype (SKY)[127] and gene microarray[128] analysis are promising avenues for understanding the key biological and morphological steps in the pathogenesis of HCC.

Hepatocellular carcinoma

Hepatocellular carcinoma (HCC) ranks fifth among malignant tumours worldwide.[100] Epidemiological and other studies of HCC have defined geographical variations in the incidence and prevalence of this tumour, as well as a multifactorial aetiology.[129] Chronic necrosis and inflammation of the liver are important driving forces in the multistep process of hepatocarcinogenesis[130,131] in the context of underlying risk factors such as hepatitis B and C viral infections,[100] iron overload,[132] aflatoxin exposure[133] and the presence of fatty liver disease.[134–136] At the molecular level, identification of genetic changes that control cell cycling and apoptosis,[137] as well as oncogene expression,[138] mutation of tumour suppressor genes such as *p53*,[139] expression of vascular and cellular growth factors[140–145] and proliferation of hepatic stem cells or their progeny[146,147] constitute a large and growing literature on this subject.

The majority of HCCs develop in cirrhotic liver.[148] The cause of the cirrhosis is usually known, even in many cases labelled as 'cryptogenic' where risk factors for non-alcoholic fatty liver disease (**see Ch. 7**) become apparent.[135] The non-cirrhotic setting accounts

**Figure 11.11
Hepatocellular
carcinoma.**
Note the trabecular–
sinusoidal structure
and resemblance of
the tumour cells to
normal hepatocytes.
(Needle biopsy, H&E.)

for a substantial number of cases from North America[149] and elsewhere[150] and can be seen in hepatitis B virus carriers[151,152] or in those with suspected occult hepatitis B[150] and in individuals infected with hepatitis C virus.[153] HCC may even develop within ectopic liver.[154] The cirrhosis associated with carcinoma is often macronodular in pattern, except for the micronodular cirrhosis seen in genetic haemochromatosis and chronic hepatitis C. The cirrhosis is usually inactive, although inflammation and necrosis may be seen near the tumour itself. Tumours may be multifocal.[155] Intrahepatic tumour spread is both portal (via portal-vein branches) and lobular.[156] Rarely, HCC may spontaneously regress.[100,157,158] Following transplantation, cirrhotic explant livers require careful examination for small carcinomas and precursor lesions which are clinically undetected.[159] Pathology reports on explants or partial resections with HCC should specify the number of lesions and their sizes, as well as the histological grade and evidence of vascular invasion[160] since these factors affect TNM staging and other prognostic classifications.[161]

The outstanding histological features of HCC are the resemblance of the tumour cells to normal hepatocytes, and of their arrangement to the trabeculae of normal liver (**Fig. 11.11**). However, the trabeculae are for the most part thicker and reticulin is often scanty or even absent (**Fig. 11.12**). This paucireticulin pattern is helpful in fine-needle aspiration biopsies (see Cytopathological diagnosis). In exceptional cases where there may be an increase in reticulin, other histological features and/or the clinical behaviour of the tumour must be used as diagnostic criteria of malignancy. Rarely, the trabecular pattern and even bile production is mimicked by primary tumours ('hepatoid carcinomas') of the stomach, ovary and other sites[162] (see section on Metastatic tumour). Between the tumour trabeculae in HCC there is a network of vascular channels lined by endothelium which is positive with immunostains for CD34,[140,141] factor VIII-related antigen and *Ulex europaeus* lectin.[163] The endothelial lining of these channels is a particularly helpful diagnostic feature in fine-needle aspirates (**see Fig. 11.36**). The absence of portal tracts and a cohesive connective tissue framework in the tumour results in a characteristic fragmentation of needle biopsy specimens with separation of tumour trabeculae that is readily observed at low

Figure 11.12 Hepatocellular carcinoma.

Reticulin is scanty in this example. (Needle biopsy, reticulin.)

magnification. Although connective tissue stroma is uncommon except in **fibrolamellar carcinoma** (described below), focal areas of fibrosis may follow tumour necrosis. A form of HCC designated as **sclerosing carcinoma**[164] is often associated with hypercalcaemia; some of these tumours appear to be of bile duct rather than hepatocellular origin. The **adenoid** (acinar) variant of HCC (**Fig. 11.13**) should not be confused with adenocarcinoma of the biliary tree. Bile-duct carcinomas are usually scirrhous, mucin-secreting tumours, whereas the characteristic secretion of HCCs is bile, seen in a minority of tumours in spaces homologous with normal bile canaliculi. Mixed or combined tumours designated **hepatocellular–cholangiocarcinoma** are also well described, with special stains and immunohistochemical features representative of both hepatocellular and bile-duct epithelial derivation. Progenitor/stem cell constituents are sometimes present[165] as shown by cytokeratin 7 or 19 positivity (discussed below). Occasionally HCC is infiltrated by T lymphocytes and shows an improved prognosis.[166]

At a cellular level variants include giant-cell forms with multinucleated tumour cells (a bad prognostic sign[167]) (**Fig. 11.14**), spindle-cell or sarcomatoid tumours[168,169] and clear-cell carcinomas. The last must be distinguished from metastatic renal adenocarcinoma.[170,171] Fine-needle aspiration yields diagnostic material in a high proportion of patients.[172–175] Histological grading of HCC from 1 to 4 is based on nuclear features, with grade 1 HCC resembling normal hepatocytes and grade 2 showing prominent nucleoli, hyperchromatism and nuclear membrane irregularities.[176] Grades 3 and 4 show progressively greater nuclear pleomorphism, the latter featuring anaplastic and giant tumour cells (**Fig. 11.14**).

When there is doubt about the hepatocellular origin of a carcinoma, further evidence can sometimes be gained from the characteristics of the tumour cells. In hepatocellular carcinoma these often contain fat and glycogen, and may also contain α_1-antitrypsin globules, even in patients without genetic α_1-antitrypsin deficiency. Mallory bodies are commonly found in the cytoplasm of the tumour cells.[177] Evidence of hepatocellular

Figure 11.13 Hepatocellular carcinoma. Adenoid pattern. Other areas of this tumour showed a more typical trabecular structure. (Post-mortem liver, H&E.)

origin is also provided when immunohistochemical stains of paraffin sections are positive for albumin, fibrinogen, liver-cell cytokeratins (8 and 18), α_1-antitrypsin or α_1-antichymotrypsin.[178–182]

There are several possible immunohistochemical strategies for confirming the diagnosis of HCC (**Table 11.4**). One established approach is to use the quartet of cytokeratin 7 (CK7), cytokeratin 20 (CK20), Hep Par 1 ('hepatocyte') and polyclonal carcinoembryonic antigen (pCEA). HCC typically is negative for both CK7 and CK20,[183] while Hep Par 1 stains normal and malignant hepatocytes (and, rarely, several extrahepatic tumours[184]). Hep Par 1 staining may be only patchy in needle biopsies of HCC or negative with more poorly differentiated tumours, liabilities which can be surmounted using more recently recommended immunostains (described below). Polyclonal carcinoembryonic antigen (CEA) provides positive staining of the carbohydrate moiety of biliary glycoprotein on the apical surfaces or canalicular structures of the HCC cells (**see Fig. 11.15**) and on bile canaliculi in non-neoplastic liver tissue. CD10 shows similar results to pCEA but is far less sensitive.[185] α-Fetoprotein is an unreliable immunostain for HCC,[186] in contrast to hepatoblastoma where most cases stain positively. Interestingly, the immunostain for thyroid transcription factor-1 (TTF-1), often used in the diagnosis of lung carcinomas, showed positive cytoplasmic (not nuclear) staining in the majority of HCCs in one study,[187] which may be helpful in specific diagnostic settings.

The trio of glypican-3 (GPC-3), glutamine synthetase (GS) and heat shock protein 70 (HSP70) immunostains is proving to be an exceptionally robust combination for the diagnosis of HCC, particularly when any two of the three are positive.[188] GPC-3, a cell-surface heparan sulphate proteoglycan, usually shows cytoplasmic positivity in the tumour cells, but may also be membranous or canalicular. It has particular value in staining poorly differentiated HCCs that are negative with Hep Par 1 and is also applicable to fine-needle aspiration specimens.[189] However, cirrhotic nodules and hepatocytes in chronic hepatitis

Figure 11.14 Hepatocellular carcinoma: cytological grading.
Grades 1–4 are illustrated in the respective panels. Grade 1 (well differentiated) tumours have small, round nuclei similar to those of normal and cirrhotic liver. Grades 2 and upwards show progressive alterations in nuclear contour, chromatin coarseness and chromaticity. Grade 4 shows marked anaplasia with giant, multinucleated tumour cells and atypical mitotic figures. (Needle biopsies, H&E.)

C with high-grade necroinflammatory activity may also show strong GPC-3 positivity.[190,191] Positive GPC-3 staining may also be seen in certain germ cell tumours,[192] ovarian clear-cell carcinoma[193] and in squamous cell carcinoma of the lung.[194] GS staining in non-neoplastic liver is restricted to the cytoplasm of perivenular hepatocytes, but HCC shows diffuse strong lesional staining.[97,188] HSP70 shows focal nucleocytoplasmic positivity in HCC.[97] This panel of three immunostains also helps distinguish dysplastic lesions from HCC.[188]

Fibrolamellar carcinoma

This tumour usually develops in non-cirrhotic liver in older children and adults and carries a better prognosis (because of its resectability[195] and absence of cirrhosis[195a]) than typical HCC.[196–199] The lesions are solitary or multiple and occasionally resemble focal nodular hyperplasia macroscopically in having a central fibrous scar.[200] The unique histological

Table 11.4 Immunohistochemical stains in the evaluation of hepatic tumours

Tumour	Recommended immunostain(s)
Heptatocellular carcinoma	Hep Par 1 (hepatocyte) Polyclonal CEA* Cytokeratin 7/20 pair (−/− staining)** GPC-3/GS/HSP70 trio***
Hepatoblastoma	α-Fetoprotein (AFP) Hep Par 1 (hepatocyte) Polyclonal CEA
Cholangiocarcinoma	Cytokertain 7/19 pair (+/+ staining) Cytokeratin 7/20 pair (+/+ staining)**
Angiomyolipoma	HMB-45
Solitary fibrous tumour	CD34 Vimentin
Epithelioid	CD34
Haemangioendothelioma	CD31 Factor VIII
Metastatic carcinoma Neuroendocrine	 Chromogranin Synaptophysin Neuron-specific enolase
Pancreas	Cytokeratin 7/20 pair (+/+ staining)**
Colorectal	Cytokeratin 7/20 pair (−/+ staining)**
Breast	Cytokeratin 7/20 pair (+/− staining)**
Lung (non-small cell)	Cytokeratin 7/20 pair (+/− staining)**

*Staining is canalicular or apical.
**See Ref. 183.
***GPC-3: glypican-3; GS: glutamine synthetase; HSP70: heat shock protein 70. At least 2 of the 3 should be positive (see Ref. 188).

features distinguish this tumour from routine hepatocellular carcinoma. Fibrous lamellae arranged in parallel separate groups of large, densely eosinophilic tumour cells[198,201] which produce transforming growth factor-β[202] (**Fig. 11.16**). The eosinophilia is due to the presence of abundant mitochondria.[197,203] Tumour cells commonly contain eosinophilic, diastase–PAS-negative globules which stain immunohistochemically for C-reactive protein, fibrinogen and α$_1$-antitrypsin, as well as cytoplasmic 'pale bodies' which are reactive for fibrinogen.[198] Additional features include bile production (as in other forms of hepatocellular carcinoma), copper and copper-associated protein within tumour cells,[204,205] and stainable CEA in bile canaliculi.[206] Some fibrolamellar carcinomas have neuroendocrine features,[207,208] mucicarmine-positive pseudoglands[208a] or show features of both fibrolamellar and typical hepatocellular carcinoma.[209] Despite isolated reports such as the association of Fanconi's anaemia with fibrolamellar carcinoma,[210] the pathogenesis of this tumour is uncertain and risk factors are not apparent.

Bile-duct carcinoma (cholangiocarcinoma)

Carcinoma of the bile ducts can arise anywhere between the papilla of Vater and the smaller branches of the biliary tree within the liver. It is not usually associated with cirrhosis. There are two major anatomic types:[211] one arising either from extrahepatic bile ducts or at the birfurcation of right and left hepatic ducts (the latter perihilar

Figure 11.15 Immunohistochemical demonstration of bile canalicular structures in a hepatocellular carcinoma. The branching spaces are here outlined by the use of polyclonal anti-CEA.

Figure 11.16 Hepatocellular carcinoma: fibrolamellar type. Groups of large, eosinophilic tumour cells are surrounded by fibrous septa in parallel arrays. (Needle biopsy, H&E.) *Inset*: Tumour cells contain 'pale bodies' (top centre). Several hyaline bodies are also evident in tumour cells at top, left of centre. (Explant liver, H&E.)

Figure 11.17 Bile-duct carcinoma. There are islands of adenocarcinoma in the connective tissue. The appearances are different from those of the hepatocellular carcinoma of adenoid pattern shown in **Fig. 11.13**. (Operative specimen, H&E.)

cholangiocarcinoma sometimes referred to as a **Klatskin tumour**[212]), and a second type presenting as an intrahepatic mass.[213] Carcinoma of the hepatic ducts is an important cause of biliary obstruction, which may be missed at laparotomy unless the intrahepatic bile ducts are explored or visualised. The commonest known predisposing factors to bile-duct cancer are infestation with oriental flukes, primary sclerosing cholangitis[214] and congenital cystic lesions of the biliary tree.[215] Of these, Caroli's disease and choledochal cysts are important precursors, but carcinoma may also arise in von Meyenburg complexes (bile-duct microhamartomas)[216] and in congenital hepatic fibrosis.[217] Development of carcinoma in bile-duct adenoma is also reported.[218] In Japan, hepatitis C virus infection has been suggested as a risk factor[219] and intrahepatic cholangiocarcinoma is a known consequence of hepatolithiasis.[220] Investigations at the molecular level indicate pathogenetic roles for K-*ras* and *p53* mutations, increased expression of receptor tyrosine kinase c-erB-2 and c-met and expression of human telomerase reverse transcriptase (hTERT).[211]

Microscopically, bile-duct carcinomas are mucin-secreting adenocarcinomas with a reactive, desmoplastic fibrous stroma (**Fig. 11.17**). A fairly uniform gland size (medium to small) is often maintained within these tumours, in comparison with the wide size variations seen in glands of metastatic pancreatic carcinoma. The *cholangiolocellular carcinoma* subtype shows interanastomosing duct-like structures composed of small cuboidal cells with scant cytoplasm that appear to evolve from progenitor cells in the region of the canal of Hering.[221] The tumour cells are cuboidal or columnar and may assume a papillary pattern. Adenosquamous, squamous, mucinous,[222] clear-cell[223] and anaplastic histological types are less common.[224] Intraneural and perineural invasion is common. The presence of free stromal mucin, small groups and isolated tumour cells in fibrous stroma and the concurrence of apparently normal epithelium and abnormal tumour cells within a duct-like structure all help to distinguish cholangiocarcinoma from metastatic tumour.[225] Cholangiocarcinoma must be distinguished from the acinar type of hepatocellular carcinoma, a distinction usually made with confidence on the basis of mucin or bile secretion, respectively. In difficult cases positive staining for epithelial membrane antigen,[226] tissue polypeptide antigen,[227] biliary cytokeratins[179] (7 and 19), Lewis(x) and Lewis(y) blood group-related antigens[228] and α-amylase[229] helps to exclude hepatocellular carcinoma. In the uncommon tumour which shows combined hepatocellular–cholangiocarcinoma, cytokeratins 7 and 19 and epithelial membrane antigen immunostaining is positive in the cholangiocellular component.[230,231] Other rare mixed tumours show sarcomatoid[232] or fibrolamellar regions.[233] The differential diagnosis of bile-duct cancer includes epithelioid haemangioendothelioma. Bile-duct tumours are very occasionally of neuroendocrine type, with characteristic neurosecretory granules in their cytoplasm.

Cystadenocarcinomas are rare malignant tumours which sometimes develop from benign cystadenomas.[68,70] Although these have been considered distinct from the more aggressive carcinomas arising from pre-existing congenital cystic lesions,[234] occasional tumours with features of cystadenocarcinoma develop in fibropolycystic disease.[235]

Angiosarcoma

This uncommon, highly malignant tumour forms multiple or, less often, solitary haemorrhagic masses. Predisposing factors include treatment with arsenic,[236] injection of the radioactive contrast medium Thorotrast[237–239] and industrial exposure to vinyl chloride.[240] Other postulated factors include copper-containing vineyard sprays,[241] steroid hormones,[242-244] phenelzine[245] and urethane.[246] Positive staining of tumour cells for factor VIII-related antigen and other endothelial markers is evidence of their endothelial origin.[247,248] Their growth is characteristically along sinusoids and around surviving hyperplastic hepatocytes (**Fig. 11.18**). The presence of the latter may lead to confusion with hepatocellular carcinoma, with which angiosarcoma, however, occasionally coexists. Infiltration of sinusoids beyond the main tumour mass makes the outlines of the tumour indistinct. Both cavernous and solid areas may be present. Other features include islands of haemopoietic cells, and areas of thrombosis and infarction.

Figure 11.18
Angiosarcoma.
Elongated tumour cells surround islands of hepatocytes (centre) in this highly vascular tumour. *Inset*: Pleomorphic endothelial cells line the vascular spaces. (Operative specimen, H&E.)

The non-neoplastic liver tissue is usually not cirrhotic, but may show fibrosis and other changes attributable to the predisposing factors listed above, including deposits of refractile Thorotrast granules in macrophages. Features seen irrespective of the cause include focal dilatation of sinusoids, hyperplasia of hepatocytes, sinusoid-lining cells and perisinusoidal cells, and increased perisinusoidal reticulin.[249] These changes may precede the development of the tumour.[250]

Epithelioid haemangioendothelioma

This endothelial tumour of soft tissues or the lung (intravascular bronchioloalveolar tumour) may uncommonly present as a primary liver tumour. In the liver it is seen in patients from the second to eighth decades of life, with women more commonly affected.[251-253] Its prognosis varies very widely, some patients surviving for decades while others die within months of diagnosis.[254] Histologically, it may be confused with adenocarcinoma or with veno-occlusive disease. Its causes are unknown, but a relationship to oral contraceptive use has been postulated.[255]

The lesion consists of proliferated endothelial cells with pleomorphic nuclei, arranged in clusters or singly, some of them with rounded lumens (**Fig. 11.19**). The lumens may be mistaken for lipid or for mucin droplets in a signet-ring cell adenocarcinoma. Two types of tumour cells have been described,[251,253] dendritic and epithelioid, the latter giving rise to the adenocarcinoma-like appearance. The tumour cells should be positive on immunostaining for one or more endothelial markers (CD34, CD31, factor VIII[253]). CD34 immunostaining is more sensitive than factor VIII.[256] Further evidence of vascular differentiation is seen ultrastructurally where Weibel–Palade bodies in tumour cells and a tumour tissue component of pericytes have been noted.[257] High cellularity is a predictor of unfavourable prognosis, whereas nuclear pleomorphism and mitotic count are not.[253]

Vascular occlusion by dense fibrous tissue containing tumour cells, a characteristic feature, is seen in both portal and hepatic vein branches. This is best seen with connective tissue stains. The problem of confusion with veno-occlusive disease or even steatohepatitis

Figure 11.19 Epithelioid haemangio-endothelioma. Individual tumour cells and small groups are set in a dense fibrous stroma. Some of the tumour cells have formed vascular lumens (arrow). (Operative specimen, H&E.)

Figure 11.20 Epithelioid haemangioendothelioma.
In this example the tumour has a zonal distribution, mimicking the fibrosis of venous outflow obstruction. The tumour stroma is predominantly seen in the perivenular and mid-zonal regions, while surviving periportal hepatocytes and ductular reaction are evident at left and at lower right. (Operative specimen, H&E.)

is compounded by the fact that the tumour sometimes has a zonal distribution, affecting perivenular regions of each lobule in a more or less regular fashion (**Fig. 11.20**).

Extrahepatic malignancy and the liver

Patients with extrahepatic tumour may have biochemical evidence of hepatic dysfunction in the absence of liver metastases, particularly when the tumour is a renal adenocarcinoma. Liver biopsies in such patients have shown Kupffer-cell proliferation, hepatocellular swelling, focal necrosis, fatty change and mild inflammation.[258,259] Granulomas are occasionally found and there may be cholestasis, especially in Hodgkin's disease (see below).

Metastatic tumour

Blind percutaneous needle biopsy may reveal metastatic tumour, but the yield of correct diagnoses is increased if the needle is guided by means of an imaging method. Multiple punctures may be needed to sample the tumour. Guided fine-needle aspiration is a helpful diagnostic procedure,[260,261] and cytological examination of aspiration fluid and touch preparations of biopsy specimens increase the yield of positive results.[262] Step sections of biopsy specimens should be examined if tumour is suspected clinically but initial sections are negative. The primary site of a tumour can sometimes be determined histologically. Some metastases, notably from renal adenocarcinoma, can mimic hepatocellular carcinoma, and metastatic tumour may invade liver-cell plates, giving a false impression of

Figure 11.21
Metastatic tumour.
Cells of a carcinoid tumour (arrows) have invaded liver-cell plates (L), giving a false impression of origin from the latter. (Needle biopsy, H&E.)

primary carcinoma arising within them (**Fig. 11.21**). Primary extrahepatic carcinomas of the stomach, sex cord-stromal tumours of the ovary and other sites[162] may closely resemble hepatocellular carcinoma in both their primary sites and in metastatic foci. These 'hepatoid carcinomas' may produce bile or be positive with pCEA or α-fetoprotein immunostains.

Biopsy specimens from the vicinity of a metastasis typically show portal oedema, ductular reaction and infiltration by neutrophils, as well as focal sinusoidal dilatation[263] (**see Fig. 1.5**). The ductular structures sometimes have abnormal epithelium with atypical, hyperchromatic nuclei. The portal changes are reminiscent of those seen in biliary obstruction.

Lymphomas and leukaemias

Hodgkin's disease

Liver biopsy plays an important part in staging; wedge biopsies are more likely than multiple needle biopsies to reveal deposits, and either may be positive in spite of normal macroscopic appearances of the liver at laparotomy.[264] Negative biopsy does not rule out liver involvement. Hepatic involvement by Hodgkin's disease is usually associated with splenic involvement.[265] Step sections of initially negative small biopsies should be examined because the infiltrates of Hodgkin's disease are unevenly distributed and may be sparse. Correct diagnosis of an infiltrate may be difficult because Reed–Sternberg cells are often very scanty, so that the correct diagnosis must be suspected on the basis of other features. These include an abnormal population of cells with deeply stained angular nuclei or vesicular nuclei with prominent nucleoli (**Fig. 11.22**), irregular infiltration beyond portal tracts with destruction of hepatocytes and abundant reticulin fibres. There is a variable component of reactive lymphoid cells, eosinophils and histiocytes. The differential diagnosis of Hodgkin's disease in the liver includes reactive infiltrates and other lymphomas, especially of the T-cell type.

**Figure 11.22
Hodgkin's disease.**
The portal infiltrate is composed of a variety of cells, including large tumour cells with angular, hyperchromatic nuclei. (Needle biopsy, H&E.)

A variety of non-specific changes may be seen in parts of the liver adjacent to the malignant deposits. Even in the absence of malignant deposits there may be lobular lymphoid aggregates with some degree of cellular atypia[266] or epithelioid-cell granulomas.[267] Sinusoidal dilatation with or without Hodgkin's infiltrates in the liver has been reported, most often in patients with general symptoms.[268] The lesion is most severe in acinar zones 2 and 3. **Cholestasis** in Hodgkin's disease is uncommon, seen in the absence of hepatic infiltration in some patients[269] but more often as a feature of advanced disease. In some cases cholestasis is explained by destruction of interlobular bile ducts (ductopenia) related directly to the malignant infiltrates or resembling that seen in ductopenic rejection after liver transplantation.[270,271]

Non-Hodgkin's lymphoma and other haemopoietic malignancies

Non-Hodgkin's lymphomas primarily involve portal tracts, but may spread to periportal parenchyma and sinusoids.[272] Predominantly sinusoidal infiltration is also recognised.[273] Tumour deposits and fibrosis may cause portal hypertension[274] and, rarely, massive infiltration presents clinically as liver failure.[275] Vasculitis is another rare presentation. Malignant infiltrates can usually be distinguished from inflammatory ones by their dense and homogeneous appearance, and by the total or near-total involvement of portal tracts. Substantial apoptosis and necrotic debris may also be seen in lymphoma (**Fig. 11.23**) but are not characteristic of benign infiltrates. Immunohistochemical stains are important in establishing the type of lymphoma.[276] The disease is usually systemic, with involvement of lymphoid tissues as well as liver. **Primary hepatic lymphoma** is quite rare, representing less than 1% of extranodal lymphomas.[277-279] Both B-cell lymphomas, including **MALT (mucosa-associated lymphoid tissue) lymphoma**,[280,281] and T-cell lymphomas are seen, with B-cell tumours predominating.[278,282] Many B-cell lymphomas and proliferative diseases (mixed cryoglobulinaemia, monoclonal gammopathy) and, rarely, T-cell

**Figure 11.23
Non-Hodgkin's lymphoma.**
Tumour cells are seen irregularly infiltrating the adjacent periportal liver parenchyma. Extensive tumour cell necrosis is apparent. (Wedge biopsy, H&E.)

lymphoma[283] are associated with underlying chronic hepatitis C virus infection.[284] Chronic hepatitis C with concomitant B-cell lymphoma and hepatocellular carcinoma may also occur.[285] **Peripheral γ-δ**[286] and rare **α-β**[287] **T-cell lymphomas** with hepatic sinusoidal infiltration and splenic involvement have also been described. Primary hepatic lymphomas present as solitary or multiple masses, as diffuse hepatic involvement with hepatomegaly, or as liver failure with elevated serum lactate dehydrogenase activity.[278]

The liver may be diffusely or focally infiltrated in **multiple myeloma**.[288] Solitary primary hepatic plasmacytoma has also been reported.[289] In **macroglobulinaemia**,[290] mononuclear cells, some with pyroninophilic cytoplasm, may be found in portal tracts and sinusoids. Both diseases are sometimes complicated by amyloid deposition. **Langerhans' cell histiocytosis** involving only the liver may rarely occur.[291,292] The infiltrating Langerhans' cells, positive on immunostains for S-100 and CD1a, may invade and destroy interlobular bile ducts, leading to ductopenia, chronic cholestasis and features resembling primary sclerosing cholangitis.[293] In **systemic mast cell disease** with liver involvement, infiltration of portal tracts by mast cells is associated with fibrosis.[294] Parenchymal infiltrates are also seen. The infiltrating cells may be rounded, histiocyte-like or spindle shaped. Their nature may not be suspected on routine stains of paraffin sections; plastic sections or special mast cell stains make the diagnosis clear.

The infiltrates of various **leukaemias** are often seen in the liver and are frequently accompanied by steatosis and/or fibrosis.[295] Schwartz and co-workers[296] reported hepatic involvement in nearly all cases of **chronic lymphocytic leukaemia** examined, and noted marked widening of portal tracts with portal–portal linking and a variable degree of fibrosis. In **hairy cell leukaemia** the hepatic sinusoids are infiltrated by the leukaemic cells, often identifiable by the halo-like, clear cytoplasm around rounded or indented nuclei.[297] However, these are not always present.[298] Another histological characteristic is the formation of angiomatous lesions, in which vascular channels in portal tracts or acini are lined by leukaemic cells rather than by endothelium. Endothelial disruption with communication of sinusoids with the perisinusoidal space of Disse is seen by electron microscopy.[299]

Staining for tartrate-resistant acid phosphatase in paraffin sections has sometimes been helpful in diagnosis.[300]

Neoplasms and nodules in children

Benign lesions

Rarely, **liver-cell adenoma** may develop spontaneously in children with no underlying disease or exposure to hormones.[301] In this age group it has also been associated with Fanconi's anaemia,[15] type I glycogen storage disease, Hurler's disease, severe combined immunodeficiency,[302] the antiepileptic agent oxcarbazepine[303] and mutations in hepatocyte nuclear factor-1α (see Liver-cell adenoma in adults). The vast majority pursue a benign course, but transformation to hepatocellular carcinoma after many years of observation has been reported.[304] The identification of **focal nodular hyperplasia** in infancy as well as adulthood has been taken as additional evidence that it is a tumour-like malformation rather than a true neoplasm. **Nodular regenerative hyperplasia** is unusual in childhood. It occurs as early as 7 months of age and shows the same histological features as in adults.[305] Hepatosplenomegaly and portal hypertension may be present and in some patients there is a history of prior chemotherapy or anticonvulsant medication.

Mesenchymal hamartoma

This is an uncommon lesion of infancy and childhood, rarely seen in older subjects. Loose, oedematous connective tissue rich in blood vessels contains lymphangioma-like cystic spaces, bile ducts and hepatocytes[306,307] (**Fig. 11.24**). Haemopoietic cells are often present. The edge of the lesion is irregular, gradually merging with adjacent normal liver. In adults the bile-duct elements may be difficult to find and the collagenous stroma is densely

Figure 11.24 Mesenchymal hamartoma.
Loose connective tissue (left and right) containing bile ducts and blood vessels is separated by intervening hepatocellular parenchyma. (Operative specimen, H&E.)

Figure 11.25 Infantile haemangio-endothelioma. The tumour is composed of vascular channels lined by plump endothelium. Entrapped bile ducts are often present (arrow). (Operative specimen, H&E.)

hyalinised.[308] An undifferentiated embryonal sarcoma arising in mesenchymal hamartoma has been reported.[309]

Infantile haemangioendothelioma

This solitary or multicentric tumour is composed of capillary-like vascular channels lined by plump endothelium (**Fig. 11.25**), which with time undergo progressive maturation, scarring and eventual involution.[76,310,311] Central portions of the tumour may show increased fibrous stroma, and thrombosis and dystrophic calcification are sometimes present. The margin of the tumour often merges into adjacent liver parenchyma. Dehner and Ishak[310] described type I tumours with cytologically bland endothelium and type II tumours capable of aggressive behaviour and metastasis, with atypical, hyperchromatic endothelium and intravascular budding. The latter are now considered angiosarcomas.[312] Most cases present in the first 6 months of life with hepatomegaly, abdominal mass or diffuse abdominal enlargement.[76,310,313] There may be high-output cardiac failure due to shunting through the tumour, liver failure or tumour rupture. The possibility that some of these tumours will pursue a malignant course should be kept in mind in evaluating the histopathology of individual cases.

Malignant lesions

Hepatoblastoma

Hepatoblastoma is the most common liver tumour in childhood,[314] usually presenting at less than 2 years of age. The prognosis depends on surgical resectability and histological type. These tumours are usually solitary and histologically classified as **epithelial, mixed epithelial–mesenchymal** and **anaplastic (undifferentiated)** types.[315–318]

The epithelial type consists of fetal or embryonal liver cells, or both. Fetal cells somewhat resemble adult hepatocytes in appearance but are smaller (**Fig. 11.26**). The fat and

**Figure 11.26
Hepatoblastoma,
fetal epithelial
type.**
The tumour grows
in cords of small
hepatocytes with
a 'light-and-dark'
herringbone pattern
due to the admixed
clear (glycogenated)
and eosinophilic
liver cells. Foci of
extramedullary
haemopoiesis,
including several
megakaryocytes
and clusters of
erythrocyte
precursors, are
seen at upper left.
(Operative specimen,
H & E.)

glycogen content in some fetal cells gives them a pale appearance, thereby rendering a 'light-and-dark' pattern to fetal areas at low magnification. These areas are also characterised by foci of extramedullary haemopoiesis and an absence of mitoses. By histological pattern, the purely fetal type has the best prognosis.[319] Embryonal cells have less cytoplasm, higher nucleus–cytoplasm ratios, higher cell proliferative indices,[320] poorly defined cellular margins and mitotic activity (**Fig. 11.27**). They may form rosettes, acini or tubules. Squamous differentiation may be present in epithelial hepatoblastomas. The anaplastic type shows sheets of cells resembling neuroblastoma cells with little cytoplasm, hyperchromatic nuclei and no mitoses. Gonzalez-Crussi et al.[321] described a **'macrotrabecular'** pattern reminiscent of hepatocellular carcinoma but containing fetal or embryonal cells. Anaplastic and macrotrabecular variants have the worst prognosis.[315] Mixed epithelial–mesenchymal hepatoblastomas contain mesenchymal elements such as osteoid and cartilage in addition to epithelium. Staining for α-fetoprotein is common in hepatoblastoma and, depending on the type of histological differentiation, immunohistochemistry may also be positive for α_1-antitrypsin, cytokeratins, vimentin and CEA.[322]

Sarcoma and lymphoma

Undifferentiated sarcomas with a poor prognosis occasionally develop in the liver in children.[323] Epithelium trapped within the tumour may give rise to confusion. Light microscopic and ultrastructural features suggest malignant fibrous histiocytoma[324,325] or myoblastic differentiation.[325] Immunohistochemical results are inconsistent, with reports of staining for histiocytic markers, desmin, vimentin, and even cytokeratin.[325,326] Another form of sarcoma, arising in the biliary tract, is the **embryonal rhabdomyosarcoma** or **sarcoma botryoides**.[319] The histologically distinctive **calcifying nested stromal–epithelial tumour** is a mixed stromal and epithelial low-grade malignant neoplasm with foci of calcification or ossification.[327–329] This tumour usually grows indolently and shows nests of small, round spindled and large eosinophilic epithelioid cells arranged in irregular zig-zag patterns surrounded by desmoplastic stroma with interspersed bile ducts

Figure 11.27
Hepatoblastoma, embryonal epithelial type. Tumour cells grow in tubules and show an increased nucleus–cytoplasm ratio. Darkly stained mitotic figures can be identified in some cells. (Operative specimen, H&E.)

(**Fig. 11.28**). Exceptionally rare **primary non-Hodgkin's lymphoma** in the liver has been reported in childhood.[330]

Hepatocellular carcinoma

Hepatocellular carcinoma in children resembles the adult type histologically, but cirrhosis is usually absent.[319] Predisposing causes include tyrosinaemia and type I glycogenosis. The fibrolamellar type of carcinoma has been described in older children, with better prognosis than hepatocellular carcinoma in general.[197]

Cytopathological diagnosis

Fine-needle aspiration biopsy (FNAB) is often used to investigate hepatic masses, particularly for patients with cirrhosis in whom HCC is suspected.[331] This technique may demonstrate lesional tissue as well as components of normal or non-neoplastic liver. In the latter regard, the interpreter must be familiar with the cytological appearances of normal liver, cirrhosis or dysplasia, which are discussed below.

Normal or reactive liver

Aspirates from non-neoplastic liver will contain **normal** or **reactive hepatocytes,** which are present as single cells, clusters or two-dimensional monolayer sheets (**Fig. 11.29**). Normal hepatocytes may be arranged in trabeculae, but these should consist of three or fewer cells, without enveloping endothelium (**Fig. 11.30**). Individual hepatocytes are polygonal cells with well-defined borders and centrally placed, round nuclei which often have conspicuous nucleoli and occasionally show intranuclear cytoplasmic pseudoinclusions (vesicular inclusions). The latter may also be seen in HCC and are therefore not diagnostic. The nuclei of benign hepatocytes may vary considerably in size (not shape)

Figure 11.28 Calcifying nested stromal–epithelial tumour.
The desmoplastic stroma contains epithelial nests arranged in a 'zig-zag' pattern. The epithelium varies from larger eosinophilic cells (nest at right) to more basophilic and spindled. Bile-duct structures are in close proximity to the nests. (Partial hepatectomy, H&E.)

Figure 11.29 Normal hepatocytes.
A cluster of normal liver cells includes several binucleated hepatocytes and an enlarged, polyploid cell at top. Prominent nucleoli are visible. (Papanicolaou.)

Figure 11.30
Normal hepatocyte trabeculae.
Normal trabeculae of hepatocytes on aspirate contain up to two or three cells. (Papanicolaou.)

and this is a helpful diagnostic sign which contrasts with the more monomorphic nuclei seen in HCC.[332] The appearance of pigment in the liver varies according to the staining method used.[332,333] The presence of lipofuscin in hepatocytes is indicative of a benign process.

Benign aspirates may also contain **bile-duct epithelium**, which is usually not present in specimens from liver-cell adenoma and HCC.[334] Bile-duct epithelial cells are smaller than hepatocytes, are arranged in monolayers with a 'honeycomb' glandular pattern (**Fig. 11.31**) and have eccentrically located nuclei in a pale, non-granular cytoplasm. The nuclei have fine chromatin and no prominent nucleoli. Aspirates may also contain sheets of benign **mesothelium** derived from the peritoneum (**Fig. 11.32**).

Cirrhosis and liver-cell dysplasia

Aspirates from cirrhotic liver may contain portions of connective tissue and fibroblasts (**Fig. 11.33**), bile-duct epithelium, reactive hepatocytes arranged in clusters with jagged edges (rather than smooth-edged trabeculae as in HCC) and mixed chronic inflammatory cells (mostly lymphocytes). A definitive diagnosis of cirrhosis based only on FNAB is usually not possible.[335]

Large-cell and small-cell dysplasia (**Ch. 10**) can also be identified on FNAB. The type and degree of nuclear atypia distinguish dysplastic hepatocytes from normal or reactive liver cells. In large-cell dysplasia, nuclei are enlarged, hyperchromatic and pleomorphic, with one or more prominent nucleoli (**Fig. 11.34**). Coarse nuclear chromatin and pseudo-inclusions of invaginated cytoplasm are often present. The presence of cellular enlargement with ample cytoplasm maintains a relatively normal nucleus–cytoplasm ratio. In small-cell dysplasia this ratio is increased because the atypical nuclei are found in cells that are smaller than normal hepatocytes (**Fig. 11.35**). The aspirated cell clusters in which dysplastic hepatocytes may be found are accompanied by normal or reactive hepatocytes with heterogeneous nuclear features and cell sizes, an important distinction from aspirates of HCC which typically show a relatively monomorphous population of hepatocytes.[336]

Figure 11.31 Bile-duct epithelium.
Clusters of bile-duct epithelial cells are distinguishable from the group of hepatocytes near the centre by their smaller size and round, nondescript nuclei. Microglandular structures are also focally present. (Papanicolaou.)

Figure 11.32 Mesothelium.
A sheet of mesothelial cells from the peritoneum shows a characteristic clear 'window' at right. (Papanicolaou.)

**Figure 11.33
Cirrhosis.**
The aspirate includes interweaving spindled fibroblasts, stroma and the round nuclei of lymphocytes. (Diff-Quick.)

**Figure 11.34
Large-cell dysplasia.**
Two groups of hepatocytes (top and centre) contain large dysplastic cells intermixed with smaller reactive hepatocytes. The dysplastic cells have hyperchromatic nuclei, coarse chromatin and prominent nucleoli. Normal hepatocytes are seen at left and at bottom. (Papanicolaou.) (Illustration kindly provided by Dr Alastair Deery, London, UK.)

**Figure 11.35
Small-cell
dysplasia.**
The cluster of small
hepatocytes slightly
below centre shows
hyperchromatic
atypical nuclei.
(Papanicolaou.)
(Illustration kindly
provided by Dr
Alastair Deery,
London, UK.)

Liver-cell adenoma

The cytological diagnosis rendered from the FNAB smear of liver-cell adenoma is typically 'compatible with' this tumour, since the specimen usually shows single hepatocytes or clusters which resemble benign, normal liver cells.[334] Bile-duct epithelium and connective tissue should be absent, in contrast to focal nodular hyperplasia.

Focal nodular hyperplasia

Establishing the cytological diagnosis of focal nodular hyperplasia is based on finding one or more of the several cellular elements constituting this lesion (hepatocytes, fibrous tissue, bile-duct epithelium) within the smear. The presence of bile-duct epithelium in duct-like structures or clusters effectively rules out liver-cell adenoma and hepatocellular carcinoma. The bile-duct epithelium may show nuclear variation and conspicuous nucleoli.[337] Fibrous tissue and bile-duct epithelium are not always present in the aspirate but the bland appearance of the hepatocytes – with small, round nuclei lacking prominent nucleoli – implies a benign lesion. The hepatocytes are arranged in clusters with irregular or jagged edges without traversing or peripheral endothelium.

Haemangioma

Aspirates of haemangiomas are bloody, and numerous red blood cells are seen on the smear. Fragments of fibrous tissue[338] and/or single or clustered spindle-shaped endothelial cells may also be present (**see Fig. 11.36**).

Hepatocellular carcinoma

The low-power microscopic appearance of smears from HCC provides several important diagnostic features, especially the rounded edges of tumour cells in clusters or trabeculae

**Figure 11.36
Haemangioma.**
A focus of stromal cells is present with an extensive background of red blood cells. Scattered spindle-shaped endothelial or fibroblast nuclei are seen amid the erythrocytes. (Papanicolaou.)

(in contrast to the ragged edges of normal or reactive hepatocyte clusters) and endothelial cells which traverse clusters of tumour cells as well as wrap around the periphery of clusters or trabeculae (**Figs 11.37, 11.38**). The paucireticulin pattern of HCC is helpful in FNABs where low-power examination of glass slides shows a finely granular smear (in contrast to the preserved cores or larger tissue fragments seen with benign liver diseases and masses[339]). Tumour cells are polygonal with central nuclei that may have either coarse or fine chromatin and prominent nucleoli or macronucleoli (**Fig. 11.39**). There is usually less variability in the features of HCC cells on smear than in normal or reactive hepatocytes.

Atypical naked nuclei[340] (exceptionally large and irregular nuclei without visible cytoplasm) are also an important diagnostic feature (**Fig. 11.40**). A stepwise logistic regression study showed that the three features which best differentiate HCC from normal or reactive liver are: increased nucleus–cytoplasm ratio; a trabecular pattern of tumour cells enclosed by endothelium; and atypical naked nuclei.[332,341] **Table 11.5** summarises some of the major FNAB cytological features of HCC. The presence of bile within or between tumour cells is indicative of their hepatocellular origin, but bile may be seen in only half the cases[342] and can also be present in smears from non-neoplastic liver.

Table 11.5 Major fine-needle aspiration biopsy features of hepatocellular carcinoma

Polygonal cells with central or paracentral nuclei
Relative homogeneity of tumour cells
High nucleus–cytoplasm ratio
Cell nests and trabeculae with smooth edges
Traversing and/or peripheral endothelium
Atypical naked nuclei

Variants of HCC which may be present include acinar, clear-cell and fibrolamellar carcinoma. As with typical HCC, the presence of peripheral endothelial wrapping or traversal of endothelium across tumour cell clusters favours HCC. When **clear cells** are identified, there are also usually non-clear-cell HCC cells present which help distinguish the tumour from renal, adrenal and ovarian neoplasms.[343] **Fibrolamellar carcinoma** can be diagnosed if the smear includes fibrous tissue or fibroblasts and the distinctive polygonal cells with granular, eosinophilic cytoplasm[344] (**Fig. 11.41**). The tumour cells

**Figure 11.37
Hepatocellular
carcinoma.**
Malignant
hepatocytes in
clusters are traversed
by slender strings
of endothelium.
(Papanicolaou.)

**Figure 11.38
Hepatocellular
carcinoma.**
Flattened
endothelium is seen
peripherally at the
edge of a trabecula
of hepatocellular
carcinoma.
(Papanicolaou.)

of fibrolamellar carcinoma are often dispersed or dishesive, in comparison with the cell clusters and trabeculae of typical HCC.[345]

When metastatic carcinoma must be differentiated from HCC on FNAB, the cytopathologist should bear in mind that nearly all HCCs will have two or three of the following key diagnostic criteria:[332] polygonal cells with centrally placed nuclei; malignant cells traversed by sinusoidal capillaries; and bile.

**Figure 11.39
Hepatocellular
carcinoma.**
Malignant
hepatocytes have
fairly uniform nuclei
which are centrally
or peripherally
located. Prominent
nucleoli are seen
throughout and a
mitotic figure is
present at right
centre.
(Papanicolaou.)

**Figure 11.40
Hepatocellular
carcinoma.**
A cluster of
malignant
hepatocytes is
present along with
'naked nuclei'.
(Diff-Quick.)

Figure 11.41 Fibrolamellar carcinoma.
The malignant hepatocytes in this aspirate have ample granular cytoplasm and prominent nucleoli. (Papanicolaou.) (Illustration kindly provided by Dr Alastair Deery, London, UK.)

Hepatoblastoma

The **epithelial type** of hepatoblastoma cytologically resembles HCC and on smear shows cohesive nests, sheets or trabeculae of malignant hepatocytes (**Fig. 11.42**). The tumour cells have hyperchromatic nuclei which may overlap and show prominent nucleoli. Fetal and embryonal subtypes are difficult to distinguish on FNAB alone.[346] There may be extramedullary haemopoiesis, formation of acini and naked tumour cell nuclei.[346,347] The **mesenchymal type** of hepatoblastoma, or the mixed epithelial–mesenchymal variant, may be represented by spindle cells in the smear.

Cholangiocarcinoma

Aspirate smears from cholangiocarcinoma demonstrate three-dimensional clusters of atypical cells having a small amount of cytoplasm and nuclei with granular chromatin and one or more prominent nucleoli. Tumour cells may also be arranged in acini and cannot be readily distinguished on routine stains from metastatic pancreatic or other adenocarcinomas.[344]

Angiosarcoma

The smear of this tumour is typically bloody, and features a necrotic background with dishesive, pleomorphic spindle cells. Factor VIII and CD34 immunostains are diagnostically helpful.[348]

Lymphoma

Lymphoid proliferations in the liver, including lymphoma and post-transplant lympho-proliferative disease,[349] can be diagnosed on FNAB according to cytological criteria used

Figure 11.42 Hepatoblastoma. The cell cluster is packed with malignant epithelium. Nuclear features resemble those seen in hepatocellular carcinoma. (Papanicolaou.)

for aspirates from extrahepatic sites. Smears show dispersed single, monomorphous lymphoid cells with 'blue blobs' of stripped cytoplasm (lymphoglandular bodies[350]) in the background (**Fig. 11.43**). Blue blobs may also be present in smears containing non-neoplastic lymphocytes.

Metastatic tumours

Adenocarcinoma from the colon and pancreas on aspirate smears presents as cell clusters with round or oval vesicular nuclei, prominent nucleoli and delicate cytoplasm. The presence of columnar cells with cigar-shaped, palisaded nuclei and apical cytoplasm or vacuoles (goblet cells) is characteristic of **colon carcinoma (Fig. 11.44)**. The cytological features of **breast carcinoma** include the tendency to smear as dishesive cell groups or single cells with eccentric nuclei and cone-shaped cytoplasm. Relative uniformity of cell size and shape, prominent small nucleoli and the absence of marked atypia are seen in infiltrating duct carcinoma. Lobular carcinoma may show single-file lines of cells with nuclear moulding. **Neuroendocrine carcinomas** on smear feature organoid nests (carcinoid tumours) or loose groups or sheets (islet cell carcinoma). The coarse 'salt and pepper' chromatin pattern is characteristic of these neoplasms, with islet cell carcinomas often showing more nuclear pleomorphism with prominent nucleoli than carcinoid tumours (**Fig. 11.45**). **Malignant melanoma** often metastasises to the liver and may be confused with HCC on FNAB because of features in common, including eosinophilic macronucleoli, nuclear pseudoinclusions, polygonal cell shape and cohesive cell groups. However, in contrast to HCC, aspirates of melanoma are more likely to show single, dishesive cells with eccentric nuclei and intracellular melanin pigment (**Fig. 11.46**). If cell grouping is present, it is unlikely to be accompanied by the traversing or peripheral endothelium seen in HCC. Immunostains for HMB-45 and S-100 should be undertaken if melanoma is a possible diagnosis, particularly if pigment is absent.

Figure 11.43 Lymphoma. Dissociated malignant lymphoid cells are present with a background of smaller 'blue blobs' (lymphoglandular bodies.) (Diff-Quick.)

Figure 11.44 Metastatic colonic adenocarcinoma. Several rows of columnar cells are present and the cluster at upper right contains a goblet cell with a large cytoplasmic vacuole. (Papanicolaou.)

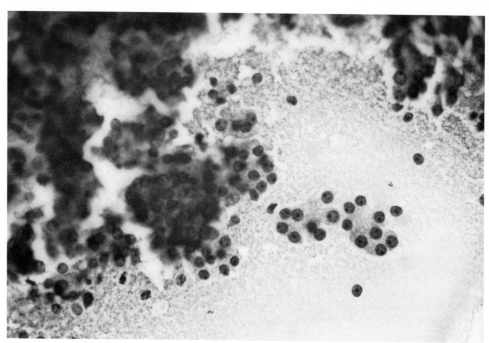

**Figure 11.45
Metastatic
neuroendocrine
carcinoma.**
Clusters of fairly
homogeneous
small cells with
regular nuclei
and substantial
cytoplasm are seen.
The patient had a
pancreatic islet cell
carcinoma. Thick
trabecular structures
are seen at left.
(Diff-Quick.)

**Figure 11.46
Metastatic uveal
melanoma.**
A cluster of
melanoma cells with
intracellular melanin
pigment is present.
Several normal
hepatocytes are seen
at upper right.
(Papanicolaou.)
(Illustration kindly
provided by Dr
Alastair Deery,
London, UK.)

References

1 Tao L-C. Oral contraceptive-associated liver cell adenoma and hepatocellular carcinoma. Cytomorphology and mechanism of malignant transformation. *Cancer* 1991; **68**: 341–347.

2 Greaves WOC, Bhattacharya B. Hepatic adenomatosis. *Arch Pathol Lab Med* 2008; **132**: 1951–1955.

3 Lepreux S, Laurent C, Blanc JF, et al. The identification of small nodules in liver adenomatosis. *J Hepatol* 2003; **39**: 77–85.

4 Hasan N, Coutts M, Portmann B. Pigmented liver cell adenoma in two male patients. *Am J Surg Pathol* 2000; **24**: 1429–1432.

5 Heffelfinger S, Irani DR, Finegold MJ. 'Alcoholic hepatitis' in a hepatic adenoma. *Hum Pathol* 1987; **18**: 751–754.

6 Le Bail B, Jouhanole H, Deugnier Y, et al. Liver adenomatosis with granulomas in two patients on long-term oral contraceptives. *Am J Surg Pathol* 1992; **16**: 982–987.

7 Bioulac-Sage P, Rebouissou S, Thomas C, et al. Hepatocellular adenoma subtype classification using molecular markers and immunohistochemistry. *Hepatology* 2007; **46**: 740–748.

8 Bioulac-Sage P, Blanc JF, Rebouissou S, et al. Genotype phenotype classification of hepatocellular adenoma. *World J Gastroenterol* 2007; **13**: 2649–2654.

9 Bioulac-Sage P, Balabaud C, Bedossa P, et al. Pathological diagnosis of liver cell adenoma and focal nodular hyperplasia: Bordeaux update. *J Hepatol* 2007; **46**: 521–527.

10 Rebouissou S, Amessou M, Couchy G, et al. Frequent in-frame somatic deletions activate gp130 in inflammatory hepatocellular tumours. *Nature* 2009; **457**: 200–204.

11 Micchelli STL, Vivekanandan P, Boitnott JK, et al. Malignant transformation of hepatic adenomas. *Mod Pathol* 2008; **21**: 491–497.

12 Rooks JB, Ory HW, Ishak KG, et al. Epidemiology of hepatocellular adenoma. The role of oral contraceptive use. *JAMA* 1979; **242**: 644–648.

13 Sánchez-Osorio M, Duarte-Rojo A, Martinez-Benitez B, et al. Anabolic–androgenic steroids and liver injury. *Liver Int* 2008; **28**: 278–282.

14 Ozenne V, Paradis V, Vullierme M-P, et al. Liver tumours in patients with Fanconi anaemia: a report of three cases. *Eur J Gastrol Hepatol* 2008; **20**: 1036–1039.

15 Velazquez I, Alter BP. Androgens and liver tumors: Fanconi's anemia and non-Fanconi's conditions. *Am J Hematol* 2004; **77**: 257–267.

16 Flejou JF, Barge J, Menu Y, et al. Liver adenomatosis. An entity distinct from liver adenoma? *Gastroenterology* 1985; **89**: 1132–1138.

17 Vetaläinen R, Erdogan D, de Graaf W, et al. Liver adenomatosis: re-evaluation of aetiology and management. *Liver Int* 2008; **28**: 499–508.

18 Bacq Y, Jacquemin E, Balabaud C, et al. Familial liver adenomatosis associated with hepatocyte nuclear factor 1α inactivation. *Gastroenterology* 2003; **125**: 1470–1475.

19 Zucman-Rossi J. Genetic alterations in hepatocellular adenomas: recent findings and new challenges. *J Hepatol* 2004; **40**: 1036–1039.

20 Kahn H, Manzarbeitia C, Theise N, et al. Danazol-induced hepatocellular adenomas. *Arch Pathol Lab Med* 1991; **115**: 1054–1057.

21 Gokhale R, Whitington PR. Hepatic adenomatosis in an adolescent. *J Pediatr Gastroenterol Nutr* 1996; **23**: 482–486.

22 Foster JH, Donohue TA, Berman MM. Familial liver-cell adenomas and diabetes mellitus. *N Engl J Med* 1978; **299**: 239–241.

23 Coire CI, Qizilbash AH, Castelli MF. Hepatic adenomata in type Ia glycogen storage disease. *Arch Pathol Lab Med* 1987; **111**: 166–169.

24 Paradis V, Laurent A, Flejou J-F, et al. Evidence for the polyclonal nature of focal nodular hyperplasia of the liver by the study of X-chromosome inactivation. *Hepatology* 1997; **26**: 891–895.

25 Wanless IR, Mawdsley C, Adams R. On the pathogenesis of focal nodular hyperplasia of the liver. *Hepatology* 1985; **5**: 1194–1200.

26 Fukukura Y, Nakashima O, Kusaba A, et al. Angioarchitecture and blood circulation in focal nodular hyperplasia of the liver. *J Hepatol* 1998; **29**: 470–475.

27 Roskams T, De Vos R, Desmet V. 'Undifferentiated progenitor cells' in focal nodular hyperplasia of the liver. *Histopathology* 1996; **28**: 291–299.

28 Scoazec J-Y, Flejou J-F, D'Errico A, et al. Focal nodular hyperplasia of the liver: composition of the extracellular matrix and expression of cell–cell and cell–matrix adhesion molecules. *Hum Pathol* 1995; **26**: 1114–1125.

29 Nime F, Pickren JW, Vana J, et al. The histology of liver tumors in oral contraceptive users observed during a national survey by the American College of Surgeons Commission on Cancer. *Cancer* 1979; **44**: 1481–1489.

30 Mathieu D, Kobeiter H, Maison P, et al. Oral contraceptive use and focal nodular hyperplasia of the liver. *Gastroenterology* 2000; **118**: 560–564.

31 Sadowski DC, Lee SS, Wanless IR, et al. Progressive type of focal nodular hyperplasia characterized by multiple tumors and recurrence. *Hepatology* 1995; **21**: 970–975.

32 Friedman LS, Gang DL, Hedberg SE, et al. Simultaneous occurrence of hepatic adenoma and focal nodular hyperplasia: report of a case and review of the literature. *Hepatology* 1984; **4**: 536–540.

33 Wanless IR, Albrecht S, Bilbao J, et al. Multiple focal nodular hyperplasia of the liver associated with vascular malformations of various organs and neoplasia of the brain: a new syndrome. *Mod Pathol* 1989; **2**: 456–462.

34 Portmann B, Stewart S, Higenbottam TW, et al. Nodular transformation of the liver associated with portal and pulmonary arterial hypertension. *Gastroenterology* 1993; **104**: 616–621.

35 Haber M, Reuben A, Burrell M, et al. Multiple focal nodular hyperplasia of the liver associated with hemihypertrophy and vascular malformations. *Gastroenterology* 1995; **108**: 1256–1262.

36 Sato Y, Harada K, Ikeda H, et al. Hepatic stellate cells are activated around central scars of focal nodular hyperplasia of the liver – a potential mechanism of central scar formation. *Hum Pathol* 2009; **40**: 181–188.

37 Butron Vila MM, Haot J, Desmet VJ. Cholestatic features in focal nodular hyperplasia of the liver. *Liver* 1984; **4**: 387–395.

38 Ahmad I, Iyer A, Marginean CE, et al. Diagnostic use of cytokeratins, CD34, and neuronal cell adhesion molecule staining in focal nodular hyperplasia and hepatic adenoma. *Hum Pathol* 2009; **40**: 726–734.

39 Ruschenburg I, Droese M. Fine needle aspiration cytology of focal nodular hyperplasia of the liver. *Acta Cytol* 1989; **33**: 857–860.

40 Makhlouf HR, Abdul-AL HM, Goodman ZD. Diagnosis of focal nodular hyperplasia of the liver by needle biopsy. *Hum Pathol* 2005; **36**: 1210–1216.

41 Schilling MK, Zimmermann A, Redaelli C, et al. Liver nodules resembling focal nodular hyperplasia after hepatic venous thrombosis. *J Hepatol* 2000; **33**: 673–676.

42 Ibarrola C, Castellano VM, Colina F. Focal hyperplastic hepatocellular nodules in hepatic venous outflow obstruction: a clinicopathological study of four patients and 24 nodules. *Histopathology* 2004; **44**: 172–179.

43 Wanless IR. Epithelioid hemangioendothelioma, multiple focal nodular hyperplasias, and cavernous hemangiomas of the liver. *Arch Pathol Lab Med* 2000; **124**: 1105–1107.

43a Ra SH, Kaplan JB, Lassman CR. Focal nodular hyperplasia after orthotopic liver transplantation. *Liver Transplant* 2010; **16**: 98–103.

44 Reshamwala PA, Kleiner DE, Heller T. Nodular regenerative hyperplasia: not all nodules are created equal. *Hepatology* 2006; **44**: 7–14.

45 Stromeyer FW, Ishak KG. Nodular transformation (nodular 'regenerative' hyperplasia) of the liver. A clinicopathologic study of 30 cases. *Hum Pathol* 1981; **12**: 60–71.

46 Thorne C, Urowitz MB, Wanless I, et al. Liver disease in Felty's syndrome. *Am J Med* 1982; **73**: 35–40.

47 Wanless IR. Micronodular transformation (nodular regenerative hyperplasia) of the liver: a report of 64 cases among 2,500 autopsies and a new classification of benign hepatocellular nodules. *Hepatology* 1990; **11**: 787–797.

48 Dubinsky MC, Vasiliauskas EA, Singh H, et al. 6-Thioguanine can cause serious liver injury in inflammatory bowel disease patients. *Gastroenterology* 2003; **125**: 298–303.

49 Paradinas FJ, Bull TB, Westaby D, et al. Hyperplasia and prolapse of hepatocytes into hepatic veins during longterm methyltestosterone therapy: possible relationships of these changes to the development of peliosis hepatis and liver tumours. *Histopathology* 1977; **1**: 225–246.

50 Baker BL, Axiotis C, Hurwitz ES, et al. Nodular regenerative hyperplasia of the liver in idiopathic hypereosinophilic syndrome. *J Clin Gastroenterol* 1991; **13**: 452–456.

51 Solis-Herruzo JA, Vidal JV, Colina F, et al. Nodular regenerative hyperplasia of the liver associated with the toxic oil syndrome: report of five cases. *Hepatology* 1986; **6**: 687–693.

52 Bloxham CA, Henderson DC, Hampson J, et al. Nodular regenerative hyperplasia of the liver in Behçet's disease. *Histopathology* 1992; **20**: 452–454.

53 Colina F, Pinedo F, Solís A, et al. Nodular regenerative hyperplasia of the liver in early histological stages of primary biliary cirrhosis. *Gastroenterology* 1992; **102**: 1319–1324.

54 Cancado ELR, Medeiros DM, Deguti MM, et al. Celiac disease associated with nodular regenerative hyperplasia, pulmonary abnormalities, and IgA anticardiolipin antibodies. *J Clin Gastroenterol* 2006; **40**: 135–139.

55 Minato H, Nakanuma Y. Nodular regenerative hyperplasia of the liver associated with metastases of pancreatic endocrine tumour: report of two autopsy cases. *Virchows Arch [A]* 1992; **421**: 171–174.

56 Kobayashi S, Saito K, Nakanuma Y. Nodular regenerative hyperplasia of the liver in hepatocellular carcinoma. *J Clin Gastroenterol* 1993; **16**: 155–159.

57 Wanless IR, Godwin TA, Allen F, et al. Nodular regenerative hyperplasia of the liver in hematologic disorders: a possible response to obliterative portal venopathy. A morphometric study of nine cases with an hypothesis on the pathogenesis. *Medicine* 1980; **59**: 367–379.

58 Wanless IR, Lentz JS, Roberts EA. Partial nodular transformation of liver in an adult with persistent ductus venosus. Review with hypothesis on pathogenesis. *Arch Pathol Lab Med* 1985; **109**: 427–432.

59 Terayama N, Terada T, Hoso M, et al. Partial nodular transformation of the liver with portal vein thrombosis. *J Clin Gastroenterol* 1995; **20**: 71–76.

60 Wanless IR. Vascular disorders. In: MacSween RNM, Anthony PP, Scheuer PJ, et al., eds. Pathology of the Liver, 3rd edn. Edinburgh: Churchill Livingstone, 1994, Ch. 14: 535–562.

61 Allaire GS, Rabin L, Ishak KG, et al. Bile duct adenoma. A study of 152 cases. *Am J Surg Pathol* 1988; **12**: 708–715.

62 Bhathal PS, Hughes NR, Goodman ZD. The so-called bile duct adenoma is a peribiliary gland hamartoma. *Am J Surg Pathol* 1996; **20**: 858–864.

63 Cho C, Rullis I, Rogers LS. Bile duct adenomas as liver nodules. *Arch Surg* 1978; **113**: 272–274.

64 Gold JH, Guzman IJ, Rosai J. Benign tumors of the liver. Pathologic examination of 45 cases. *Am J Clin Pathol* 1978; **70**: 6–17.

65 Govindarajan S, Peters RL. The bile duct adenoma. A lesion distinct from Meyenburg complex. *Arch Pathol Lab Med* 1984; **108**: 922–924.

66 Scheele PM, Bonar MJ, Zumwalt R, et al. Bile duct adenomas in heterozygous (MZ) deficiency of α1-protease inhibitor. *Arch Pathol Lab Med* 1988; **112**: 945–947.

67 Varnholt H, Vauthey J-N, Dal Cin P, et al. Biliary adenofibroma. A rare neoplasm of bile duct origin with an indolent behavior. *Am J Surg Pathol* 2003; **27**: 693–698.

68 Wheeler DA, Edmondson HA. Cystadenoma with mesenchymal stroma (CMS) in the liver and bile ducts. A clinicopathologic study of 17 cases, 4 with malignant change. *Cancer* 1985; **56**: 1434–1445.

69 Gourley WK, Kumar D, Bouton MS, et al. Cystadenoma and cystadenocarcinoma with mesenchymal stroma of the liver. Immunohistochemical analysis. *Arch Pathol Lab Med* 1992; **116**: 1047–1050.

70 Ishak KG, Willis GW, Cummins SD, et al. Biliary cystadenoma and cystadenocarcinoma: report of 14 cases and review of the literature. [Review.] *Cancer* 1977; **39**: 322–338.

71 Tung GA, Cronan JJ. Percutaneous needle biopsy of hepatic cavernous hemangioma. *J Clin Gastroenterol* 1993; **16**: 117–122.

72 Kim GE, Thung SN, Tsui WMS, et al. Hepatic cavernous hemangioma: underrecognized associated histologic features. *Liver Int* 2006; **26**: 334–338.

73 Berry CL. Solitary 'necrotic nodule' of the liver: a probable pathogenesis. *J Clin Pathol* 1985; **38**: 1278–1280.

74 Van Steenbergen W, Joosten E, Marchal G, et al. Hepatic lymphangiomatosis. Report of a case and review of the literature. *Gastroenterology* 1985; **88**: 1968–1972.

75 Peters WM, Dixon MF, Williams NS. Angiomyelolipoma of the liver. *Histopathology* 1983; **7**: 99–106.

76 Goodman ZD. Benign tumors of the liver. In: Okuda K, Ishak KG, eds. Neoplasms of the Liver. Tokyo: Springer-Verlag, 1990: 105–126.

77 Hytiroglou P, Linton P, Klion F, et al. Benign schwannoma of the liver. *Arch Pathol Lab Med* 1993; **117**: 216–218.

78 Lederman SM, Martin EC, Laffey KT, Lefkowitch JH. Hepatic neurofibromatosis, malignant schwannoma and angiosarcoma in von Recklinghausen's disease. *Gastroenterology* 1987; **92**: 234–239.

79 Andreu V, Elizalde I, Mallafré C, et al. Plexiform neurofibromatosis and angiosarcoma of the liver in Von Recklinghausen disease. *Am J Gastroenterol* 1997; **92**: 1229–1230.

80 Moran CA, Ishak KG, Goodman ZD. Solitary fibrous tumor of the liver: a clinicpathologic and immunohistochemical study of nine cases. *Ann Diagn Pathol* 1998; **2**: 19–24.

81 Fried RH, Wardzala A, Willson RA, et al. Benign cartilaginous tumor (chondroma) of the liver. *Gastroenterology* 1992; **103**: 678–680.

82 Nonomura A, Mizukami Y, Isobe M, et al. Smallest angiomyolipoma of the liver in the oldest patient. *Liver* 1993; **13**: 51–53.

83 Tsui WMS, Colombari R, Portmann BC, et al. Hepatic angiomyolipoma. A clinicopathologic study of 30 cases and delineation of unusual morphologic variants. *Am J Surg Pathol* 1999; **23**: 34–48.

84 Nonomura A, Mizukami Y, Kadoya M, et al. Multiple angiomyolipoma of the liver. *J Clin Gastroenterol* 1995; **20**: 248–251.

85 Kyokane T, Akita Y, Katayama M, et al. Multiple angiomyolipomas of the liver (case report). *Hepatol Gastroenterol* 1995; **42**: 510–515.

86 Pounder DJ. Hepatic angiomyolipoma. *Am J Surg Pathol* 1982; **6**: 677–681.

87 Goodman ZD, Ishak KG. Angiomyolipomas of the liver. *Am J Surg Pathol* 1984; **8**: 745–750.

88 Hoffman AL, Emre S, Verham RP, et al. Hepatic angiomyolipoma: two case reports of caudate-based lesions and review of the literature. *Liver Transplant Surg* 1997; **3**: 46–53.

89 Terris B, Fléjou J-F, Picot R, et al. Hepatic angiomyolipoma. A report of four cases with immunohistochemical and DNA-flow cytometric studies. *Arch Pathol Lab Med* 1996; **120**: 68–72.

90 Karhunen PJ. Hepatic pseudolipoma. *J Clin Pathol* 1985; **38**: 877–879.

91 Shek TWH, Ng IOL, Chan KW. Inflammatory pseudotumor of the liver. Report of four cases and review of the literature. *Am J Surg Pathol* 1993; **17**: 231–238.

92 Lawrence B, Perez-Atayde A, Hibbard MK, et al. TPM3-ALK and TPM4-ALK oncogenes in inflammatory myofibroblastic tumors. *Am J Pathol* 2000; **157**: 377–384.

93 Cessna MH, Zhou H, Sanger WG, et al. Expression of ALK1 and p80 in inflammatory myofibroblastic tumor and its mesenchymal mimics: a study of 135 cases. *Mod Pathol* 2002; **15**: 931–938.

94 Shek TWH, Ho FCS, Ng GOL, et al. Follicular dendritic cell tumor of the liver. Evidence for an Epstein–Barr virus-related clonal proliferation of follicular dendritic cells. *Am J Surg Pathol* 1996; **20**: 313–324.

95 Ferrell LD, Crawford JM, Dhillon AP, et al. Proposal for standardized criteria for the diagnosis of benign, borderline, and malignant hepatocellular lesions arising in chronic advanced liver disease. *Am J Surg Pathol* 1993; **17**: 1113–1123.

96 International Working Party. Terminology of nodular hepatocellular lesions. *Hepatology* 1995; **22**: 983–993.

97 International Consensus Group for Hepatocellular Neoplasia. Pathologic diagnosis of early hepatocellular carcinoma: a report of the international consensus group for hepatocellular neoplasia. *Hepatology* 2009; **49**: 658–664.

98 Park YN, Roncalli M. Large liver cell dysplasia: a controversial entity. *J Hepatol* 2006; **45**: 734–743.

99 Anthony PP, Vogel CL, Barker LF. Liver cell dysplasia: a premalignant condition. *J Clin Pathol* 1973; **26**: 217–223.

100 Anthony PP. Hepatocellular carcinoma: an overview. *Histopathology* 2001; **39**: 109–118.

101 Borzio M, Bruno S, Roncalli M, et al. Liver cell dysplasia is a major risk factor for hepatocellular carcinoma in cirrhosis: a prospective study. *Gastroenterology* 1995; **108**: 812–817.

102 Ganne-Carrié N, Chastang C, Chapel F, et al. Predictive score for the development of hepatocellular carcinoma and additional value of liver large cell dysplasia in Western patients with cirrhosis. *Hepatology* 1996; **23**: 1112–1118.

103 Thomas RM, Berman JJ, Yetter RA, et al. Liver cell dysplasia: a DNA aneuploid lesion with distinct morphologic features. *Hum Pathol* 1992; **23**: 496–503.

104 Terris B, Ingster O, Rubbia L, et al. Interphase cytogenetic analysis reveals numerical chromosome aberrations in large liver cell dysplasia. *J Hepatol* 1997; **27**: 313–319.

105 Natarajan S, Theise ND, Thung SN, et al. Large-cell change of hepatocytes in cirrhosis may represent a reaction to prolonged cholestasis. *Am J Surg Pathol* 1997; **21**: 312–318.

106 Lee RG, Tsamandas AC, Demetris AJ. Large cell change (liver cell dysplasia) and hepatocellular carcinoma in cirrhosis: matched case–control study, pathological analysis, and pathogenetic hypothesis. *Hepatology* 1997; **26**: 1415–1422.

107 Libbrecht L, Craninx M, Nevens F, et al. Predictive value of liver cell dysplasia for development of hepatocellular carcinoma in patients with non-cirrhotic and cirrhotic chronic viral hepatitis. *Histopathology* 2001; **39**: 66–71.

108 Koo JS, Kim H, Park BK, et al. Predictive value of liver cell dysplasia for development of hepatocellular carcinoma in patients with chronic hepatitis B. *J Clin Gastroenterol* 2008; **42**: 738–743.

109 Watanabe S, Okita K, Harada T, et al. Morphologic studies of the liver cell dysplasia. *Cancer* 1983; **51**: 2197–2205.

110 Adachi E, Hashimoto H, Tsuneyoshi M. Proliferating cell nuclear antigen in hepatocellular carcinoma and small cell liver dysplasia. *Cancer* 1993; **72**: 2902–2909.

111 Plentz RR, Park YN, Lechel A, et al. Telomere shortening and inactivation of cell cycle checkpoints characterize human hepatocarcinogenesis. *Hepatology* 2007; **45**: 968–976.

112 Terada T, Hoso M, Nakanuma Y. Mallory body clustering in adenomatous hyperplasia in human cirrhotic livers. *Hum Pathol* 1989; **20**: 886–890.

113 Ueno Y, Moriyama M, Uchida T, et al. Irregular regeneration of hepatocytes is an important factor in the hepatocarcinogenesis of liver disease. *Hepatology* 2001; **33**: 357–362.

114 Terada T, Nakanuma Y. Iron-negative foci in siderotic macroregenerative nodules in human cirrhotic liver. *Arch Pathol Lab Med* 1989; **113**: 916–920.

115 Deugnier YM, Charalambous P, Le Quilleuc D, et al. Preneoplastic significance of hepatic iron-free foci in genetic hemochromatosis: a study of 185 patients. *Hepatology* 1993; **18**: 1363–1369.

116 Nakanuma Y, Terada T, Ueda K, et al. Adenomatous hyperplasia of the liver as a precancerous lesion. *Liver* 1993; **13**: 1–9.

117 Furuya K, Nakamura M, Yamamoto Y, et al. Macroregenerative nodule of the liver. A clinicopathologic study of 345 autopsy cases of chronic liver disease. *Cancer* 1988; **61**: 99–105.

118 Terada T, Ueda K, Nakanuma Y. Histopathological and morphometric analysis of atypical adenomatous hyperplasia of human cirrhotic livers. *Virchows Arch [A]* 1993; **422**: 381–388.

119 Le Bail B, Bernard P-H, Carles J, et al. Prevalence of liver cell dysplasia and association with HCC in a series of 100 cirrhotic liver explants. *J Hepatol* 1997; **27**: 835–842.

120 Ferrell LD. Hepatocellular nodules in the cirrhotic liver: diagnostic features and proposed nomenclature. In: Ferrell LD, ed. Diagnostic Problems in Liver Pathology. Philadelphia, PA: Hanley & Belfus, 1994: 105–118.

121 Gastaldi M, Massacrier A, Planells R, et al. Detection by in situ hybridization of hepatitis C virus positive and negative RNA strands using digoxigenin-labeled cRNA probes in human liver cells. *J Hepatol* 1995; **23**: 509–518.

122 Terasaki S, Kaneko S, Kobayashi K, et al. Histological features predicting malignant transformation of nonmalignant hepatocellular nodules: a prospective study. *Gastroenterology* 1998; **115**: 1216–1222.

123 Theise ND, Schwartz M, Miller C, et al. Macroregenerative nodules and hepatocellular carcinoma in forty-four sequential adults liver explants with cirrhosis. *Hepatology* 1992; **16**: 949–955.

124 Eguchi A, Nakashima O, Okudaira S, et al. Adenomatous hyperplasia in the vicinity of small hepatocellular carcinoma. *Hepatology* 1992; **15**: 843–848.

125 Aihara T, Noguchi S, Sasaki Y, et al. Clonal analysis of precancerous lesion of hepatocellular carcinoma. *Gastroenterology* 1996; **111**: 455–461.

126 Donato MF, Arosio E, Del Ninno E, et al. High rates of hepatocellular carcinoma in cirrhotic patients with high liver cell proliferative activity. *Hepatology* 2001; **34**: 523–528.

127 Wong N, Lai P, Pang E, et al. A comprehensive karyotypic study on human hepatocellular carcinoma by spectral karyotyping. *Hepatology* 2000; **32**: 1060–1068.

128 Shirota Y, Kaneko S, Honda M, et al. Identification of differentially expressed genes in hepatocellular carcinoma with cDNA microarrays. *Hepatology* 2001; **33**: 832–840.

129 Di Bisceglie AM, Carithers RL, Gores GJ. Hepatocellular carcinoma. *Hepatology* 1998; **28**: 1161–1165.

130 Schirmacher P, Rogler CE, Dienes HP. Current pathogenetic and molecular concepts in viral liver carcinogenesis. *Virchows Arch [B]* 1993; **63**: 71–89.

131 Popper H, Thung SN, McMahon BJ, et al. Evolution of hepatocellular carcinoma associated with chronic hepatitis B virus infection in Alaskan eskimos. *Arch Pathol Lab Med* 1988; **112**: 498–504.

132 Mandishona E, MacPhail AP, Gordeuk VR, et al. Dietary iron overload as a risk factor for hepatocellular carcinoma in black Africans. *Hepatology* 1998; **27**: 1563–1566.

133 Sun Z, Lu P, Gail MH, et al. Increased risk of hepatocellular carcinoma in male hepatitis B surface antigen carriers with chronic hepatitis who have detectable urinary aflatoxin metabolite M1. *Hepatology* 1999; **30**: 379–383.

134 Nair S, Mason A, Eason J, et al. Is obesity an independent risk factor for hepatocellular carcinoma in cirrhosis? *Hepatology* 2002; **36**: 150–155.

135 Marrero JA, Fontana RJ, Su GL, et al. NAFLD may be a common underlying liver disease in patients with hepatocellular carcinoma in the United States. *Hepatology* 2002; **36**: 1349–1354.

136 Shimada M, Hashimoto E, Taniai M, et al. Hepatocellular carcinoma in patients with non-alcoholic steatohepatitis. *J Hepatol* 2002; **37**: 154–160.

137 Paradis V, Bièche I, Dargère D, et al. Molecular profiling of hepatocellular carcinomas (HCC) using a large-scale real-time RT-PCR approach. Determination of a molecular diagnostic index. *Am J Pathol* 2003; **163**: 733–741.

138 Chen Q, Seol D-W, Carr B, et al. Co-expression and regulation of met and ron proto-oncogenes in human hepatocellular carcinoma tissues and cell lines. *Hepatology* 1997; **26**: 59–66.

139 Tannapfel A, Wittekind C. Genes involved in hepatocellular carcinoma: deregulation in cell cycling and apoptosis. *Virchows Arch* 2002; **44**: 345–352.

140 Park YN, Yang C-P, Fernandez GJ, et al. Neoangiogenesis and sinusoidal 'capillarization' in dysplastic nodules of the liver. *Am J Surg Pathol* 1998; **22**: 656–662.

141 Kimura H, Nakajima T, Kagawa K, et al. Angiogenesis in hepatocellular carcinoma as evaluated by CD34 immunohistochemistry. *Liver* 1998; **18**: 14–19.

142 El-Assal ON, Yamanoi A, Soda Y, et al. Clinical significance of microvessel density and vascular endothelial growth factor expression in hepatocellular carcinoma and surrounding liver: possible involvement of vascular endothelial growth factor in the angiogenesis of cirrhotic liver. *Hepatology* 1998; **27**: 1554–1562.

143 Yamaguchi R, Yano H, Iemura A, et al. Expression of vascular endothelial growth factor in human hepatocellular carcinoma. *Hepatology* 1998; **28**: 68–77.

144 Torimura T, Sata M, Ueno T, et al. Increased expression of vascular endothelial growth factor is associated with tumor progression in hepatocellular carcinoma. *Hum Pathol* 1998; **29**: 986–991.

145 Nehrbass D, Klimek F, Bannasch P. Overexpression of insulin receptor substrate-1 emerges early in hepatocarcinogenesis and elicits preneoplastic hepatic glycogenosis. *Am J Pathol* 1998; **152**: 341–345.

146 Hsia CC, Evarts RP, Nakatsukasa H, et al. Occurrence of oval-type cells in hepatitis B virus-associated human hepatocarcinogenesis. *Hepatology* 1992; **16**: 1327–1333.

147 Desmet V, De Vos R. Ultrastructural characteristics of novel epithelial cell types identified in human pathologic liver specimens with chronic ductular reaction. *Am J Pathol* 1992; **140**: 1441–1450.

148 Anthony PP. Tumours and tumour-like lesions of the liver and biliary tract. In: MacSween RNM, Anthony PP, Scheuer PJ, et al., eds. Pathology of the Liver, 3rd edn. Edinburgh: Churchill Livingstone, 1994; Ch. 16: 635–712.

149 Nzeako UC, Goodman ZD, Ishak KG. Hepatocellular carcinoma in cirrhotic and noncirrhotic livers. A clinico-histopathologic study of 804 North American patients. *Am J Clin Pathol* 1996; **105**: 65–75.

150 Bralet M-P, Régimbeau J-M, Pineau P, et al. Hepatocellular carcinoma occurring in nonfibrotic liver: epidemiologic and histopathologic analysis of 80 French cases. *Hepatology* 2000; **32**: 200–204.

151 Shikata T, Yamazaki S, Uzawa T. Hepatocellular carcinoma and chronic persistent hepatitis. *Acta Pathol Japon* 1977; **27**: 297–304.

152 Tabarin A, Bioulac-Sage P, Boussarie L, et al. Hepatocellular carcinoma developed on noncirrhotic livers. *Arch Pathol Lab Med* 1987; **111**: 174–180.

153 El-Refaie A, Savage K, Bhattacharya S, et al. HCV-associated hepatocellular carcinoma without cirrhosis. *J Hepatol* 1996; **24**: 277–285.

154 Le Bail B, Carles J, Saric J, et al. Ectopic liver and hepatocarcinogenesis. *Hepatology* 1999; **30**: 585–586.

155 Miyagawa S, Kawasaki S, Makuuchi M. Comparison of the characteristics of hepatocellular carcinoma between hepatitis B and C viral infection: tumor multicentricity in cirrhotic liver with hepatitis C. *Hepatology* 1996; **24**: 307–310.

156 Kondo Y, Wada K. Intrahepatic metastasis of hepatocellular carcinoma: a histopathologic study. *Hum Pathol* 1991; **22**: 125–130.

157 van Halteren HK, Salemans JMJI, Peters H, et al. Spontaneous regression of hepatocellular carcinoma. *J Hepatol* 1997; **27**: 211–215.

158 Kaczynski J, Hansson G, Remotti H, et al. Spontaneous regression of hepatocellular carcinoma. *Histopathology* 1998; **32**: 147–150.

159 Libbrecht L, Bielen D, Verslype C, et al. Focal lesions in cirrhotic explant livers: pathological evaluation and accuracy of pretransplantation imaging examinations. *Liver Transplant* 2002; **8**: 749–761.

160 Lauwers GY, Terris B, Balis UJ, et al. Prognostic histologic indicators of curatively resected hepatocellular carcinomas. *Am J Surg Pathol* 2002; **26**: 25–34.

161 Cillo U, Bassanello M, Vitale A, et al. The critical issue of hepatocellular carcinoma prognostic classification: which is the best tool available? *J Hepatol* 2004; **40**: 124–131.

162 Lopez-Beltran A, Luque RJ, Quintero A, et al. Hepatoid adenocarcinoma of the urinary bladder. *Virchows Arch* 2003; **442**: 381–387.

163 Dhillon AP, Colombari R, Savage K, et al. An immunohistochemical study of the blood vessels within primary hepatocellular tumours. *Liver* 1992; **12**: 311–318.

164 Omata M, Peters RL, Tatter D. Sclerosing hepatic carcinoma: relationship to hypercalcemia. *Liver* 1981; **1**: 33–49.

165 Theise ND, Yao JL, Harada K, et al. Hepatic 'stem cell' malignancies in adults: four cases. *Histopathology* 2003; **43**: 263–271.

166 Wada Y, Nakashima O, Kutami R, et al. Clinicopathological study on hepatocellular carcinoma with lymphocytic infiltration. *Hepatology* 1998; **27**: 407–414.

167 Nzeako UC, Goodman ZD, Ishak KG. Comparison of tumor pathology with duration of survival of North American patients with hepatocellular carcinoma. *Cancer* 1995; **76**: 579–588.

168 Kakizoe S, Kojiro M, Nakashima T. Hepatocellular carcinoma with sarcomatous change. *Cancer* 1987; **59**: 310–316.

169 Haratake J, Horie A. An immunohistochemical study of sarcomatoid liver carcinomas. *Cancer* 1991; **68**: 93–97.

170 Buchanan TF Jr, Huvos AG. Clear-cell carcinoma of the liver. A clinicopathologic study of 13 patients. *Am J Clin Pathol* 1974; **61**: 529–539.

171 Wu PC, Lai CL, Lam KC, et al. Clear cell carcinoma of liver. An ultrastructural study. *Cancer* 1983; **52**: 504–507.

172 Ajdukiewicz A, Crowden A, Hudson E, et al. Liver aspiration in the diagnosis of hepatocellular carcinoma in the Gambia. *J Clin Pathol* 1985; **38**: 185–192.

173 Noguchi S, Yamamoto R, Tatsuta M, et al. Cell features and patterns in fine-needle aspirates of hepatocellular carcinoma. *Cancer* 1986; **58**: 321–328.

174 Pedio G, Landolt U, Zöbeli L, et al. Fine needle aspiration of the liver. Significance of hepatocytic naked nuclei in the diagnosis of hepatocellular carcinoma. *Acta Cytol* 1988; **32**: 437–442.

175 Bottles K, Cohen MB, Holly EA, et al. A step-wise logistic regression analysis of hepatocellular carcinoma. An aspiration biopsy study. *Cancer* 1988; **62**: 558–563.

176 Ishak KG, Goodman ZD, Stocker JT. Tumors of the Liver and Intrahepatic Bile Ducts. Washington, DC: Armed Forces Institute of Pathology, 2001: 199–230.

177 Nakanuma Y, Ohta G. Expression of Mallory bodies in hepatocellular carcinoma in man and its significance. *Cancer* 1986; **57**: 81–86.

178 Hurlimann J, Gardiol D. Immunohistochemistry in the differential diagnosis of liver carcinomas. *Am J Surg Pathol* 1991; **15**: 280–288.

179 Van Eyken P, Sciot R, Paterson A, et al. Cytokeratin expression in hepatocellular carcinoma: an immunohistochemical study. *Hum Pathol* 1988; **19**: 562–568.

180 Lai Y-S, Thung SN, Gerber MA, et al. Expression of cytokeratins in normal and diseased livers and in primary liver carcinomas. *Arch Pathol Lab Med* 1989; **113**: 134–138.

181 Thung SN, Gerber MA, Sarno E, et al. Distribution of five antigens in hepatocellular carcinoma. *Lab Invest* 1979; **41**: 101–105.

182 Ordonez NG, Manning JT Jr. Comparison of alpha-1-antitrypsin and alpha-1-antichymotrypsin in hepatocellular carcinoma: an immunoperoxidase study. *Am J Gastroenterol* 1984; **79**: 959–963.

183 Chu PG, Weiss LM. Keratin expression in human tissues and neoplasms. *Histopathology* 2002; **40**: 403–439.

184 Fan Z, van de Rijn M, Montgomery K, et al. Hep Par 1 antibody stain for the differential diagnosis of hepatocellular carcinoma: 676 tumors tested using tissue microarrays and conventional tissue sections. *Mod Pathol* 2003; **16**: 137–144.

185 Morrison C, Marsh W, Frankel WL. A comparison of CD10 to pCEA, MOC-31, and hepatocyte for the distinction of malignant tumors in the liver. *Mod Pathol* 2002; **15**: 1279–1287.

186 Lau SK, Prakash S, Geller SA, Alsabeh R. Comparative immunohistochemical profile of hepatocellular carcinoma, cholangiocarcinoma, and metastatic adenocarcinoma. *Hum Pathol* 2002; **33**: 1175–1181.

187 Lei J-Y, Bourne PA, diSant'Agnese PA, et al. Cytoplasmic staining of TTF-1 in the differential diagnosis of

hepatocellular carcinoma vs. cholangiocarcinoma and metastatic carcinoma of the liver. *Am J Clin Pathol* 2006; **125**: 519–525.

188 Di Tommaso L, Destro A, Seok JY, et al. The application of markers (HSP70 GPC3 and GS) in liver biopsies is useful for detection of hepatocellular carcinoma. *J Hepatol* 2009; **50**: 746–754.

189 Ligato S, Mandich D, Cartun RW. Utility of glypican-3 in differentiating hepatocellular carcinoma from other primary and metastatic lesions in FNA of the liver: an immunocytochemical study. *Mod Pathol* 2008; **21**: 626–631.

190 Shafizadeh N, Ferrell LD, Kakar S. Utility and limitations of glypican-3 expression for the diagnosis of hepatocellular carcinoma at both ends of the differentiation spectrum. *Mod Pathol* 2008; **21**: 1011–1018.

191 Abdul-AL HM, Makhlouf HR, Wang G, et al. Glypican-3 expression in benign liver tissue with active hepatitis C: implications for the diagnosis of hepatocellular carcinoma. *Hum Pathol* 2008; **39**: 209–212.

192 Zynger DL, Everton MJ, Dimov ND, et al. Expression of glypican 3 in ovarian and extragonadal germ cell tumors. *Am J Clin Pathol* 2008; **130**: 224–230.

193 Maeda D, Ota S, Takazawa Y, et al. Glypican-3 expression in clear cell adenocarcinoma of the ovary. *Mod Pathol* 2009; **22**: 824–832.

194 Aviel-Ronen S, Lau SK, Pintilie M, et al. Glypican-3 is overexpressed in lung squamous cell carcinoma, but not in adenocarcinoma. *Mod Pathol* 2008; **21**: 817–825.

195 Nagorney DM, Adson MA, Weiland LH, et al. Fibrolamellar hepatoma. *Am J Surg* 1985; **149**: 113–119.

195a Kakar S, Burgart LJ, Batts KP, Garcia J, Jain D, Ferrell LD. Clinicopathologic features and survival in fibrolamellar carcinoma: comparison with conventional hepatocellular carcinoma with and without cirrhosis. *Mod Pathol* 2005; **18**: 1417–1423.

196 Berman MM, Libbey NP, Foster JH. Hepatocellular carcinoma. Polygonal cell type with fibrous stroma – an atypical variant with a favorable prognosis. *Cancer* 1980; **46**: 1448–1455.

197 Craig JR, Peters RL, Edmondson HA, et al. Fibrolamellar carcinoma of the liver: a tumor of adolescents and young adults with distinctive clinico-pathologic features. *Cancer* 1980; **46**: 372–379.

198 Berman MA, Burnham JA, Sheahan DG. Fibrolamellar carcinoma of the liver: an immunohistochemical study of nineteen cases and a review of the literature. *Hum Pathol* 1988; **19**: 784–794.

199 El-Serag HB, Davila JA. Is fibrolamellar carcinoma different from hepatocellular carcinoma? A US population-based study. *Hepatology* 2004; **39**: 798–803.

200 Vecchio FM, Fabiano A, Ghirlanda G, et al. Fibrolamellar carcinoma of the liver: the malignant counterpart of focal nodular hyperplasia with oncocytic change. *Am J Clin Pathol* 1984; **81**: 521–526.

201 Vecchio FM. Fibrolamellar carcinoma of the liver: a distinct entity within the hepatocellular tumors. A review. *Appl Pathol* 1988; **6**: 139–148.

202 Orsatti G, Hytiroglou P, Thung SN, et al. Lamellar fibrosis in the fibrolamellar variant of hepatocellular carcinoma: a role for transforming growth factor beta. *Liver* 1997; **17**: 152–156.

203 Farhi DC, Shikes RH, Silverberg SG. Ultrastructure of fibrolamellar oncocytic hepatoma. *Cancer* 1982; **50**: 702–709.

204 Lefkowitch JH, Muschel R, Price JB, et al. Copper and copper-binding protein in fibrolamellar liver cell carcinoma. *Cancer* 1983; **51**: 97–100.

205 Vecchio FM, Federico F, Dina MA. Copper and hepatocellular carcinoma. *Digestion* 1986; **35**: 109–114.

206 Teitelbaum DH, Tuttle S, Carey LC, et al. Fibrolamellar carcinoma of the liver. Review of three cases and the presentation of a characteristic set of tumor markers defining this tumor. *Ann Surg* 1985; **202**: 36–41.

207 Payne CM, Nagle RB, Paplanus SH, et al. Fibrolamellar carcinoma of liver: a primary malignant oncocytic carcinoid? *Ultrastruct Pathol* 1986; **10**: 539–552.

208 Subramony C, Herrera GA, Lockard V. Neuroendocrine differentiation in hepatic neoplasms: report of four cases. *Surg Pathol* 1993; **5**: 17–33.

208a Torbenson M. Review of the clinicopathologic features of fibrolamellar carcinoma. *Adv Anat Pathol* 2007; **14**: 217–223.

209 Okano A, Hajiro K, Takakuwa H, et al. Fibrolamellar carcinoma of the liver with a mixture of ordinary hepatocellular carcinoma: a case report. *Am J Gastroenterol* 1998; **93**: 1144–1145.

210 LeBrun DP, Silver MM, Freedman MH, et al. Fibrolamellar carcinoma of the liver in a patient with Fanconi anemia. *Hum Pathol* 1991; **22**: 396–398.

211 Gores GJ. Cholangiocarcinoma: current concepts and insights. *Hepatology* 2003; **37**: 961–969.

212 Klatskin G. Adenocarcinoma of the hepatic duct at its bifurcation within the porta hepatis. An unusual tumor with distinctive clinical and pathological features. *Am J Med* 1965; **38**: 241–256.

213 Schlinkert RT, Nagorney DM, Van Heerden JA, et al. Intrahepatic cholangiocarcinoma: clinical aspects, pathology and treatment. *HPB Surg* 1992; **5**: 95–102.

214 Case records of the Massachusetts General Hospital. Case 29-1987. *N Engl J Med* 1987; **317**: 153–160.

215 Bloustein PA. Association of carcinoma with congenital cystic conditions of the liver and bile ducts. *Am J Gastroenterol* 1977; **67**: 40–46.

216 Burns CD, Kuhns JG, Wieman J. Cholangiocarcinoma in association with multiple biliary microhamartomas. *Arch Pathol Lab Med* 1990; **114**: 1287–1289.

217 Yamato T, Sasaki M, Hoso M, et al. Intrahepatic cholangiocarcinoma arising in congenital hepatic fibrosis: report of an autopsy case. *J Hepatol* 1998; **28**: 717–722.

218 Hasebe T, Sakamoto M, Mukai K, et al. Cholangiocarcinoma arising in bile duct adenoma with focal area of bile duct hamartoma. *Virchows Arch* 1995; **426**: 209–213.

219 Kobayashi M, Ikeda K, Saitoh S, et al. Incidence of primary cholangiocellular carcinoma of the liver in Japanese patients with hepatitis C virus-related cirrhosis. *Cancer* 2000; **88**: 2471–2477.

220 Lau GKK, Davis GL, Wu SPC, et al. Hepatic expression of hepatitis C virus RNA in chronic hepatitis C: a study by in situ reverse-transcription polymerase chain reaction. *Hepatology* 1996; **23**: 1318–1323.

221 Komuta M, Spee B, Borght SV, et al. Clinicopathological study on cholangiolocellular carcinoma suggesting hepatic progenitor cell origin. *Hepatology* 2008; **47**: 1544–1556.

222 Chow LTC, Ahuja AT, Kwong KH, et al. Mucinous cholangiocarcinoma: an unusual complication of hepatolithiasis and recurrent pyogenic cholangitis. *Histopathology* 1997; **30**: 491–494.

223 Tihan T, Blumgart L, Klimstra DS. Clear cell papillary carcinoma of the liver: an unusual variant of peripheral cholangiocarcinoma. *Hum Pathol* 1998; **29**: 196–200.

224 Nakajima T, Knodo Y, Miyazaki M, et al. A histopathologic study of 102 cases of intrahepatic cholangiocarcinoma: histologic classification and modes of spreading. *Hum Pathol* 1988; **19**: 1228–1234.

225 Weinbren K, Mutum SS. Pathological aspects of cholangiocarcinoma. *J Pathol* 1983; **139**: 217–238.

226 Bonetti F, Chilosi M, Pisa R, et al. Epithelial membrane antigen expression in cholangiocarcinoma. A useful immunohistochemical tool for differential diagnosis with hepatocarcinoma. *Virchows Arch A Pathol Anat Histopathol* 1983; **401**: 307–313.

227 Pastolero GC, Wakabayashi T, Oka T, et al. Tissue polypeptide antigen – a marker antigen differentiating cholangiolar tumors from other hepatic tumors. *Am J Clin Pathol* 1987; **87**: 168–173.

228 Jovanovic R, Jagirdar J, Thung SN, et al. Blood-group-related antigen Lewis-X and Lewis-Y in the differential diagnosis of cholangiocarcinoma and hepatocellular carcinoma. *Arch Pathol Lab Med* 1989; **113**: 139–142.

229 Terada T, Nakanuma Y. An immunohistochemical survey of amylase isoenzymes in cholangiocarcinoma and hepatocellular carcinoma. *Arch Pathol Lab Med* 1993; **117**: 160–162.

230 Maeda T, Adachi E, Kajiyama K, et al. Combined hepatocellular and cholangiocarcinoma: proposed criteria according to cytokeratin expression and analysis of clinicopathologic features. *Hum Pathol* 1995; **26**: 956–964.

231 Haratake J, Hashimoto H. An immunohistochemical analysis of 13 cases with combined hepatocellular and cholangiocellular carcinoma. *Liver* 1995; **15**: 9–15.

232 Papotti M, Sambataro D, Marchesa P, et al. A combined hepatocellular/cholangiocellular carcinoma with sarcomatoid features. *Liver* 1997; **17**: 47–52.

233 Goodman ZD, Ishak KG, Langloss JM, et al. Combined hepatocellular-cholangiocarcinoma. A histologic and immunohistochemical study. *Cancer* 1985; **55**: 124–135.

234 Azizah N, Paradinas FJ. Cholangiocarcinoma coexisting with developmental liver cysts: a distinct entity different from liver cystadenocarcinoma. *Histopathology* 1980; **4**: 391–400.

235 Theise ND, Miller F, Worman HJ, et al. Biliary cystadenocarcinoma arising in a liver with fibropolycystic disease. *Arch Pathol Lab Med* 1993; **117**: 163–165.

236 Lander JJ, Stanley RJ, Sumner HW, et al. Angiosarcoma of the liver associated with Fowler's solution (potassium arsenite). *Gastroenterology* 1975; **68**: 1582–1586.

237 Horta JS. Late effects of thorotrast on the liver and spleen, and their efferent lymph nodes. *Ann N Y Acad Sci* 1967; **145**: 676–699.

238 Visfeldt J, Poulsen H. On the histopathology of liver and liver tumours in thorium- dioxide patients. *Acta Pathol Microbiol Scand A* 1972; **80**: 97–108.

239 Winberg CD, Ranchod M. Thorotrast induced hepatic cholangiocarcinoma and angiosarcoma. *Hum Pathol* 1979; **10**: 108–112.

240 Thomas LB, Popper H, Berk PD, et al. Vinyl-chloride-induced liver disease. From idiopathic portal hypertension (Banti's syndrome) to angiosarcomas. *N Engl J Med* 1975; **292**: 17–22.

241 Pimentel JC, Menezes AP. Liver disease in vineyard sprayers. *Gastroenterology* 1977; **72**: 275–283.

242 Hoch-Ligeti C. Angiosarcoma of the liver associated with diethylstilbestrol. *JAMA* 1978; **240**: 1510–1511.

243 Falk H, Thomas LB, Popper H, et al. Hepatic angiosarcoma associated with androgenic–anabolic steroids. *Lancet* 1979; **2**: 1120–1123.

244 Monroe PS, Riddell RH, Siegler M, et al. Hepatic angiosarcoma. Possible relationship to long-term oral contraceptive ingestion. *JAMA* 1981; **246**: 64–65.

245 Daneshmend TK, Scott GL, Bradfield JW. Angiosarcoma of liver associated with phenelzine. *BMJ* 1979; **1**: 1679.

246 Cadranel JF, Legendre C, Desaint B, et al. Liver disease from surreptitious administration of urethane. *J Clin Gastroenterol* 1993; **17**: 52–56.

247 Fortwengler HP Jr, Jones D, Espinosa E, et al. Evidence for endothelial cell origin of vinyl chloride-induced hepatic angiosarcoma. *Gastroenterology* 1981; **80**: 1415–1419.

248 Manning JT Jr, Ordonez NG, Barton JH. Endothelial cell origin of thorium oxide-induced angiosarcoma of liver. *Arch Pathol Lab Med* 1983; **107**: 456–458.

249 Popper H, Thomas LB, Telles NC, et al. Development of hepatic angiosarcoma in man induced by vinyl chloride, thorotrast, and arsenic. Comparison with cases of unknown etiology. *Am J Pathol* 1978; **92**: 349–369.

250 Tamburro CH, Makk L, Popper H. Early hepatic histologic alterations among chemical (vinyl monomer) workers. *Hepatology* 1984; **4**: 413–418.

251 Ishak KG, Sesterhenn IA, Goodman ZD, et al. Epithelioid hemangioendothelioma of the liver: a clinicopathologic and follow-up study of 32 cases. *Hum Pathol* 1984; **15**: 839–852.

252 Ishak KG. Malignant mesenchymal tumors of the liver. In: Okuda K, Ishak KG, eds. Neoplasms of the Liver. Tokyo: Springer-Verlag, 1987: 159–176.

253 Makhlouf HR, Ishak KG, Goodman ZD. Epithelioid hemangioendothelioma of the liver. A clinicopathologic study of 137 cases. *Cancer* 1999; **85**: 562–582.

254 Ekfors TO, Joensuu K, Toivio I, et al. Fatal epithelioid haemangioendothelioma presenting in the lung and liver. *Virchows Arch [A]* 1986; **410**: 9–16.

255 Dean PJ, Haggitt RC, O'Hara CJ. Malignant epithelioid hemangioendothelioma of the liver in young women. Relationship to oral contraceptive use. *Am J Surg Pathol* 1985; **9**: 695–704.

256 Demetris AJ, Minervini M, Raikow RB, et al. Hepatic epithelioid hemangioendothelioma. Biological questions based on pattern of recurrence in an allograft and tumor immunophenotype. *Am J Surg Pathol* 1997; **21**: 263–270.

257 Scoazec J-Y, Degott C, Reynes M, et al. Epithelioid hemangioendothelioma of the liver: an ultrastructural study. *Hum Pathol* 1989; **20**: 673–681.

258 Utz DC, Warren MM, Gregg JA, et al. Reversible hepatic dysfunction associated with hypernephroma. *Mayo Clin Proc* 1970; **45**: 161–169.

259 Strickland RC, Schenker S. The nephrogenic hepatic dysfunction syndrome: a review. [Review.] *Am J Dig Dis* 1977; **22**: 49–55.

260 Tao LC, Donat EE, Ho CS, et al. Percutaneous fine-needle aspiration biopsy of the liver. Cytodiagnosis of hepatic cancer. *Acta Cytol* 1979; **23**: 287–291.

261 Axe SR, Erozan YS, Ermatinger SV. Fine-needle aspiration of the liver. A comparison of smear and rinse preparations in the detection of cancer. *Am J Clin Pathol* 1986; **86**: 281–285.

262 Atterbury CE, Enriquez RE, Desuto-Nagy GI, et al. Comparison of the histologic and cytologic diagnosis of liver biopsies in hepatic cancer. *Gastroenterology* 1979; **76**: 1352–1357.

263 Gerber MA, Thung SN, Bodenheimer HC Jr, et al. Characteristic histologic triad in liver adjacent to metastatic neoplasm. *Liver* 1986; **6**: 85–88.

264 Glees JP, Thomas M, Redding WH, et al. Liver biopsy at lymphoma laparotomy [letter]. *Lancet* 1978; **1**: 210–211.

265 Kim H, Dorfman RF, Rosenberg SA. Pathology of malignant lymphomas of the liver: application in staging. In: Popper H, Schaffner F, eds. Progress in Liver Diseases, Vol. V. New York: Grune & Stratton, 1976; Ch. 40: 683–698.

266 Leslie KO, Colby TV. Hepatic parenchymal lymphoid aggregates in Hodgkin's disease. *Hum Pathol* 1984; **15**: 808–809.

267 Abt AB, Kirschner RH, Belliveau RE, et al. Hepatic pathology associated with Hodgkin's disease. *Cancer* 1974; **33**: 1564–1571.

268 Bruguera M, Caballero T, Carreras E, et al. Hepatic sinusoidal dilatation in Hodgkin's disease. *Liver* 1987; **7**: 76–80.

269 Perera DR, Greene ML, Fenster LF. Cholestasis associated with extrabiliary Hodgkin's disease. Report of three cases and review of four others. *Gastroenterology* 1974; **67**: 680–685.

270 Hubscher SG, Lumley MA, Elias E. Vanishing bile duct syndrome: a possible mechanism for intrahepatic cholestasis in Hodgkin's lymphoma. *Hepatology* 1993; **17**: 70–77.

271 Lefkowitch JH, Falkow S, Whitlock RT. Hepatic Hodgkin's disease simulating cholestatic hepatitis with liver failure. *Arch Pathol Lab Med* 1985; **109**: 424–426.

272 De Wolf-Peeters C. Liver involvement in lymphomas. *Ann Diagn Pathol* 1998; **2**: 363–369.

273 Trudel M, Aramendi T, Caplan S. Large-cell lymphoma presenting with hepatic sinusoidal infiltration. *Arch Pathol Lab Med* 1991; **115**: 821–824.

274 Dubois A, Dauzat M, Pignodel C, et al. Portal hypertension in lymphoproliferative and myeloproliferative disorders: hemodynamic and histological correlations. *Hepatology* 1993; **17**: 246–250.

275 Saló J, Nomdedeu B, Bruguera M, et al. Acute liver failure due to non-Hodgkin's lymphoma. *Am J Gastroenterol* 1993; **88**: 774–776.

276 Verdi CJ, Grogan TM, Protell R, et al. Liver biopsy immunotyping to characterize lymphoid malignancies. *Hepatology* 1986; **6**: 6–13.

277 Freeman C, Berg JW, Cutler SJ. Occurrence and prognosis of extranodal lymphomas. *Cancer* 1972; **29**: 252–260.

278 Zafrani ES, Gaulard P. Primary lymphoma of the liver. *Liver* 1993; **13**: 57–61.

279 Stemmer S, Geffen DB, Goldstein J, et al. Primary small noncleaved cell lymphoma of the liver. *J Clin Gastroenterol* 1993; **16**: 65–69.

280 Maes M, Depardieu C, Dargent J-L, et al. Primary low-grade B-cell lymphoma of MALT-type occurring in the liver: a study of two cases. *J Hepatol* 1997; **27**: 922–927.

281 Isaacson PG, Banks PM, Best PV, et al. Primary low-grade hepatic B-cell lymphoma of mucosa-associated lymphoid tissue (MALT)-type. *Am J Surg Pathol* 1995; **19**: 571–575.

282 Scoazec J-Y, Degott C, Brousse N, et al. Non-Hodgkin's lymphoma presenting as a primary tumor of the liver: presentation, diagnosis and outcome in eight patients. *Hepatology* 1991; **13**: 870–875.

283 Kim JH, Kim HY, Kang I, et al. A case of primary hepatic lymphoma with hepatitis C liver cirrhosis. *Am J Gastroenterol* 2000; **95**: 2377–2380.

284 Rasul I, Shepherd FA, Kamel-Reid S, et al. Detection of occult low-grade B-cell non-Hodgkin's lymphoma in patient's with chronic hepatitis C infection and mixed cryoglobulinemia. *Hepatology* 1999; **29**: 543–547.

285 Lin A, Kadam JS, Bodenheimer HC, et al. Concomitant diffuse large B-cell lymphoma and hepatocellular carcinoma in chronic hepatitis C virus liver disease: a study of two cases. *J Med Virol* 2008; **80**: 1350–1353.

286 Ohshima K, Haraoka S, Harada N, et al. Hepatosplenic γδ T-cell lymphoma: relation to Epstein–Barr virus and activated cytotoxic molecules. *Histopathology* 2000; **36**: 127–135.

287 Suarez F, Wlodarski I, Rigal-Huguet F, et al. Hepatosplenic αβ T-cell lymphoma. An unusual case with clinical, histologic, and cytogenetic features of γδ hepatosplenic T-cell lymphoma. *Am J Surg Pathol* 2000; **24**: 1027–1032.

288 Thomas FB, Clausen KP, Greenberger NJ. Liver disease in multiple myeloma. *Arch Intern Med* 1973; **132**: 195–202.

289 Weichhold W, Labouyrie E, Merlio JPh, et al. Primary extramedullary plasmacytoma of the liver. A case report. *Am J Surg Pathol* 1995; **19**: 1197–1202.

290 Brooks AP. Portal hypertension in Waldenstrom's macroglobulinaemia. *BMJ* 1976; **1**: 689–690.

291 Lévy S, Capron D, Joly J-P, et al. Hepatic nodules as single organ involvement in an adult with Langerhans cell granulomatosis. *J Clin Gastroenterol* 1998; **26**: 69–73.

292 Foschini MP, Milandri GL, Dina RE, et al. Benign regressing histiocytosis of the liver. *Histopathology* 1995; **26**: 363–366.

293 Kaplan KJ, Goodman ZD, Ishak KG. Liver involvement in Langerhans' cell histiocytosis: a study of nine cases. *Mod Pathol* 1999; **12**: 370–378.

294 Yam LT, Chan CH, Li CY. Hepatic involvement in systemic mast cell disease. *Am J Med* 1986; **80**: 819–826.

295 Scheimberg IB, Pollock DJ, Collins PW, et al. Pathology of the liver in leukaemia and lymphoma. A study of 110 autopsies. *Histopathology* 1995; **26**: 311–321.

296 Schwartz JB, Shamsuddin AM. The effects of leukemic infiltrates in various organs in chronic lymphocytic leukemia. *Hum Pathol* 1981; **12**: 432–440.

297 Roquet ML, Zafrani ES, Farcet JP, et al. Histopathological lesions of the liver in hairy cell leukemia: a report of 14 cases. *Hepatology* 1985; **5**: 496–500.

298 Yam LT, Janckila AJ, Chan CH, et al. Hepatic involvement in hairy cell leukemia. *Cancer* 1983; **51**: 1497–1504.

299 Zafrani ES, Degos F, Guigui B, et al. The hepatic sinusoid in hairy cell leukemia: an ultrastructural study of 12 cases. *Hum Pathol* 1987; **18**: 801–807.

300 Grouls V, Stiens R. Hepatic involvement in hairy cell leukemia: diagnosis by tartrate-resistant acid phosphatase

enzyme histochemistry on formalin fixed and paraffin-embedded liver biopsy specimens. *Pathol Res Pract* 1984; **178:** 332–334.

301 Wheeler DA, Edmondson HA, Reynolds TB. Spontaneous liver cell adenoma in children. *Am J Clin Pathol* 1986; **85:** 6–12.

302 Resnick MB, Kozakewich HPW, Perez-Atayde AR. Hepatic adenoma in the pediatric age group. Clinicopathological observations and assessment of cell proliferative activity. *Am J Surg Pathol* 1995; **19:** 1181–1190.

303 Lautz TB, Finegold MJ, Chin AC, et al. Giant hepatic adenoma with atypical features in a patient on oxcarbazepine therapy. *J Pediatr Surg* 2008; **42:** 751–754.

304 Janes CH, McGill DB, Ludwig J, et al. Liver cell adenoma at the age of 3 years and transplantation 19 years later after development of carcinoma: a case report. *Hepatology* 1993; **17:** 583–585.

305 Moran CA, Mullick FG, Ishak KG. Nodular regenerative hyperplasia of the liver in children. *Am J Surg Pathol* 1991; **15:** 449–454.

306 Srouji MN, Chatten J, Schulman WM, et al. Mesenchymal hamartoma of the liver in infants. [Review.] *Cancer* 1978; **42:** 2483–2489.

307 Stocker JT, Ishak KG. Mesenchymal hamartoma of the liver: report of 30 cases and review of the literature. *Pediatr Pathol* 1983; **1:** 245–267.

308 Cook JR, Pfeifer JD, Dehner LP. Mesenchymal hamartoma of the liver in the adult: association with distinct clinical features and histological changes. *Hum Pathol* 2002; **33:** 893–898.

309 Lauwers GY, Grant LD, Donnelly WH, et al. Hepatic undifferentiated (embryonal) sarcoma arising in a mesenchymal hamartoma. *Am J Surg Pathol* 1997; **21:** 1248–1254.

310 Dehner LP, Ishak KG. Vascular tumors of the liver in infants and children. A study of 30 cases and review of the literature. *Arch Pathol* 1971; **92:** 101–111.

311 Selby DM, Stocker JT, Waclawiw MA, et al. Infantile hemangioendothelioma of the liver. *Hepatology* 1994; **20:** 39–45.

312 Dimashkieh HH, Mo JQ, Wyatt-Ashmead J, et al. Pediatric hepatic angiosarcoma: case report and review of the literature. *Pediatr Dev Pathol* 2004; **7:** 527–532.

313 Dachman AH, Lichtenstein JE, Friedman AC, et al. Infantile hemangioendothelioma of the liver: a radiologic–pathologic–clinical correlation. *AJR Am J Roentgenol* 1983; **140:** 1091–1096.

314 Darbari A, Sabin KM, Shapiro CN, et al. Epidemiology of primary hepatic malignancies in US children. *Hepatology* 2003; **38:** 560–566.

315 Stocker JT, Ishak KG. Hepatoblastoma. In: Okuda K, Ishak KG, eds. Neoplasms of the Liver. Tokyo: Springer-Verlag, 1987; Ch. 9: 127–136.

316 Ishak KG, Glunz PR. Hepatoblastoma and hepatocarcinoma in infancy and childhood. Report of 47 cases. *Cancer* 1967; **20:** 396–422.

317 Lack EE, Neave C, Vawter GF. Hepatoblastoma. A clinical and pathologic study of 54 cases. *Am J Surg Pathol* 1982; **6:** 693–705.

318 Kasai M, Watanabe I. Histologic classification of liver cell carcinoma in infancy and childhood and its clinical evaluation. *Cancer* 1970; **25:** 551–563.

319 Weinberg AG, Finegold MJ. Primary hepatic tumors of childhood. [Review.] *Hum Pathol* 1983; **14:** 512–537.

320 Rugge M, Sonego F, Pollice L, et al. Hepatoblastoma: DNA nuclear content, proliferative indices, and pathology. *Liver* 1998; **18:** 128–133.

321 Gonzalez-Crussi F, Upton MP, Maurer HS. Hepatoblastoma. Attempt at characterization of histologic subtypes. *Am J Surg Pathol* 1982; **6:** 599–612.

322 Abenoza P, Manivel JC, Wick MR, et al. Hepatoblastoma: an immunohistochemical and ultrastructural study. *Hum Pathol* 1987; **18:** 1025–1035.

323 Stocker JT, Ishak KG. Undifferentiated (embryonal) sarcoma of the liver: report of 31 cases. *Cancer* 1978; **42:** 336–348.

324 Keating S, Taylor GP. Undifferentiated (embryonal) sarcoma of the liver: ultrastructural and immunohistochemical similarities with malignant fibrous histiocytoma. *Hum Pathol* 1985; **16:** 693–699.

325 Aoyama C, Hachitanda Y, Sato JK, et al. Undifferentiated (embryonal) sarcoma of the liver. A tumor of uncertain histogenesis showing divergent differentiation. *Am J Surg Pathol* 1991; **15:** 615–624.

326 Lack EE, Schloo BL, Azumi N, et al. Undifferentiated (embryonal) sarcoma of the liver. Clinical and pathologic study of 16 cases with emphasis on immunohistochemical features. *Am J Surg Pathol* 1991; **15:** 1–16.

327 Heerema-McKenney A, Leuschner I, Smith N, et al. Nested stromal epithelial tumor of the liver. Six cases of a distinctive pediatric neoplasm with frequent calcifications and association with Cushing syndrome. *Am J Surg Pathol* 2005; **29:** 10–20.

328 Hill DA, Swanson PE, Anderson K, et al. Desmoplastic nested spindle cell tumor of liver. Report of four cases of a proposed new entity. *Am J Surg Pathol* 2005; **29:** 1–9.

329 Makhlouf HR, Abdul-AL HM, Wang G, et al. Calcifying nested stromal–epithelial tumors of the liver. A clinicopathologic, immunohistochemical, and molecular genetic study of 9 cases with a long-term follow-up. *Am J Surg Pathol* 2009; **33:** 976–983.

330 Mills AE. Undifferentiated primary hepatic non-Hodgkin's lymphoma in childhood. *Am J Surg Pathol* 1988; **12:** 721–726.

331 Caturelli E, Solmi L, Anti M, et al. Ultrasound guided fine needle biopsy of early hepatocellular carcinoma complicating liver cirrhosis: a multicentre study. *Gut* 2004; **53:** 1356–1362.

332 Bottles K, Cohen MB. An approach to fine-needle aspiration biopsy diagnosis of hepatic masses. *Diagn Cytopathol* 1991; **7:** 204–210.

333 Frias-Hidvegi D. Guides to Clinical Aspiration Biopsy. Liver and Pancreas. New York & Tokyo: Igaku-Shoin, 1988: 27–42.

334 Suen KC. Diagnosis of primary hepatic neoplasms by fine needle aspiration cytology. *Diagn Cytopathol* 1986; **2:** 99–109.

335 Perry MD, Johnson WW. Needle biopsy of the liver for the diagnosis of nonneoplastic liver disease. *Acta Cytol* 1985; **29:** 385–390.

336 Tao L-C. Are oral contraceptive-associated liver cell adenomas premalignant? *Acta Cytol* 1992; **36:** 338–344.

337 Ruschenberg I, Droese M. Fine needle aspiration cytology of focal nodular hyperplasia of the liver. *Acta Cytol* 1989; **33:** 857–860.

338 Taavitsainen M, Airaksinin T, Kreula J, et al. Fine-needle aspiration biopsy of liver hemangioma. *Acta Radiol* 1990; **31:** 69–71.

339 Yang GCH, Yang G-Y, Tao L-C. Distinguishing well-differentiated hepatocellular carcinoma from benign liver by the physical features of fine-needle aspirates. *Mod Pathol* 2004; **17**: 798–802.

340 Pedio G, Landolt U, Zobeli L, et al. Fine needle aspiration of the liver. Significance of hepatocytic naked nuclei in the diagnosis of hepatocellular carcinoma. *Acta Cytol* 1988; **32**: 437–442.

341 Cohen MB, Haber MM, Holly EA, et al. Cytologic criteria to distinguish hepatocellular carcinoma from non-neoplastic liver. *Am J Clin Pathol* 1991; **95**: 125–130.

342 Wee A, Nilsson B, Chan-Wilde C, et al. Fine needle aspiration biopsy of hepatocellular carcinoma: some unusual features. *Acta Cytol* 1991; **35**: 661–670.

343 Donat EE, Anderson V, Tao L-C. Cytodiagnosis of clear cell hepatocellular carcinoma. A case report. *Acta Cytol* 1991; **35**: 671–675.

344 Nguyen G-K. Fine-needle aspiration biopsy cytology of hepatic tumors in adults. *Pathol Annu* 1986; **21**: 321–349.

345 Davenport RD. Cytologic diagnosis of fibrolamellar carcinoma of the liver by fine-needle aspiration. *Diagn Cytopathol* 1990; **6**: 275–279.

346 Wakely PEJ, Silverman JF, Geisinger KR, et al. Fine needle aspiration cytology of hepatoblastoma. *Mod Pathol* 1990; **3**: 688–693.

347 Dekmezian R, Sneigi N, Papok S, et al. Fine needle aspiration cytology of pediatric patients with primary hepatic tumors. *Diagn Cytopathol* 1988; **4**: 162–168.

348 Saleh HA, Tao LC. Hepatic angiosarcoma: aspiration biopsy cytology and immunocytochemical contribution. *Diagn Cytopathol* 1998; **18**: 208–211.

349 Siddiqui MT, Reddy VB, Castelli MJ, et al. Role of fine-needle aspiration in clinical management of transplant patients. *Diagn Cytopathol* 1997; **17**: 429–435.

350 Flanders E, Kornstein M, Wakely P, et al. Lymphoglandular bodies in fine-needle aspiration cytology smears. *Am J Clin Pathol* 1993; **99**: 566–569.

General reading

Blechacz B, Gores GJ. Cholangiocarcinoma: advances in pathogenesis, diagnosis, and treatment. *Hepatology* 2008; **48**: 308–321.

DeMay RM. Practical Principles of Cytopathology. Chicago, IL: ASCP Press, 1999: 307–320.

El-Serag HB, Rudolph KL. Hepatocellular carcinoma: epidemiology and molecular carcinogenesis. *Gastroenterology* 2007; **132**: 2557–2576.

Goodman ZD, Terracciano L. Tumours and tumour-like lesions of the liver. In: Burt AD, Portmann BC, Ferrell LD, eds. Pathology of the Liver, 5th edn. Edinburgh: Churchill Livingstone/Elsevier, 2007: 761–814.

Kakar S, Gown AM, Goodman ZD, Ferrell LD. Best practices in diagnostic immunohistochemistry. Hepatocellular carcinoma versus metastatic neoplasms. *Arch Pathol Lab Med* 2007; **131**: 1648–1654.

Okuda K, Ishak KG, eds. Neoplasms of the Liver. Tokyo: Springer-Verlag, 1987.

Pitman MB, Szyfelbein WM, eds. Fine Needle Aspiration Biopsy of the Liver. A Color Atlas. Boston: Butterworth-Heinemann, 1994.

Tao L-C. Liver and pancreas. In: Bibbo M, ed. Comprehensive Cytopathology, 2nd edn. Philadelphia, PA: WB Saunders, 1997: 827–864.

Vascular Disorders 12

The hepatic arteries

The effects of occlusion of hepatic artery branches are unpredictable because of the liver's double blood supply and variable collateral flow. Potential effects of thrombotic or other occlusion include infarction, and ischaemic damage to the biliary tree leading to stricture formation, cholangitis or duct rupture.[1-3] The branches of the hepatic artery are sometimes involved in **polyarteritis nodosa**,[2,4] the arteritis of **systemic lupus erythematosus**,[5] **Schön-lein–Henoch purpura**[3] and **giant-cell arteritis**.[6] In the last the liver may contain granulomas of classical[7] or fibrin-ring type.[8] The arterial lesions of these systemic diseases are not often seen in needle biopsies of the liver. Vasculitis affecting small intrahepatic vessels is sometimes a manifestation of infection or neoplasia.

In some older patients, especially those with systemic hypertension, small arteries and arterioles in portal tracts appear thickened and hyaline. **Amyloidosis** can give rise to thickening of arterial walls in the absence of sinusoidal deposits.

The arteriovenous malformations and telangiectases of **hereditary haemorrhagic telangiectasia** are sometimes found in the liver, with or without surrounding fibrosis.[9] The presentation is as portal hypertension (accompanied by hepatic encephalopathy and nodular regeneration[10,11]), biliary disease (sometimes resembling primary sclerosing cholangitis or Caroli's disease) or cardiac failure due to arteriovenous shunting.[12] Patients with liver involvement may have raised serum alkaline phosphatase levels without jaundice ('anicteric cholestasis'), attributed to abnormal blood supply to the biliary tree.[13] Severely damaged medium-sized bile ducts are occasionally seen histologically.

Infarcts of the liver result from arteritis, aneurysms, thrombosis, embolism or surgical ligation. They may complicate pregnancy or liver transplantation. Infarction can also follow occlusion of portal-vein branches,[14] and may even be found in the absence of demonstrable vascular obstruction. The pathological features are as in other organs: there are well-defined zones of coagulative necrosis with congested and inflamed borders (**Fig. 12.1**). Portal tracts may survive within the infarcted areas. Coagulative necrosis of the centres of cirrhotic nodules following hypoperfusion is sometimes called nodular infarction.

Shock, heart failure and heatstroke

Severe hypoperfusion of the hepatic parenchyma leads to necrosis, usually in perivenular regions (acinar zone 3) but also, additionally or alternatively, in mid-zonal regions (zone 2).[15] Portal tracts and the periportal parenchyma typically remain normal. In contrast to

©2010 Elsevier Ltd
DOI: 10.1016/B978-0-7020-3410-7.00018-6

Figure 12.1
Infarct.
The dead parenchyma to the right is intensely congested. Surviving liver tissue (left) is fatty. (Post-mortem liver, H&E.)

the necrosis of acute hepatitis there is usually little or no inflammation, but in some patients neutrophils accumulate in limited numbers, particularly if the individual has received pressor support for 1 or more days.[16] Affected areas may be congested, and contain large, ceroid-laden macrophages. There may be cholestasis and evidence of regenerative hyperplasia in the surviving parenchyma. The reticulin network shows regular condensation in the necrotic areas. Similar changes are seen in patients with heatstroke (**Fig. 12.2**). There may be steatosis in the surviving parenchyma. Inflammation ranges from absent in mild cases[17] to severe when the damage is extensive.[18] Systemic candidiasis is a complication.

One of the most important causes of this type of necrosis is heart failure with consequent hypoperfusion of the liver. The term ischaemic hepatitis is commonly used for the viral hepatitis-like clinical picture which may ensue.[19] Congestive heart failure leads to sinusoidal dilatation (see Venous congestion and outflow obstruction).

The portal veins

Thrombosis of the main portal veins may result from infection (local or in the portal venous drainage area), cirrhosis,[20] liver transplantation, disorders of coagulation and venous outflow obstruction.[21] Invasion by hepatocellular carcinoma is a common cause. In some patients no reason for the thrombosis can be discovered, but an underlying thrombophilic condition should always be excluded.[20] In the acute phase of pylephlebitis, septic thrombi may be seen in portal-vein branches in portal tracts (**Fig. 12.3**).

Possible results of portal-vein thrombosis include diffuse or focal parenchymal atrophy, increase in the number of apoptotic hepatocytes,[22] parenchymal nodularity (see Nodular regenerative hyperplasia, **Ch. 11**), and a mild degree of portal fibrosis. Focal atrophy, also known as Zahn's infarction, is often found at the margins of tumour nodules. Occasionally portal venous obstruction leads to true infarction of the hepatic parenchyma.[14] In many patients with thrombosis of the main portal veins the liver remains histologically normal.

**Figure 12.2
Heatstroke.**
There has been confluent necrosis in acinar zone 3. (Needle biopsy, H&E.) (Section kindly provided by Professor Helmut Denk, Graz, Austria.)

**Figure 12.3
Pylephlebitis.**
Thrombus with inflammatory cells, outlined by arrowheads, fills a portal-vein branch. The surrounding portal tract is also inflamed. (Wedge biopsy, H&E.)

Portal hypertension

Portal hypertension is most often the result of cirrhosis. Other causes include schisto-somiasis, alcohol-related liver disease, non-alcoholic steatohepatitis, congenital hepatic fibrosis, the tropical splenomegaly syndrome, hepatic venous outflow obstruction and portal venous thrombosis. The last probably contributes to portal hypertension in

Figure 12.4 Non-cirrhotic portal hypertension.
The portal-vein branches in the two portal tracts are widely dilated and appear to have herniated into the parenchyma. (Needle biopsy, H&E.) (Section kindly provided by Professor Helmut Denk, Graz, Austria.)

polycythaemia and other haematological diseases.[23] In lymphoproliferative and myelo-proliferative disorders, the portal infiltration may be a further pathogenetic factor.[24] The anatomical subdivision of portal hypertension into pre-hepatic, intra-hepatic and post-hepatic forms should be considered in conjunction with specific structural alterations in classifying the individual case.[25]

There remains a somewhat ill-defined group of patients with portal hypertension not attributable to cirrhosis or to the other causes mentioned above (**non-cirrhotic portal hypertension**). In a few cases the condition is attributable to a toxin or toxins such as arsenic,[26] vinyl chloride[27,28] or cytotoxic drugs,[29] but in the majority no cause can be found. Several different labels have been used to describe aspects of this group (**hepatoportal sclerosis, non-cirrhotic portal fibrosis, idiopathic portal hypertension**). The term **obliterative portal venopathy** indicates that there may be demonstrable thrombosis or narrowing of portal-vein branches, but this is not always the case, and it is not clear whether the portal venous narrowing or occlusion is primary or secondary.

Needle liver biopsies from patients with non-cirrhotic portal hypertension are often normal or show only non-specific changes. Abnormalities are more likely to be seen in operative wedge biopsies. Portal-vein branches are sometimes thickened and narrowed, unusually inconspicuous or replaced by multiple small, thin-walled channels. Their overall area is reduced, while portal tract lymphatics increase in number.[30] Dilated venules appear to herniate into the adjacent parenchyma[31,32] (**Fig. 12.4**). There may be portal fibrosis and enlargement, with or without inflammatory-cell infiltration (**Fig. 12.5**). Slender fibrous septa extending from the portal tracts give an appearance indistinguishable from incomplete septal cirrhosis.[33] These septa sometimes connect with bridge-like zones of necrosis.[31] There may be randomly distributed thin-walled vessels in the lobules ('megasinusoids'), and sclerosis or dilatation of efferent veins.[31]

Diffuse or localised nodular hyperplasia of the parenchyma is commonly seen in these patients. There is thus overlap between hepatoportal sclerosis, nodular regenerative hyperplasia, incomplete septal cirrhosis[33,34] and, rarely, partial nodular transformation.[35] Nodular

Figure 12.5 Non-cirrhotic portal hypertension. An enlarged, sclerotic portal tract contains arteries (a) and bile ducts (b), but portal-vein branches are inconspicuous. (Wedge biopsy, H&E.)

regenerative hyperplasia, however, is also found in the absence of clinically evident portal hypertension.

In patients exposed to vinyl chloride monomer and other carcinogens there may be, in addition to the above features, perisinusoidal fibrosis and an increase in the number and size of sinusoidal cells.[27,28] Perisinusoidal fibrosis may also contribute to the portal hypertension which develops in some patients after renal transplantation.[36] Prolonged drug therapy has been suggested as a possible mechanism.

The hepatic sinusoids

The width of the sinusoids in liver biopsy specimens is very variable. It is influenced not only by the state of the patient's circulation at the time of biopsy, but also by fixation and tissue processing. Slight variations in width are therefore of doubtful significance.

The amount of connective tissue in sinusoidal walls should also be assessed critically, since its appearance varies with section thickness. A definite increase in fibres is characteristic of chronic venous outflow obstruction and of steatohepatitis. In the former the pattern of fibrosis is usually linear (peri- or parasinusoidal fibrosis), while in steatohepatitis the fibrosis surrounds hepatocytes (pericellular fibrosis). Increased sinusoidal type IV collagen in diabetic hepatosclerosis[37] is also in the differential diagnosis (**see Ch. 7**). Other causes and associations, some of them already mentioned above, include congenital syphilis, vinyl chloride toxicity, heroin addiction,[38] hypervitaminosis A,[39] diabetes,[40] renal transplantation, myeloid metaplasia[41] and thrombocytopenic purpura.[42] Endothelial cells lining the hepatic sinusoids sometimes contain iron-rich granules of uncertain significance, especially in viral hepatitis[43] and alcoholic liver disease. Immunoglobulin-containing eosinophilic granules have been reported, particularly in chronic hepatitis[44,45] (**see Fig. 9.12**).

**Figure 12.6
Sinusoidal
dilatation.**
Dilated periportal
and midzonal
sinsuoids are seen to
the left, and a
terminal hepatic
venule to the right.
The dilatation was
attributed to an oral
contraceptive
steroid. (Needle
biopsy, H&E.)
(Section kindly
provided by
Professor Hemming
Poulsen,
Copenhagen,
Denmark.)

**Figure 12.6
Sinusoidal
dilatation.**
Dilated periportal
and midzonal
sinsuoids are seen to
the left, and a
terminal hepatic
venule to the right.
The dilatation was
attributed to an oral
contraceptive
steroid. (Needle
biopsy, H&E.)
(Section kindly
provided by
Professor Hemming
Poulsen,
Copenhagen,
Denmark.)

Definite and regular **dilatation** of the sinusoidal network is associated with several conditions, the most important being venous outflow obstruction (see below). It has been reported in patients with tumours or granulomas, even when these did not involve the liver,[46] in Crohn's disease,[47] in patients with anti-cardiolipin antibodies and features of the antiphospholipid syndrome,[48] haemophagocytic syndrome[49] and in heroin addicts.[50] Sinusoidal dilatation and congestion in the absence of venous outflow obstruction may also be seen with portal-vein thrombosis and congenital absence, rheumatoid arthritis, Still's disease, and in wedge biopsies taken during abdominal surgery.[51] Dilatation of peri-portal and mid-zonal sinusoids has been described in a small number of patients taking oral contraceptives[52,53] (**Fig. 12.6**). In some patients with renal cell carcinoma there is focal dilatation of mid-zonal sinusoids.[54]

Peliosis hepatis

The borderline between regular diffuse dilatation and the focal dilatation known as pelio-sis hepatis is not always sharp.[54,55] In peliosis, blood-filled cysts are found in the paren-chyma (**Fig. 12.7**), ranging in size from less than 1 to several millimetres in diameter. The endothelial lining is usually incomplete.[56] Peliosis is found in association with many different conditions and circumstances including wasting diseases, asphyxia,[57] neoplasia,[58] liver and renal transplantation,[59,60] drug therapy[61,62] and bacterial infection.[63] The lesion is often discovered incidentally, but rupture leading to haemoperitoneum has been reported.[63,64] Bacillary peliosis hepatis (**see Ch. 15**) is a different lesion, and is attributed to the bacteria which cause cutaneous bacillary angiomatosis in patients with AIDS. Their presence in silver preparations distinguishes the condition from simple peliosis.

Disseminated intravascular coagulation

This commonly involves the liver.[65] Sinusoids and small portal vessels contain fibrin thrombi (**Fig. 12.8**), but the fibrin is often difficult to identify with certainty in

Figure 12.7
Peliosis.
There are blood-
filled spaces within
the parenchyma.
(Needle biopsy,
H&E.)

Figure 12.8
Disseminated
intravascular
coagulation.
Periportal sinusoids
are filled with fibrin
and neutrophils.
(Needle biopsy,
H&E.)

**Figure 12.9
Sickle-cell disease.**
Clumped and sickled erythrocytes are seen in distended sinusoids. (Needle biopsy, H&E.)

conventional sections. Similar changes are seen in eclampsia, in association with periportal necrosis and acute inflammation. In congestive cardiac failure thrombi may form in the sinusoids.[66]

Sickle-cell disease

In most patients with sickle-cell disease clumps of sickled erythrocytes are found in dilated sinusoids[67] (**Fig. 12.9**). Lesions of peliosis may develop, and there is often some degree of perisinusoidal fibrosis. There is erythrophagocytosis, and hypertrophied Kupffer cells and hepatocytes contain iron. Hepatocytes may show atrophy and ischaemic necrosis[68] as well as evidence of regeneration. The degree of sickling seen does not correlate with biochemical or clinical evidence of liver damage, and some hepatic manifestations in patients with sickle-cell disease are thought to be the result of complications such as transfusion-related hepatitis,[69] siderosis, cholelithiasis and venous outflow obstruction. Cirrhosis occasionally develops, possibly as a consequence of viral hepatitis.

Venous congestion and outflow obstruction

Interference with the venous outflow of the liver results from a multitude of causes ranging from congestive cardiac failure to occlusion of the smallest tributaries of the hepatic veins within the liver. Space-occupying lesions such as tumours may cause localised obstruction affecting only parts of the liver. The term **Budd–Chiari syndrome** is often used to describe the clinical findings when the inferior vena cava or main hepatic veins are obstructed, and is sometimes extended to obstruction at the level of the heart.[70] Further classification should be based on the nature and location of the obstruction.[71] The pathologist faced with a severely congested liver biopsy is often unsure about the level and nature of the block. Use of the term **venous outflow obstruction** is then appropriate.

Figure 12.10 Venous congestion. Perivenular sinusoids are dilated. The pale zone of necrosis indicates an element of hypoperfusion. Kupffer cells in and around this area are loaded with brown ceroid pigment. (Needle biopsy, H&E.)

Congestive cardiac failure

The terminal hepatic venules and adjacent sinusoids show variable combinations of dilatation and congestion in patients with congestive failure.[72] The degree of dilatation or congestion can vary from lobule to lobule in a given tissue section. As already noted, the congestion may be accompanied by hepatocellular necrosis if there is also a significant element of hypoperfusion (**Fig. 12.10**), as in the combination of right- and left-sided heart failure. Sinusoidal and venous thrombosis may also contribute to hepatocellular damage.[66] Blood may infiltrate the liver-cell plates.[73] Canalicular cholestasis is sometimes seen, and must be distinguished from the commonly found ceroid pigment in Kupffer cells. Inflammation is typically mild or absent, and portal tracts usually remain normal. Periportal necrosis occurs rarely.[72] There may be regenerative hyperplasia of hepatocytes; chronic venous congestion is one cause of nodular regenerative hyperplasia and, very rarely, cirrhosis.[72] Perivenular and perisinusoidal fibrosis ('cardiac sclerosis') reflects prior episodes of failure.[16,72] In some patients hepatocytes contain periodic acid–Schiff (PAS)-positive globules which probably represent phagosomes containing imbibed plasma proteins.[74] The globules are usually located in or near the congested areas. They can be distinguished from the globules of α_1-antitrypsin deficiency by their location and, if necessary, by immunochemical staining.

Obstruction to large veins

Obstruction of the inferior vena cava or the main hepatic veins typically causes severe congestion. The many causes include thrombosis related to myeloproliferative disorders,[9,75] predisposing coagulopathies[76] and other haematological diseases. Disorders characterised by vasculitis, such as Behçet's disease, may be complicated by either venous outflow obstruction[77,78] or portal-vein obstruction.[79] An association of outflow obstruction with the use of oral contraceptives lacks conclusive proof.[80] Fibrous webs may represent a late consequence of thrombosis,[81,82] but there is some evidence to support an alternative,

Figure 12.11 Acute venous outflow obstruction.

In this example, owing to obstruction of major veins (Budd–Chiari syndrome), much of the parenchyma has been replaced by blood. A few hepatocytes have survived around the portal tract (below right). (Wedge biopsy, H&E.)

non-thrombotic pathogenesis.[83] Occasionally the obstruction results from adminstration of chemotherapeutic agents[9] or infection.[84] In some patients no cause can be discovered. While in Western countries primary hepatic vein thrombosis is commoner than obliterative disease of the inferior vena cava ('obliterative cavopathy'), the reverse is true in the developing world.[85] Caval obstruction is often complicated by hepatocellular carcinoma.

In the acute stages much of the parenchyma may be replaced by blood. Sinusoids at the border between the haemorrhagic zones and the surviving parenchyma are dilated and empty (**Fig. 12.11**). Small efferent veins may be narrowed or blocked, depending on the cause of the obstruction (see discussion of veno-occlusive disease, below). Portal-vein branches may also be thrombosed.[86] In acute or chronic venous outflow obstruction it is common to find normal-appearing portal tracts, but there may also be portal features that mimic biliary tract disease, including a ductular reaction, inflammation, and portal and/or periportal fibrosis, typically unassociated with cholestasis.[87] Eventually the haemorrhage and congestion lead to fibrosis or even cirrhosis (**Fig. 12.12**). The pattern of cirrhosis following venous outflow obstruction is influenced by the presence or absence of concomitant portal venous thrombosis; this is associated with extensive portal–central–portal bridging, with presence of portal tracts within the fibrous septa.[21] In some cases parenchymal nodularity is due to nodular regenerative hyperplasia rather than true cirrhosis, and isolated nodules resembling focal nodular hyperplasia (**see Ch. 11**) can develop as a result of locally increased arterial blood flow.[86]

Fibrosis is often difficult to distinguish from simple acute condensation of pre-existing reticulin and collagen. Stains for elastic fibres are then sometimes helpful, as in the distinction between bridging necrosis and fibrosis (**see Ch. 4**). Two further diagnostic problems should be noted. First, blocked veins may be missed in haematoxylin and eosin stained sections so that a collagen stain should be examined if venous outflow obstruction is suspected. Thin-walled bypass channels should not be mistaken for patent veins. Second, the obstruction may not affect all the hepatic veins, so that parts of the liver escape serious congestion. As a result, biopsy samples may show considerable regional variability, which

Figure 12.12
Chronic venous outflow obstruction.
Late in the disease fibrous tissue has been laid down in the congested areas, top left. Surviving parenchyma shows 'reversed lobulation' around a portal tract. (Needle biopsy, H&E.)

can lead to diagnostic confusion. It follows that a near-normal liver biopsy does not exclude a diagnosis of venous outflow obstruction.

Sinusoidal obstruction syndrome/veno-occlusive disease

The recent term **sinusoidal obstruction syndrome** (SOS) has been used to describe the spectrum of sinusoidal congestion, dilatation, thrombosis and fibrous occlusion of efferent venules which develop due to injury to sinusoidal endothelial injury of varying aetiology, often chemical.[9,88] **Veno-occlusive disease** (VOD) – in which the smallest tributaries of the hepatic veins, the terminal hepatic venules and sublobular veins are occluded by fibrous tissue (**Fig. 12.13**) – is a manifestation of SOS. The venous lesions can thus be detected in needle biopsies. There is often associated fibrosis of sinusoidal walls (perisinusoidal fibrosis), probably mediated by hepatic stellate cells.[89] Apart from these lesions the changes are as for obstruction of large veins. As already noted, the borderline between obstruction to large and small veins is not sharp, since both may be affected by thrombosis, for example in patients with coagulation disorders. Furthermore, thrombosis of large or medium-sized hepatic veins may lead to fibrous intimal thickening of smaller vessels. Rarely, an exuberant form of fibrous obliteration involves veins of all calibres and has been shown to recur after liver transplantation.[90] Careful inspection of the congested sinusoids in SOS in liver biopsy specimens may disclose loss or discontinuity of endothelium from the vascular lining, endothelial and/or hepatocyte extrusion into the sinusoidal lumen and intravasation of red blood cells into the space of Disse (**see Fig. 16.21**).

As in the case of obstruction to larger veins, there are many causes of SOS and VOD. The classical cause, ingestion of pyrrolizidine alkaloids, remains a hazard.[91] Sinusoidal endothelium in general is also susceptible to similar toxic injury, particularly in individuals receiving chemotherapy or myeloablative conditioning therapy prior to haematopoietic cell transplantation.[9,92] Among these agents are 6-thioguanine, busulfan, gemtuzimab–ozogamicin and oxaliplatin.[9] Venous occlusion is also seen following renal or liver transplantation.[89,93-95] Other associations and causes are irradiation of the liver,[96] AIDS,[97]

**Figure 12.13
Veno-occlusive
disease.**

A terminal hepatic
venule has been
occluded by recently
formed collagen and
cells, following liver
transplantation.
(Needle biopsy,
chromotrope–aniline
blue). (Section kindly
provided by
Professor A. P.
Dhillon, London, UK.)

heroin addiction,[38] primary vascular disease,[98] Hodgkin's disease,[99,100] drug therapy[62,101] and arsenic poisoning.[102] Epithelioid haemangioendothelioma of the liver can mimic VOD because of the characteristic vascular occlusions produced by tumour invasion, and can also give rise to clinical and histological features of the Budd–Chiari syndrome.[103] Finally, careful examination of connective tissue stains may reveal occluded veins in the livers of patients with alcoholic and non-alcoholic fatty liver disease[104,105] and indeed in cirrhosis from any cause.[106]

References

1 Valente JF, Alonso MH, Weber FL, et al. Late hepatic artery thrombosis in liver allograft recipients is associated with intrahepatic biliary necrosis. *Transplantation* 1996; **61:** 61–65.

2 Goritsas CP, Repanti M, Papadaki E, et al. Intrahepatic bile duct injury and nodular regenerative hyperplasia of the liver in a patient with polyarteritis nodosa. *J Hepatol* 1997; **26:** 727–730.

3 Viola S, Meyer M, Fabre M, et al. Ischemic necrosis of bile ducts complicating Schönlein–Henoch purpura. *Gastroenterology* 1999; **117:** 211–214.

4 Parangi S, Oz MC, Blume RS, et al. Hepatobiliary complications of polyarteritis nodosa. *Arch Surg* 1991; **126:** 909–912.

5 Matsumoto T, Yoshimine T, Shimouchi K, et al. The liver in systemic lupus erythematosus: pathologic analysis of 52 cases and review of Japanese autopsy registry data. *Hum Pathol* 1992; **23:** 1151–1158.

6 Rousselet M-C, Kettani S, Rohmer V, et al. A case of temporal arteritis with intrahepatic arterial involvement. *Pathol Res Pract* 1989; **185:** 329–331.

7 Heneghan MA, Feeley KM, DeFaoite N, et al. Granulomatous liver disease and giant-cell arteritis. *Dig Dis Sci* 1998; **43:** 2164–2167.

8 De Bayser L, Roblot P, Ramassamy A, et al. Hepatic fibrin-ring granulomas in giant cell arteritis. *Gastroenterology* 1993; **105:** 272–273.

9 DeLeve LD, Valla D-C, Garcia-Tsao G. Vascular disorders of the liver. *Hepatology* 2009; **49:** 1729–1764.

10 Martini GA. The liver in hereditary haemorrhagic telangiectasia: an inborn error of vascular structure with multiple manifestations: a reappraisal. *Gut* 1978; **19:** 531–537.

11 Wanless IR, Gryfe A. Nodular transformation of the liver in hereditary hemorrhagic telangiectasia. *Arch Pathol Lab Med* 1986; **110:** 331–335.

12 Larson AM. Liver disease in hereditary hemorrhagic telangiectasia. *J Clin Gastroenterol* 2003; **36:** 149–158.

13 Bernard G, Mion F, Henry L, et al. Hepatic involvement in hereditary hemorrhagic telangiectasia: clinical, radiological, and hemodynamic studies of 11 cases. *Gastroenterology* 1993; **105:** 482–487.

14 Saegusa M, Takano Y, Okudaira M. Human hepatic infarction: histopathological and postmortem angiological studies. *Liver* 1993; **13**: 239–245.

15 de la Monte SM, Arcidi JM, Moore GW, et al. Midzonal necrosis as a pattern of hepatocellular injury after shock. *Gastroenterology* 1984; **86**: 627–631.

16 Lefkowitch JH, Mendez L. Morphologic features of hepatic injury in cardiac disease and shock. *J Hepatol* 1986; **2**: 313–327.

17 Sort P, Mas A, Salmeron JM, et al. Recurrent liver involvement in heatstroke. *Liver* 1996; **16**: 334–337.

18 Hassanein T, Perper JA, Tepperman L, et al. Liver failure occurring as a component of exertional heatstroke. *Gastroenterology* 1991; **100**: 1442–1447.

19 Gitlin N, Serio KM. Ischemic hepatitis: widening horizons.. *Am J Gastroenterol* 1992; **87**: 831–836.

20 Amitrano L, Guardascione MA, Brancaccio V, et al. Risk factors and clinical presentation of portal vein thrombosis in patients with liver cirrhosis. *J Hepatol* 2004; **40**: 736–741.

21 Tanaka M, Wanless IR. Pathology of the liver in Budd–Chiari syndrome: portal vein thrombosis and the histogenesis of veno-centric cirrhosis, veno-portal cirrhosis, and large regenerative nodules. *Hepatology* 1998; **27**: 488–496.

22 Shimamatsu K, Wanless IR. Role of ischemia in causing apoptosis, atrophy, and nodular hyperplasia in human liver. *Hepatology* 1997; **26**: 343–350.

23 Wanless IR, Peterson P, Das A, et al. Hepatic vascular disease and portal hypertension in polycythemia vera and agnogenic myeloid metaplasia: a clinicopathological study of 145 patients examined at autopsy. *Hepatology* 1990; **12**: 1166–1174.

24 Dubois A, Dauzat M, Pignodel C, et al. Portal hypertension in lymphoproliferative and myeloproliferative disorders: hemodynamic and histological correlations. *Hepatology* 1993; **17**: 246–250.

25 Roskams T, Baptista A, Bianchi L, et al. Histopathology of portal hypertension: a practical guideline. *Histopathology* 2003; **42**: 2–13.

26 Nevens F, Fevery J, Van Steenbergen W, et al. Arsenic and non-cirrhotic portal hypertension. A report of eight cases. *J Hepatol* 1990; **11**: 80–85.

27 Thomas LB, Popper H, Berk PD, et al. Vinyl-chloride-induced liver disease. From idiopathic portal hypertension (Banti's syndrome) to angiosarcomas. *N Engl J Med* 1975; **292**: 17–22.

28 Popper H, Thomas LB, Telles NC, et al. Development of hepatic angiosarcoma in man induced by vinyl chloride, thorotrast, and arsenic. Comparison with cases of unknown etiology. *Am J Pathol* 1978; **92**: 349–369.

29 Shepherd P, Harrison DJ. Idiopathic portal hypertension associated with cytotoxic drugs. *J Clin Pathol* 2004; **43**: 206–210.

30 Oikawa H, Masuda T, Sato S-I, et al. Changes in lymph vessels and portal veins in the portal tract of patients with idiopathic portal hypertension: a morphometric study. *Hepatology* 1998; **27**: 1607–1610.

31 Ludwig J, Hashimoto E, Obata H, et al. Idiopathic portal hypertension: a histopathological study of 26 Japanese cases. *Histopathology* 1993; **22**: 227–234.

32 Ohbu M, Okudaira M, Watanabe K, et al. Histopathological study of intrahepatic aberrant vessels in cases of noncirrhotic portal hypertension. *Hepatology* 1994; **20**: 302–308.

33 Nakanuma Y, Hoso M, Sasaki M, et al. Histopathology of the liver in non-cirrhotic portal hypertension of unknown etiology. *Histopathology* 1996; **28**: 195–204.

34 Bernard P-H, Le Bail B, Cransac M, et al. Progression from idiopathic portal hypertension to incomplete septal cirrhosis with liver failure requiring liver transplantation. *J Hepatol* 2004; **22**: 495–499.

35 Ibarrola C, Colina F. Clinicopathological features of nine cases of non-cirrhotic portal hypertension: current definitions and criteria are inadequate. *Histopathology* 2003; **42**: 251–264.

36 Nataf C, Feldmann G, Lebrec D, et al. Idiopathic portal hypertension (perisinusoidal fibrosis) after renal transplantation. *Gut* 1979; **20**: 531–537.

37 Harrison SA, Brunt EM, Goodman ZD, et al. Diabetic hepatosclerosis: a novel entity or a rare form of nonalcoholic fatty liver disease? *Arch Pathol Lab Med* 2006; **130**: 27–32.

38 Trigueiro de Araújo MS, Gerard F, Chossegros P, et al. Vascular hepatotoxicity related to heroin addiction. *Virchows Arch [A]* 1990; **417**: 497–503.

39 Bioulac-Sage P, Quinton A, Saric J, et al. Chance discovery of hepatic fibrosis in patient with asymptomatic hypervitaminosis A. *Arch Pathol Lab Med* 1988; **112**: 505–509.

40 Latry P, Bioulac-Sage P, Echinard E, et al. Perisinusoidal fibrosis and basement membrane-like material in the livers of diabetic patients. *Hum Pathol* 1987; **18**: 775–780.

41 Degott C, Capron J, Bettan L, et al. Myeloid metaplasia, perisinusoidal fibrosis, and nodular regenerative hyperplasia of the liver. *Liver* 1985; **5**: 276–281.

42 Lafon ME, Bioulac-Sage P, Grimaud JA, et al. Perisinusoidal fibrosis of the liver in patients with thrombocytopenic purpura. *Virchows Arch [A]* 1987; **411**: 553–559.

43 Bardadin KA, Scheuer PJ. Endothelial cell changes in acute hepatitis. A light and electron microscopic study. *J Pathol* 1984; **144**: 213–220.

44 Iwamura S, Enzan H, Saibara T, et al. Appearance of sinusoidal inclusion-containing endothelial cells in liver disease. *Hepatology* 1994; **20**: 604–610.

45 Iwamura S, Enzan H, Saibara T, et al. Hepatic sinusoidal endothelial cells can store and metabolize serum immunoglobulin. *Hepatology* 1995; **22**: 1456–1461.

46 Bruguera M, Aranguibel F, Ros E, et al. Incidence and clinical significance of sinusoidal dilatation in liver biopsies. *Gastroenterology* 1978; **75**: 474–478.

47 Capron JP, Lemay JL, Gontier MF, et al. Hepatic sinusoidal dilatation in Crohn's disease. *Scand J Gastroenterol* 1979; **14**: 987–992.

48 Saadoun D, Cazals-Hatem D, Denninger M-H, et al. Association of idiopathic hepatic sinusoidal dilatation with the immunological features of the antiphospholipid syndrome. *Gut* 2004; **53**: 1516–1519.

49 de Kerguenec C, Hillaire S, Molinié V, et al. Hepatic manifestations of hemophagocytic syndrome: a study of 30 cases. *Am J Gastroenterol* 2001; **96**: 852–857.

50 Trigueiro de Araújo MS, Gerard F, Chossegros P, et al. Lack of hepatocyte involvement in the genesis of the sinusoidal dilatation related to heroin addiction: a morphometric study. *Virchows Arch [A]* 1992; **420**: 149–153.

51 Kakar S, Kamath PS, Burgart LJ. Sinusoidal dilatation and congestion in liver biopsy. Is it always due to venous

outflow impairment? *Arch Pathol Lab Med* 2004; **128:** 901–904.

52 Winkler K, Poulsen H. Liver disease with periportal sinusoidal dilatation. A possible complication to contraceptive steroids. *Scand J Gastroenterol* 1975; **10:** 699–704.

53 Winkler K, Christoffersen P. A reappraisal of Poulsen's disease (hepatic zone 1 sinusoidal dilatation). *APMIS* 1991; **(Suppl. 23):** 86–90.

54 Aoyagi T, Mori I, Ueyama Y, et al. Sinusoidal dilatation of the liver as a paraneoplastic manifestation of renal cell carcinoma. *Hum Pathol* 1989; **20:** 1193–1197.

55 Oligny LL, Lough J. Hepatic sinusoidal ectasia. *Hum Pathol* 1992; **23:** 953–956.

56 Wold LE, Ludwig J. Peliosis hepatis: two morphologic variants? *Hum Pathol* 1981; **12:** 388–389.

57 Selby DM, Stocker JT. Focal peliosis hepatis, a sequela of asphyxial death? *Pediatr Pathol Lab Med* 1995; **15:** 589–596.

58 Fine KD, Solano M, Polter DE, et al. Malignant histiocytosis in a patient presenting with hepatic dysfunction and peliosis hepatis. *Am J Gastroenterol* 1995; **90:** 485–488.

59 Degott C, Rueff B, Kreis H, et al. Peliosis hepatis in recipients of renal transplants. *Gut* 1978; **19:** 748–753.

60 Scheuer PJ, Schachter LA, Mathur S, et al. Peliosis hepatis after liver transplantation. *J Clin Pathol* 1990; **43:** 1036–1037.

61 Soe KL, Soe M, Gluud C. Liver pathology associated with the use of anabolic-androgenic steroids. *Liver* 1992; **12:** 73–79.

62 Modzelewski JRJ, Daeschner C, Joshi VV, et al. Veno-occlusive disease of the liver induced by low-dose cyclophosphamide. *Mod Pathol* 1994; **7:** 967–972.

63 Jacquemin E, Pariente D, Fabre M, et al. Peliosis hepatis with initial presentation as acute hepatic failure and intraperitoneal hemorrhage in children. *J Hepatol* 1999; **30:** 1146–1150.

64 Takiff H, Brems JJ, Pockros PJ, et al. Focal hemorrhagic necrosis of the liver. A rare cause of hemoperitoneum. *Dig Dis Sci* 1992; **37:** 1910–1914.

65 Shimamura K, Oka K, Nakazawa M, et al. Distribution patterns of microthrombi in disseminated intravascular coagulation. *Arch Pathol Lab Med* 1983; **107:** 543–547.

66 Wanless IR, Liu JJ, Butany J. Role of thrombosis in the pathogenesis of congestive hepatic fibrosis (cardiac cirrhosis). *Hepatology* 1995; **21:** 1232–1237.

67 Banerjee S, Owen C, Chopra S. Sickle cell hepatopathy. *Hepatology* 2001; **33:** 1021–1028.

68 Charlotte F, Bachir D, Nénert M, et al. Vascular lesions of the liver in sickle cell disease. A clinicopathological study in 26 living patients. *Arch Pathol Lab Med* 1995; **119:** 46–52.

69 Comer GM, Ozick LA, Sachdev RK, et al. Transfusion-related chronic liver disease in sickle cell anemia. *Am J Gastroenterol* 1991; **86:** 1232–1234.

70 Valla D-C. Budd Chiari syndrome and veno-occlusive disease/sinusoidal obstruction syndrome. *Gut* 2008; **57:** 1469–1478.

71 Ludwig J, Hashimoto E, McGill DB, et al. Classification of hepatic venous outflow obstruction: ambiguous terminology of the Budd–Chiari syndrome. *Mayo Clin Proc* 1990; **65:** 51–55.

72 Myers RP, Cerini R, Sayegh R, et al. Cardiac hepatopathy: clinical, hemodynamic, and histologic characteristics and correlations. *Hepatology* 2003; **37:** 393–400.

73 Kanel GC, Ucci AA, Kaplan MM, et al. A distinctive perivenular hepatic lesion associated with heart failure. *Am J Clin Pathol* 1980; **73:** 235–239.

74 Klatt EC, Koss MN, Young TS, et al. Hepatic hyaline globules associated with passive congestion. *Arch Pathol Lab Med* 1988; **112:** 510–513.

75 Boughton BJ. Hepatic and portal vein thrombosis. Closely associated with chronic myeloproliferative disorders. *BMJ* 1991; **302:** 192–193.

76 Valla D-C. The diagnosis and management of the Budd–Chiari syndrome: consensus and controversies. *Hepatology* 2003; **38:** 793–803.

77 Bismuth E, Hadengue A, Hammel P, et al. Hepatic vein thrombosis in Behçet's disease. *Hepatology* 1990; **11:** 969–974.

78 Bayraktar Y, Balkanci F, Bayraktar M, et al. Budd–Chiari syndrome: a common complication of Behcet's disease. *Am J Gastroenterol* 1997; **92:** 858–862.

79 Bayraktar Y, Balkanci F, Kansu E, et al. Cavernous transformation of the portal vein: a common manifestation of Behcet's syndrome. *Am J Gastroenterol* 1995; **90:** 1476–1479.

80 Maddrey WC. Hepatic vein thrombosis (Budd–Chiari syndrome): possible association with the use of oral contraceptives. *Semin Liver Dis* 1987; **7:** 32–39.

81 Blanshard C, Dodge G, Pasi J, et al. Membranous obstruction of the inferior vena cava in a patient with factor V Leiden: evidence for a post-thrombotic aetiology. *J Hepatol* 1997; **26:** 731–735.

82 Valla D, Hadengue A, el Younsi M, et al. Hepatic venous outflow block caused by short-length hepatic vein stenoses. *Hepatology* 1997; **25:** 814–819.

83 Riemens SC, Haagsma EB, Kok T, et al. Familial occurrence of membranous obstruction of the inferior vena cava: arguments in favor of a congenital etiology. *J Hepatol* 1995; **22:** 404–409.

84 Vallaeys JH, Praet MM, Roels HJ, et al. The Budd–Chiari syndrome caused by a zygomycete. A new pathogenesis of hepatic vein thrombosis. *Arch Pathol Lab Med* 1989; **113:** 1171–1174.

85 Okuda K, Kage M, Shrestha SM. Proposal of a new nomenclature for Budd–Chiari syndrome: hepatic vein thrombosis versus thrombosis of the inferior vena cava at its hepatic portion. *Hepatology* 1998; **28:** 1191–1198.

86 Cazals-Hatem D, Vilgrain V, Genin P, et al. Arterial and portal circulation and parenchymal changes in Budd–Chiari syndrome: a study in 17 explanted livers. *Hepatology* 2003; **37:** 510–519.

87 Kakar S, Batts KP, Poterucha JJ, Burgart LJ. Histologic changes mimicking biliary disease in liver biopsies with venous outflow impairment. *Mod Pathol* 2004; **17:** 874–878.

88 DeLeve LD, Shulman HM, McDonald GB. Toxic injury to hepatic sinusoids: sinusoidal obstruction syndrome (veno-occlusive disease). *Semin Liver Dis* 2002; **22:** 27–42.

89 Sato Y, Asada Y, Hara S, et al. Hepatic stellate cells (Ito cells) in veno-occlusive disease of the liver after allogeneic bone marrow transplantation. *Histopathology* 1999; **34:** 66–70.

90 Fiel MI, Schiano TD, Klion FM, et al. Recurring fibro-obliterative venopathy in liver allografts. *Am J Surg Pathol* 1999; **23:** 734–737.

91 Chojkier M. Hepatic sinusoidal-obstruction syndrome: toxicity of pyrrolizidine alkaloids. *J Hepatol* 2003; **39**: 437–446.

92 Sakai M, Strasser SI, Shulman HM, et al. Severe hepatocellular injury after hematopoietic cell transplant: incidence, etiology and outcome. *Bone Marrow Transplant* 2009; **56**: 1–7.

93 Katzka DA, Saul SH, Jorkasky D, et al. Azathioprine and hepatic venocclusive disease in renal transplant patients. *Gastroenterology* 1986; **90**: 446–454.

94 Shulman HM, FIsher LB, Schoch HG, et al. Venooclusive disease of the liver after marrow transplantation: histological correlates of clinical signs and symptoms. *Hepatology* 1994; **19**: 1171–1180.

95 Dhillon AP, Burroughs AK, Hudson M, et al. Hepatic venular stenosis after orthotopic liver transplantation. *Hepatology* 1994; **19**: 106–111.

96 Lawrence TS, Robertson JM, Anscher MS, et al. Hepatic toxicity resulting from cancer treatment. *Int J Radiat Oncol Biol Phys* 1995; **31**: 1237–1248.

97 Buckley JA, Hutchins GM. Association of hepatic veno-occlusive disease with the acquired immunodeficiency syndrome. *Mod Pathol* 1995; **8**: 398–401.

98 Ito N, Kimura A, Nishikawa M, et al. Veno-occlusive disease of the liver in a patient with allergic granulomatous angiitis. *Am J Gastroenterol* 1988; **83**: 316–319.

99 Lohse AW, Dienes HP, Wolfel T, et al. Veno-occlusive disease of the liver in Hodgkin's disease prior to and resolution following chemotherapy (Letter). *J Hepatol* 1995; **22**: 378.

100 Palladino M, Miele L, Pompili M, et al. Severe veno-occlusive disease after autologous peripheral blood stem cell transplantation for high-grade non-Hodgkin lymphoma: report of a successfully managed case and a literature review of veno-occlusive disease. *Clin Transplant* 2008; **22**: 837–841.

101 Nakhleh RE, Wesen C, Snover DC, et al. Venoocclusive lesions of the central veins and portal vein radicles secondary to intraarterial 5-fluoro-2′-deoxyuridine infusion. *Hum Pathol* 1989; **20**: 1218–1220.

102 Labadie H, Stoessel P, Callard P, et al. Hepatic venoocclusive disease and perisinusoidal fibrosis secondary to arsenic poisoning. *Gastroenterology* 1990; **99**: 1140–1143.

103 Walsh MM, Hytiroglou P, Thung SN, et al. Epithelioid hemangioendothelioma of the liver mimicking Budd–Chiari syndrome. *Arch Pathol Lab Med* 1998; **122**: 846–848.

104 Burt AD, MacSween RN. Hepatic vein lesions in alcoholic liver disease: retrospective biopsy and necropsy study. *J Clin Pathol* 1986; **39**: 63–67.

105 Wanless IR, Shiota K. The pathogenesis of nonalcoholic steatohepatitis and other fatty liver diseases: a four-step model including the role of lipid release and hepatic venular obstruction in the progression to cirrhosis. *Semin Liver Dis* 2004; **24**: 99–106.

106 Nakanuma Y, Ohta G, Doishita K. Quantitation and serial section observations of focal venocclusive lesions of hepatic veins in liver cirrhosis. *Virchows Arch [A]* 1985; **405**: 429–438.

General reading

Cazals-Hatem D, Vilgrain V, Genin P, et al. Arterial and portal circulation and parenchymal changes in Budd–Chiari syndrome: a study in 17 explanted livers. *Hepatology* 2003; **37**: 510–519.

DeLeve LD, Shulman HM, McDonald GB. Toxic injury to hepatic sinusoids: sinusoidal obstruction syndrome (veno-occlusive disease). *Semin Liver Dis* 2002; **22**: 27–42.

DeLeve LD, Valla D-C, Garcia-Tsao G. Vascular disorders of the liver. *Hepatology* 2009; **49**: 1729–1764.

Okudaira M, Ohbu M, Okuda K. Idiopathic portal hypertension and its pathology. *Semin Liver Dis* 2002; **22**: 59–72.

Roskams T, Baptista A, Bianchi L, et al. Histopathology of portal hypertension: a practical guideline. *Histopathology* 2003; **42**: 2–13.

Wanless IR. Vascular disorders. In: Burt AD, Portmann BC, Ferrell LD, eds. MacSween's Pathology of the Liver, 5th edn. Edinburgh: Churchill Livingstone/Elsevier, 2007: 613–648.

Childhood Liver Disease and Metabolic Disorders

Introduction

Paediatric liver biopsies present a unique set of diagnostic problems for the pathologist, many of which become clinically apparent in the first few months of life as **neonatal cholestasis**.[1] Among the important disorders one must consider in evaluating neonatal liver biopsies are **extrahepatic biliary atresia**, **paucity of intrahepatic bile ducts** (syndromatic and non-syndromatic types), **metabolic diseases**, **viral hepatitis** and the hepatic effects of **parenteral nutrition (Table 13.1)**. Common to many of these conditions are the histological features of **cholestasis** and **giant-cell hepatitis** (formation of multinucleated hepatocytes). Because these features are not specifically diagnostic of any one neonatal liver disease, the pathologist must be acquainted with other biopsy changes by which to establish or suggest the diagnosis. In many instances, assays of metabolic enzymes and products in serum and liver tissue take diagnostic precedence over routine histopathological interpretation. Electron microscopy may be required to assess the structure of organelles or storage material in hepatocytes or Kupffer cells, particularly when lysosomal storage disorders are being considered. Consultation with investigators dealing with mitochondriopathies,[2,3] mutations of bile-salt transport proteins[4] and expression of proteins involved in blood vessel and bile-duct morphogenesis (e.g. Jagged proteins and Notch receptors) should be considered if special studies are needed to determine the cause of neonatal cholestasis. Childhood liver tumours are discussed in **Chapter 11**.

Diagnostic approach to neonatal liver biopsy

Histopathological examination of neonatal liver biopsies may benefit from a systematic checklist of questions by which the major diagnostic concerns in neonatal liver disease can be evaluated. A simplified, stepwise set of seven questions can be asked:

1 *Is the acinar structure normal for age?* As described in **Chapter 3**, the hepatic plates are two cells thick until 5 or 6 years of age and should not be misconstrued as a pathological change. As with adult biopsies, the presence of fibrosis, nodularity or cirrhosis should be noted early in the biopsy evaluation and correlated with other histological features which may define the aetiology.

2 *Are cholestasis and giant cells present?* As indicated above, neither of these is diagnostically specific. If present, the next interpretive steps should be examination

©2010 Elsevier Ltd
DOI: 10.1016/B978-0-7020-3410-7.00019-8

Table 13.1 Liver biopsy interpretation in neonatal cholestasis*

Aetiology	Histological features
Extrahepatic biliary atresia	Ductular reaction; ductular cholestasis; portal and periportal fibrosis
Paucity of intrahepatic bile ducts	Loss of interlobular bile ducts (bile duct–hepatic artery ratio <1)
Neonatal hepatitis	Portal and lobular mononuclear cell inflammation; apoptotic bodies
Metabolic disorders	Steatosis; fibrosis or cirrhosis; storage product in liver cells or Kupffer cells (see specific disorder)
Parenteral nutrition	Ductular reaction; portal fibrosis or cirrhosis

* Many of the conditions shown in **Table 13.1** are associated with histological cholestasis and formation of giant multinucleated hepatocytes, in addition to the diagnostic features listed.

of portal tracts for evidence of biliary tract obstruction (atresia, etc.) and of portal tracts and parenchyma for evidence of hepatitis.

3 *Are histological changes of hepatitis present?* Mononuclear cell infiltrates within acini and portal tracts associated with liver-cell degeneration should be sought when considering cytomegalovirus, Epstein–Barr virus, rubella or hepatitis virus infections.

4 *Are the interlobular bile ducts normal?* This question has three major ramifications. **Abundance of bile ducts** usually signifies some form of biliary obstruction, such as extrahepatic atresia or choledochal cyst. **Paucity of bile ducts (ductopenia, vanishing bile-duct syndrome)** may be due to developmental, metabolic, or infectious causes. Last, **malformations of bile ducts** comprise a spectrum of problems related to abnormal remodelling of the embryonic bile-duct plate (fibropolycystic diseases).

5 *Does the biopsy specimen contain iron or copper?* Although rare, neonatal haemochromatosis[5] and Indian childhood cirrhosis (copper toxicosis in young children) are serious liver diseases with high mortality rates that must be excluded. In the older child and adolescent, Wilson's disease (**Ch. 14**) must not be overlooked. It should be noted, however, that fetal and neonatal liver contains much higher copper levels than adults, with an irregular tissue distribution.[6] Mild siderosis is also within the spectrum of normal findings in the fetal and neonatal liver.[7]

6 *Has the biopsy specimen been studied by diastase–periodic acid–Schiff (PAS) or immunoperoxidase staining to exclude α_1-antitrypsin deficiency?* The expression of α_1-antitrypsin deficiency is variable, and biopsies may not show diagnostic staining of retained enzyme within liver cells prior to 13–15 weeks of age. This condition should be histologically excluded whenever possible.

7 *Are storage cells present?* Abnormal storage products in liver cells or Kupffer cells may be seen in various metabolic diseases which cause hepatomegaly and failure to thrive. These should be sought on routine haematoxylin and eosin (H&E) as well as special stains.

Neonatal hepatitis

Inflammation and hepatocellular damage in the neonatal period may result from infections and from inborn errors of metabolism. The former include type B hepatitis, cytomegalovirus infection and rubella among others, the latter α_1-antitrypsin deficiency,

Figure 13.1 Neonatal (giant cell) hepatitis. Fibrosis extends from portal tracts into the acini and architecture is distorted. (Wedge biopsy, reticulin.)

galactosaemia and bile acid synthetic defects.[8] Disorders at the ultrastructural or molecular level may also need to be considered, such as neonatal hepatitis due to depletion of mitochondrial DNA.[9] A diagnosis of neonatal hepatitis is therefore a signal for further investigation. The histological picture is broadly similar whatever the cause. There is a variable degree of hepatocellular swelling and multinucleation, cholestasis and portal inflammation. Lobular inflammation may be mild. Liver-cell necrosis and swelling result in collapse and distortion of the reticulin framework (**Fig. 13.1**). Fibrosis is sometimes already well developed, as in neonatal haemochromatosis (**see Ch. 14**) or the severe perinatal liver disease which may rarely be seen in Down's syndrome.[10] Giant multinucleated hepatocytes are commonly seen, whatever the cause of the hepatitis (**Fig. 13.2**). The outcome of neonatal giant-cell hepatitis is resolution, liver failure, cirrhosis or a chronic cholestatic course. The variety of different outcomes is well illustrated in α_1-antitrypsin deficiency.[11]

From a histological point of view, the main differential diagnosis of neonatal hepatitis is extrahepatic biliary obstruction, which may require surgical treatment. Giant multinucleated hepatocytes and an altered reticulin structure are more prominent in hepatitis than in biliary obstruction, while cholestasis is usually more severe in atresia and there is typically a ductular reaction.

Extrahepatic biliary atresia

Extracellular biliary atresia results from inflammation and destruction of all or part of the extrahepatic bile-duct system *in utero* or in the perinatal period.[12] Pathological studies of atretic bile-duct segments[13-15] show chronic inflammation and obliterative fibrosis, sometimes with a few remaining bile-duct cells[16] seen on routine stains or cytokeratin immunostaining. Satisfactory bile drainage and an improved outcome after the Kasai portoenterostomy[17] have sometimes been associated with identification of bile ducts with lumens of 150 μm or greater at the proximal resection margin.[14] Optimal surgical results

**Figure 13.2
Neonatal (giant
cell) hepatitis.**
The parenchyma
consists of
multinucleated giant
liver cells and the
portal tract shown
is infiltrated by
lymphocytes.
(Wedge biopsy,
H&E.)

are obtained if the Kasai procedure (hepatic portoenterostomy) is performed within the first 8 weeks of life.[18] Many patients, nevertheless, later require liver transplantation.[19]

The trigger for the destructive process in extrahepatic atresia is unknown, but considerations have included viral infections (reovirus type 3, rotavirus), exposure to toxins, abnormal remodelling of the embryonic bile-duct plate and disorders of Jagged protein/Notch receptor signalling.[12] DNA microarray studies suggest a gene profile of abnormal cell signalling and transcription regulation.[20] There may be associated congenital abnormalities, including polysplenia[21] and intrahepatic biliary cysts,[22] in approximately 20% of cases with more severe and earlier disease (the 'embryonic' form of biliary atresia). In contrast, the majority of patients have the 'perinatal' form without such anomalies. Expression of various regulatory genes appears to differentiate the two types.[23] The process of biliary atresia is a dynamic one which may also involve the intrahepatic bile ducts,[24,25] even after Kasai surgery.[26]

Liver biopsy shows cholestasis and portal tract changes resembling those of large bile-duct obstruction in the adult (**see Ch. 5**). Portal tracts are enlarged by oedema, a striking ductular reaction and infiltrating neutrophils with fewer chronic inflammatory cells (**Fig. 13.3**). Native interlobular bile ducts are usually intact and can be identified near hepatic arterioles. Bile-containing portal macrophages are often also present. Ductular structures may contain inspissated bile ('ductular cholestasis') and occasionally resemble the embryonic bile-duct plate described by Jörgensen[27] (**Figs 13.4, 13.5**). A prominent ductular reaction is the major histological point of distinction from neonatal hepatitis.[28] There is panlobular cholestasis with accentuation in zone 3. Giant cells are common, but not as numerous or as striking as in neonatal hepatitis. The degree of portal fibrosis[29] depends on the duration of the obstruction and the age at diagnosis. The overall lobular architecture remains intact except in patients diagnosed late in the disease who may then show secondary biliary cirrhosis (**see Fig. 5.11**). The differential diagnosis includes biliary obstruction by a choledochal cyst, chronic injury associated with parenteral nutrition and various inborn errors of metabolism.

Figure 13.3
Extrahepatic biliary atresia.
An expanded, inflamed portal tract at left contains many proliferated bile ducts, some of which are filled with inspissated bile. There is also panacinar cholestasis. (Wedge biopsy, H&E.)

Figure 13.4
Extrahepatic biliary atresia with bile-duct plate-like structures.
The proliferating bile-duct structures in this case resemble the embryonic bile-duct plate. (Wedge biopsy, H&E.)

**Figure 13.5
Extrahepatic biliary
atresia with
bile-duct plate-like
structures.**
The field shown in
Fig. 13.4 stained
with antibodies
to cytokeratin
highlights the
circumferential
portal bile-duct
structures
resembling the
embryonic bile-duct
plate. (Wedge
biopsy, specific
immunoperoxidase.)

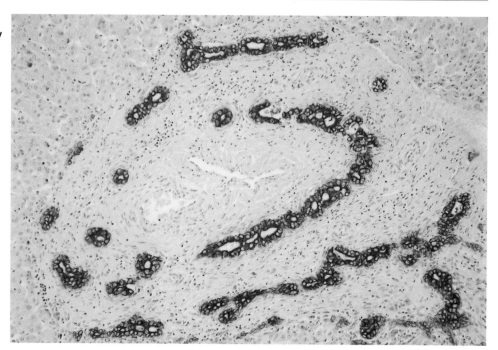

Paucity of intrahepatic bile ducts in childhood

Two varieties of intrahepatic bile duct paucity (formerly called intrahepatic biliary atresia) are recognised in childhood: **syndromatic** and **non-syndromatic**.[30] In syndromatic paucity[31,32] (Alagille's syndrome, arteriohepatic dysplasia), loss of small intrahepatic bile ducts is associated with abnormal facies, vertebral anomalies and various other malformations. The pathogenesis is linked to mutations in the *Jagged 1* gene that produce a structurally abnormal ligand for binding to the Notch 1 receptor which is involved in cell–cell interactions in differentiation and the development of intrahepatic bile ducts.[33] There is associated impairment of branching and elongation of hilar ducts distally into the liver periphery.[34] Increased mortality in these patients is linked to the presence of intracardiac congenital heart disease.[35] In non-syndromatic paucity, duct loss is not associated with facial or other anomalies. In some patients it may be related to a definable cause such as α_1-antitrypsin deficiency or cytomegalovirus infection,[36] while in others there is no detectable aetiological factor. The exact time of onset of bile-duct injury is difficult to establish accurately and probably varies from case to case. Some patients have active destruction of ducts in the first few weeks of life[32] and later stabilise, potentially with few symptoms or only mild chronic cholestasis, into young adulthood. In others, cirrhosis and liver failure may develop within months or many years later.[37] It has been speculated that there may be a small subgroup of patients with non-syndromatic paucity in which cholestatic disease first presents in adulthood[37] ('**idiopathic adulthood ductopenia**').[38]

Histologically, in both forms of intrahepatic duct paucity there is canalicular cholestasis and chronic periportal cholestasis. Portal tracts show a variable degree of fibrosis and small bile ducts are scanty or absent[39] (**Fig. 13.6**). Step sections and cytokeratin 7 or 19 immunostaining may be needed for thorough assessment of duct numbers which, as in primary biliary cirrhosis, should approximately correspond to the number of arteries of similar size. A ductular reaction is usually not a prominent feature, in contrast to extrahepatic biliary atresia[40] (**see Fig. 1.8**). Inflammation is often slight or even absent, but lymphoid

Figure 13.6
Paucity of bile ducts in childhood. The portal tract shows an artery (left arrow) but no corresponding bile duct of similar calibre. There is periportal cholestasis (right arrow). (Needle biopsy, H&E.)

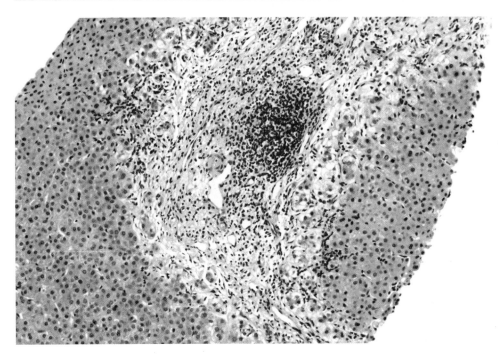

Figure 13.7
Paucity of bile ducts in childhood. A lymphoid aggregate is present at the former site of the bile duct. (Needle biopsy, H&E.)

aggregates may be seen in the place of bile ducts (**Fig. 13.7**). Secondary biliary cirrhosis develops in some patients.[37,41] α_1-Antitrypsin deficiency should be looked for in all patients with paucity of ducts. Duct paucity has also been described in association with Langerhans' cell histiocytosis.[42,43] As primary sclerosing cholangitis can also present in childhood,[44] it should be considered in the differential diagnosis.

Fibropolycystic diseases

The term fibropolycystic diseases covers a number of congenital abnormalities involving bile ducts, many of them related to an abnormal remodelling of the embryonic 'bile-duct plate'.[45-48] They include congenital hepatic fibrosis, Caroli's disease (congenital dilatation of the intrahepatic bile ducts), microhamartoma (von Meyenburg complex), choledochal cyst, and both infantile and adult forms of polycystic disease. The first four of these carry an increased risk of carcinoma of the biliary tree.[49-52] The bile-duct plate, first seen at approximately 8 weeks of gestation, is a layer of primitive small cells encircling the portal tract mesenchyme (**see Figs 13.4, 13.5**). Progressive involution of most of these cells, with acquisition of strong cytokeratin 7 and 19 positivity in those remaining, is the process by which mature interlobular bile ducts of the portal tracts are formed.[46] Persistence of portions of the ductal plate and abnormal remodelling (the 'ductal plate malformation' described by Jörgensen[27]) lead to ectatic and irregularly shaped bile ducts set in dense fibrous stroma, the basic histopathological feature common to all fibropolycystic diseases.

Congenital hepatic fibrosis

Congenital hepatic fibrosis is a recessively inherited condition, which presents as hepatomegaly or the effects of portal hypertension, usually in childhood but occasionally in adults.[53] Some cases have been associated with phosphomannose isomerase deficiency in which the resultant hypoglycosylation may affect remodelling of the bile-duct plate.[54] The liver is enlarged and very hard. Islands of normal liver parenchyma with unaltered vascular relationships are separated by broad and narrow septa of dense, mature fibrous tissue containing elongated or cystic spaces lined by regular biliary epithelium (**Fig. 13.8**). These

Figure 13.8 Congenital hepatic fibrosis.

Several portal tracts are interconnected by bridging fibrous septa containing ductal plate malformations. The fibrosis surrounds normal parenchyma with a terminal venule (short arrow) preserved in a central position. *Inset*: Higher magnification of the abnormal duct structures seen at lower left (long arrow). (Explant liver, H&E.)

represent cross-sections of the hollow structures constituting the ductal plate malformation. Two separate sets of duct-like structures can often be identified, one lying centrally in the septa, the other near the parenchyma. The lumens may contain inspissated bile. Portal-vein branches are small and inconspicuous in some cases. There is usually no cholestasis, necrosis, inflammation or hepatocellular regeneration. In older patients with congenital hepatic fibrosis, the abnormal duct-like structures may be less apparent because of atrophy.

Congenital hepatic fibrosis must be differentiated from cirrhosis, in which there is nodular regeneration and often inflammation and necrosis, and in which the abnormal biliary channels are not seen. The shape of the parenchymal islands in congenital hepatic fibrosis is very similar to that seen in secondary biliary cirrhosis (**see Fig. 5.11**). In this condition the septa contain irregular, newly proliferated bile ducts rather than congenitally abnormal plates; the connective tissue of the septa is loose and inflamed and there may be cholestatic features. Histological cholangitis, other types of inflammation or cholestasis in a liver with the characteristic features of congenital hepatic fibrosis should raise the possibility of coexisting Caroli's disease. The combination constitutes Caroli's syndrome.

Caroli's disease (congenital dilatation of the intrahepatic bile ducts)

This cystic malformation can affect different parts of the intrahepatic biliary tree and is seen alone or in combination with other congenital abnormalities, notably congenital hepatic fibrosis.[55] Because the cysts communicate with the rest of the biliary tree, there is a risk of ascending bacterial infection. Liver biopsy then shows the changes of cholangitis, with or without associated congenital hepatic fibrosis. The lesion of Caroli's disease must be distinguished from the acquired cholangiectases sometimes found in primary sclerosing cholangitis.[56]

Microhamartoma

Microhamartomas (von Meyenburg complexes, bile-duct malformations) are rounded nodules closely related to portal tracts, containing multiple biliary channels lined by regular epithelium and set in a stroma of dense fibrous tissue (**Fig. 13.9**). They may be grossly visible on the liver surface as white nodules 1–2 mm across. The lumens of the biliary structures sometimes contain inspissated bile. Serial sectioning shows that they are interconnected.[57] Microhamartomas are usually found incidentally and do not normally give rise to symptoms or abnormalities of liver function. They are often multiple, in which case they may very occasionally be associated with portal hypertension; distinction from congenital hepatic fibrosis is then difficult. If a small nodule on the liver surface is seen during surgery, frozen section may occasionally be requested in order to exclude metastatic carcinoma. The irregularly dilated duct structures, inspissated bile, and circumscription seen in microhamartomas are helpful in making this distinction.

Polycystic disease

The infantile type of polycystic disease is regularly associated with renal involvement.[46,58] Portal tracts contain multiple cystic channels set in a fibrous stroma. In the adult type the cysts are lined by epithelium of biliary type (**Fig. 13.10**) but are not connected with the rest of the biliary tree. Solitary congenital cysts are histologically similar. The cuboidal or flattened epithelial lining helps distinguish these cysts from **ciliated hepatic foregut cysts** which are lined by ciliated cells and mucin-secreting goblet cells.[59] The presence of microhamartomas and features of Caroli's disease in individuals with polycystic disease favours a continuum in the expression of fibropolycystic disease.[60-62]

Figure 13.9 Microhamartoma. A cluster of duct-like structures with irregular contours and focal dilatations is seen in a portal tract. Note resemblance to congenital hepatic fibrosis, shown in **Fig. 13.8**. (Wedge biopsy, H&E.)

Figure 13.10 Cystic liver. A cyst (top left) is lined by a single layer of low cuboidal epithelium. (Wedge biopsy, H&E.)

Inherited metabolic disorders

Cystic fibrosis

Cystic fibrosis is an inherited disease in which abnormally viscous exocrine secretions are present in the pancreas, salivary glands, alimentary tract and lungs; the prevalence of liver disease is variable and in part age-dependent.[63–65] Subclinical liver disease may be significant.[64] Jaundice in the neonatal period has been attributed to bile-duct obstruction by abnormally viscous bile and to gastrointestinal obstruction by meconium. Intercurrent hepatitis may also be responsible. Steatosis is common, although not always related to malnutrition.[66] Paucity of intrahepatic bile ducts in cystic fibrosis has also been reported.[67] In a proportion of older children a characteristic lesion of intrahepatic bile ducts is found.[68] Dense plugs of PAS-positive material are seen within dilated, proliferated ducts (**Fig. 13.11**). Bile-duct cells may undergo degeneration and necrosis.[66] There is surrounding fibrosis[69] and a variable degree of inflammatory infiltration which may be associated with abnormal intrahepatic ducts on cholangiography.[64] Eventually the fibrous areas may join, separating parenchymal islands. The term **focal biliary fibrosis** expresses the uneven involvement of the intrahepatic bile ducts in this process, with parts of the liver remaining unaffected. In some patients the disease evolves to secondary biliary cirrhosis.[68]

Storage disorders: general remarks

Inherited metabolic defects leading to the abnormal accumulation of lipids, proteins and carbohydrates in the liver are many and varied; for a full description of the morphological changes, recent reviews should be consulted.[70–72] Ishak[70] helpfully discusses the differential diagnosis of individual histological features. Liver biopsy is sometimes useful in diagnosis, though by no means always decisive. The following points are offered as practical sugges-

**Figure 13.11
Cystic fibrosis.**
Proliferated bile ducts in an enlarged, fibrosed portal tract contain dense inspissated material (arrows). (Post-mortem liver, H&E.)

tions for occasions when biopsy is contemplated in children suspected of having storage disorders.

1   Storage disorders can involve hepatocytes (e.g. glycogenoses, α_1-antitrypsin deficiency), macrophages (e.g. Gaucher's disease), or both (e.g. Niemann–Pick disease, mucopolysaccharidoses,[73] cholesterol ester storage disease). When Kupffer cells are involved, they may swell to the size of hepatocytes and their involvement may not at first be apparent; the use of stains other than haematoxylin and eosin (H&E), especially PAS and trichrome stains, then usually makes the Kupffer-cell involvement obvious.

2   Suspicion of a possible storage disorder is one of the few indications for electron microscopy of part of the biopsy specimen as a diagnostic procedure, because characteristic ultrastructural appearances sometimes enable a correct diagnosis to be established quickly.[74] Even when the changes are not diagnostic they can direct attention to a particular group of diseases, and suggest the next line of investigation. Arrangements for electron microscopy should be made beforehand, so that part of the specimen can be put into the correct fixative without delay. In centres wtihout facilities for electron microscopy, part of the specimen should still be correctly fixed and/or embedded, and sent to a referral centre later if light microscopic findings warrant this.

3   Arrangements should also be made to freeze part of the specimen and to store it in liquid nitrogen for possible biochemical analysis and histochemical staining of frozen sections. Speed is essential to avoid loss of enzyme activity. Again, a specialist centre may need to be consulted, because few centres or pathologists have the necessary expertise to investigate the rarer metabolic diseases.

Many inherited metabolic diseases affect the liver and several may lead to **cirrhosis**[70] (glycogenosis types III, IV and VI, galactosaemia, tyrosinaemia type I, α_1-antitrypsin deficiency, Wilson's disease, hereditary haemochromatosis). Liver transplantation may be indicated in some patients.[19,75,76] The discussion in this chapter will be limited primarily to the disorders mentioned under point 1 above. Haemochromatosis and Wilson's disease are described in **Chapter 14**.

Glycogen storage diseases (glycogenoses)

Most forms of glycogen storage disease involve the liver.[77] In type I glycogenosis (von Gierke's disease), fat and glycogen accumulate in the cytoplasm of hepatocytes. These appear swollen, pale-staining and sometimes vacuolated with H&E and have centrally placed nuclei (**Fig. 13.12**). Mallory bodies may be found in the cytoplasm.[78] The abundant glycogen displaces the organelles of affected cells to the periphery, giving them a plant-cell-like appearance. Some liver-cell nuclei also contain glycogen. Sinusoids are compressed. The overall appearance has been described as a uniform mosaic pattern.[77] Slender periportal fibrous scars often develop. Liver-cell adenomas[79,80] or even, rarely, carcinomas[81] may develop. Rapid fixation in buffered formal saline usually enables abundant glycogen to be demonstrated in hepatocytes in paraffin sections, but it should be noted that the diagnosis does not rest only on the demonstration of glycogen, which is plentiful in normal liver. Features closely resembling type I glycogenosis can be seen in poorly controlled diabetics as **Mauriac syndrome (see Ch. 7)**.

In type II glycogenosis (Pompe's disease), the highly soluble storage material is contained in enlarged lysosomes, visible as vacuoles in hepatocytes and Kupffer cells by light microscopy. Many other tissues are involved. Type III glycogenosis has been subdivided into several biochemical subtypes. Histological appearances are like those of type I, but fat is less abundant and there may be fibrosis or cirrhosis.[82] Type IV (amylopectinosis) is characterised by abnormal glycogen in the form of well-defined cytoplasmic inclusions in hepatocytes[83] (**see Ch. 4**). The glycogen is only incompletely removed by diastase diges-

Figure 13.12
Glycogenosis.
In this example of type I glycogen storage disease, hepatocytes are swollen and resemble plant cells. (Wedge biopsy, H&E.)

tion. The inclusions have a ground-glass appearance and must be distinguished from hepatitis B virus surface antigen and other similar cytoplasmic inclusions[84] (**see Fig. 4.8 and Table 4.1**). In other types of glycogenosis there is often much variation in the degree of hepatocellular swelling in different areas, in contrast to the regular distribution of the changes in type I.[77]

α_1-Antitrypsin deficiency

Individuals with decreased levels of the serum protease inhibitor α_1-antitrypsin (α_1-antitrypsin deficiency) may present with liver disease as neonates (neonatal cholestasis), in adolescence or in adulthood, even beyond 60 years of age.[85–87] There are over 100 different alleles of the α_1-antitrypsin (AAT) gene,[88] two of which determine an individual's phenotype. The most common phenotype, PiMM, is associated with normal serum levels of AAT. Individuals with heterozygous (PiMZ) and homozygous (PiZZ) deficiency have moderately and profoundly reduced serum levels of AAT, respectively. The accumulation of characteristic PAS-positive, diastase-resistant globules in the hepatocytes of AAT-deficient individuals (**Fig. 13.13**) is based on a structural change in the glycoprotein which is encoded by the mutant Z gene.[89] An amino acid substitution (lysine for glutamic acid at position 342) results in abnormal folding and polymerisation[90] of the protein and failure of both its secretion from the endoplasmic reticulum[89] and its subsequent degradation. In this regard AAT deficiency is conceptually similar to Alzheimer's and Parkinson's diseases where inclusions result from conformational disorders of serine proteases ('serpinopathies').[91]

The globules of AAT which accumulate range from less than 1 μm to 10 μm or more in diameter. They are mainly found in periportal hepatocytes, a similar distribution to the much smaller granules of copper-associated protein and haemosiderin, from which they need to be distinguished. In doubtful cases, immunohistochemical staining enables AAT to be identified with certainty (**Fig. 13.14**). Moreover, immunohistochemical staining is more sensitive than diastase–PAS positivity, and is helpful when diastase–PAS-positive globules are scanty or unevenly distributed. Conversely, immunohistochemically positive

**Figure 13.13
α₁-Antitrypsin
deficiency.**
Hepatocytes near a
fibrous septum
contain many
magenta globules of
different sizes.
(Post-mortem liver,
diastase–PAS.)

**Figure 13.14
α₁-Antitrypsin
deficiency.**
Periportal
hepatocytes contain
numerous globules
of α₁-antitrypsin,
stained brown
by the
immunoperoxidase
method. Each
globule typically is
stained around the
perimeter, with a
central unstained
region. (Needle
biopsy, specific
immunoperoxidase.)

material is found in some patients without the genetic deficiency, usually with a panlobular or perivenular rather than a periportal distribution[92,93] and particularly in livers with sinusoidal congestion and hypoxia.[94] From a practical point of view, it is wise to regard the presence of diastase-resistant PAS-positive globules in periportal liver cells as evidence for α₁-antitrypsin deficiency until proved otherwise.[95] Intracellular AAT globules have been vividly demonstrated in a transgenic mouse model of the disease.[96]

Some children with homozygous AAT deficiency develop neonatal cholestasis. Histological changes include a ductular reaction and fibrosis, but the typical globules may not be seen until the age of 3 or 4 months.[97] The subsequent course varies: many children improve, while others develop a chronic cholestatic syndrome with paucity of bile ducts or cirrhosis.[11,87,98] Cirrhosis in children with AAT deficiency often has 'biliary' features, such as a ductular reaction and partial preservation of lobular architecture.

Adults carrying two Z alleles present with pulmonary emphysema or liver disease, but may also be symptom-free and healthy. Liver biopsy may show little apart from the PAS-positive globules, or varying degrees of fibrosis. Cirrhosis develops in approximately one-third of homozygotes[88] and is either inactive or shows features of chronic hepatitis. An increased prevalence of hepatitis B and C viral infections in AAT deficiency may contribute to this picture.[99] The characteristic globules are found predominantly in periportal or periseptal hepatocytes. They are seen most easily in sections stained with diastase–PAS, phosphotungstic acid–haematoxylin or specific immunoperoxidase, but are also seen in trichrome preparations and, when large and abundant, are faintly visible with H&E. Similar globules are seen in some hepatocellular carcinomas in patients with or without the Z allele.[100,101] Furthermore, an increased risk of hepatocellular carcinoma has been reported in male patients with AAT deficiency.[102] Chronic hepatitis, cirrhosis, large-cell liver-cell dysplasia and hepatocellular carcinoma may also be seen in heterozygous (PiMZ) AAT deficiency[103] and in individuals with other allelic variants such as Mmalton.[104–106]

Brief mention should be made of several other endoplasmic reticulum inclusions found in hepatocytes in patients who may have chronic hepatitis or cirrhosis. Diastase–PAS-negative periportal granules of α_1-antichymotrypsin can be identified by specific immunohistochemical staining in **partial α_1-antichymotrypsin deficiency**.[107,108] In **fibrinogen storage disease** there are diastase–PAS-negative intracellular pale inclusions resembling ground-glass hepatocytes.[107,109]

Gaucher's disease (glycosyl ceramide lipidosis)

Cerebrosides accumulate in Kupffer cells and portal macrophages, which are enlarged, moderately diastase–PAS-positive and have a finely striated appearance (**Fig. 13.15**). The affected cells compress hepatocytes and sinusoids and may give rise to portal hypertension. Pericellular fibrosis is a common finding.[110]

Niemann–Pick disease (sphingomyelin lipidosis)

There are several variants of Niemann–Pick disease, and the clinical features range from severe and fatal neurological disease in infancy to symptomless hepatosplenomegaly in adults. The typical morphological feature of this disorder is the accumulation of sphingomyelin in both hepatocytes and macrophages. The latter are greatly swollen, foamy and diastase–PAS-positive to a variable extent. They can readily be distinguished from glycogen-rich liver cells in sections stained by the PAS method (**Fig. 13.16**). In addition to sphingomyelin, portal phagocytes, especially in the adult form, may also contain a brown lipofuscin-like pigment; these, as well as similar cells in bone marrow, stain a sea-blue colour by the Giemsa method. Niemann–Pick disease is thus one cause of the so-called sea-blue histiocyte syndrome.[111] Type B Niemann–Pick disease may progress to cirrhosis.[76,112]

Wolman's disease and cholesterol ester storage disease

In these apparently related conditions – the first a severe and usually fatal disease of infants, the second a milder disease of older children – cholesterol esters accumulate in hepatocytes and macrophages.[113,114] Hepatocytes also contain much triglyceride. The

Figure 13.15 Gaucher's disease. Pale-staining, striated Kupffer cells containing stored lipid are present within sinusoids. (Wedge biopsy, H&E.)

Figure 13.16 Niemann–Pick disease. The darker cells are glycogen-rich PAS-positive hepatocytes. Between them are large, pale-staining Kupffer cells filled with lipid. (Wedge biopsy, PAS.)

diagnosis may be suspected from the bright-orange colour of the liver biopsy core. By light microscopy, hepatocytes appear fat-laden, and macrophages are enlarged and foamy. Crystalline deposits may be seen within affected cells, particularly in frozen sections. The excess lipid is birefringent. Other features which may be found include ductular proliferation, pericellular fibrosis and even cirrhosis.[114]

Galactosaemia

Severe fatty change appears early in children with an inherited deficiency of galactose-1-phosphate uridyl transferase. Ductular reaction and cholestasis may also be present. Within a few weeks, liver-cell plates become transformed into tubular, duct-like structures (cholestatic rosettes) which dominate the histological picture, and there is siderosis and extramedullary haemopoiesis. Fibrosis and cirrhosis then develop. Institution of a galactose-free diet may result in substantial histological improvement.[115]

Histologically, the differential diagnosis includes **hereditary fructose intolerance**, in which the changes are somewhat similar but less severe. Also similar but more severe are the histological changes of **tyrosinaemia**. In this condition adenoma-like nodules are often seen, containing much fat.[70,71] Siderosis is also prominent. Hepatocellular carcinoma can develop, particularly in children over the age of 2 years, and liver transplantation is an important therapeutic option to forestall this event.[116]

Disorders of ureagenesis

Deficiencies in enzymes of the urea cycle, including ornithine transcarbamylase and carbamyl-phosphate synthase, may produce fatal hyperammonaemia in children and, rarely, in adults.[117] In these disorders the liver shows microvesicular steatosis which may be accompanied by aggregates of clear hepatocytes (**focal glycogenosis**[118]) (**Fig. 13.17**). These glycogen-enriched regions stain brightly with PAS and are diagnostically helpful in excluding other causes of paediatric microvesicular fatty liver such as Reye's syndrome (see below).

Figure 13.17 Focal glycogenosis.
Two foci of glycogen-containing hepatocytes with clear cytoplasm are seen near the portal tract. The patient had undergone partial hepatectomy for metastatic adenocarcinoma. In individuals with deficiencies of urea cycle enzymes, this lesion is accompanied by microvesicular steatosis. (Partial hepatectomy, H&E.)

Reye's syndrome

This is a serious and often fatal condition of encephalopathy and fatty change in the viscera of children under the age of 18 years. Viral infections (influenza B or A, varicella), salicylate ingestion and endotoxaemia have been implicated in the pathogenesis.[119-121] The incidence of Reye's syndrome declined throughout the 1980s, parallel with a decrease in the use of salicylates for childhood viral illnesses, but it is still seen in some parts of the world.

Liver biopsy is an important part of the investigation. The specimen is abnormally pale or yellow on naked-eye examination, and on light microscopy there is fine-droplet fatty change. This is panlobular in distribution and may be difficult to see without specific staining for fat, because of the small size of the vacuoles. Droplets are smaller in perivenular regions than elsewhere. Necrosis and inflammation are usually slight or absent, but in a few patients there is periportal ballooning or necrosis of hepatocytes.[122,123] Electron microscopy shows characteristic degenerative changes in liver-cell mitochondria; these are swollen and irregular in shape, with flocculent, electron-lucent matrix and reduced numbers of granules.[124] Succinic dehydrogenase activity is reduced. The differential diagnosis includes other conditions with microvesicular fat such as drug hepatotoxicity, urea cycle defects and mitochondrial hepatopathies associated with respiratory chain[125] and fatty acid oxidation defects.[3]

Parenteral nutrition

The effects of parenteral nutrition have been briefly mentioned in **Chapters 7 and 8**. It is pertinent to note here that in infants **cholestasis** is the major lesion associated with parenteral nutrition;[126,127] this may occasion diagnostic difficulties when other causes of cholestasis such as sepsis or biliary obstruction are also under clinical consideration. These difficulties are compounded by the fact that with prolonged administration of parenteral nutrition the portal tracts show progressive changes which are very similar to those of bile-duct obstruction (**Fig. 13.18**). A ductular reaction may be present after 3 weeks of parenteral nutrition[128] followed by portal fibrosis at 8–12 weeks and cirrhosis after 12 weeks.[129] Correlation of biopsy features with detailed clinical information regarding the duration of parenteral nutrition is clearly paramount in establishing the cause of jaundice in this population.

Hyperbilirubinaemias

In **Gilbert's syndrome**, a common form of familial unconjugated hyperbilirubinaemia,[130] the liver is histologically normal by light microscopy except for small amounts of stainable iron which are often seen in hepatocytes. In the **Dubin–Johnson syndrome**, in which the serum bilirubin is mainly conjugated, canalicular excretion of bilirubin and some other organic substances is defective[131] because of a mutation in the gene for canalicular multi-specific-organic-anion transporter.[132] Other constituents of bile are excreted normally and there is no cholestasis. A complex dark brown pigment accumulates in hepatocytes, especially in perivenular areas, giving the liver a dark, speckled appearance to the naked eye. The pigment granules somewhat resemble normal lipofuscin pigment and occupy a similar pericanalicular site in hepatocytes, but are darker, more abundant, larger and more variable in size (**Fig. 13.19**). When the pigment is very abundant, its pericanalicular location is no longer evident. Simple histochemical characteristics such as PAS-positivity and acid-fastness do not reliably distinguish between Dubin–Johnson pigment and lipofuscin

**Figure 13.18
Parenteral
nutrition.**
An irregular, fibrotic
portal tract shows
proliferated bile
ductules and a
mixed inflammatory
cell infiltrate of
neutrophilic
leucocytes and
lymphocytes. Many
cholestatic rosettes
are present. (Needle
biopsy, H&E.)

**Figure 13.19
Dubin–Johnson
syndrome.**
Hepatocytes contain
abundant coarse,
dark-brown pigment
granules. (Needle
biopsy, H&E.)

because both stain variably (**see Table 3.1**), but the distinction is usually clear on the basis of the above morphological features. When there is doubt, this may be resolved by electron microscopy, which shows the Dubin–Johnson pigment granules to be composed of characteristic strands of electron-dense material in an electron-lucent background, together with scanty lipid droplets (**see Fig. 17.2**).

Inherited cholestatic syndromes

Consideration of this group of disorders should be prompted when bland canalicular or canalicular and hepatocellular cholestasis with or without giant-cell transformation are the predominant histological features. This picture may develop owing to a variety of mutations of bile transport proteins or inborn errors of bile acid synthesis. The morphological assessment should take into account not only the presence or absence of giant cells, but also whether native bile ducts are injured or absent and whether a mild ductular reaction and/or portal/periportal fibrosis are present, since such features may help to distinguish among aetiologies.[1] Electron microscopy to assess the appearance of the bile and immunohistochemical staining to evaluate preservation or absence of specific bile transport proteins (e.g. bile-salt export pump; BSEP[133]) provide additional diagnostic information.

The cholestatic group of diseases termed **progressive familial intrahepatic cholestasis** (**PFIC**) – currently subdivided into three types: PFIC-1, -2, and -3 – are autosomal recessive disorders in which gene mutations result in defective bile-salt transporter proteins on the canalicular membrane.[132,134,135] Affected infants have jaundice, pruritus and intrahepatic cholestasis which progress to cirrhosis in childhood. The best known of these is **Byler disease** (PFIC-1), which affects kindred of the Amish settler Jacob Byler.[136,137] A clinically similar subgroup of PFIC-1 in non-Amish individuals is designated **Byler syndrome**. PFIC-1 is caused by mutations in *ATP8B1* on chromosome 18q21–22 that encode FIC-1 protein, which is expressed on bile canaliculi and intestinal epithelium. The presence of normal to low levels of serum γ-glutamyl transferase relative to the degree of cholestasis is an important diagnostic feature of Byler disease and syndrome. In both, the liver shows canalicular and sometimes hepatocellular bile plugs (**Fig. 13.20**). The bland cholestasis of Byler disease, however, contrasts with the features of 'neonatal hepatitis' (giant cells, chronic inflammation) and intrahepatic bile-duct paucity seen in Byler syndrome and in PFIC-2 caused by mutations in *ABCB11*, which encodes the BSEP. Electron microscopy

Figure 13.20 Byler syndrome.
Canalicular bile (arrow) and multinucleated giant hepatocytes are present in this specimen from a non-Amish patient. (Explant liver, H&E.)

Figure 13.21
Benign recurrent intrahepatic cholestasis.
Bile canalicular cholestasis is diffusely prominent (arrowheads). (Needle biopsy, H&E.)

shows distinctive coarsely granular bile in Byler disease and filamentous or amorphous bile in Byler syndrome[136] (**see Fig. 17.10**). Portal fibrosis, ductular reaction and cirrhosis eventually develop. Hepatocellular carcinoma[133] and cholangiocarcinoma[138] are other reported sequelae. Many of these patients develop graft steatosis after liver transplantation, possibly because of the continued expression of dysfunctional FIC-1 protein on intestinal epithelium.[139,140] Steatohepatitis with cirrhosis are additional complications[141].

Two subtypes of **benign recurrent intrahepatic cholestasis** (BRIC) are recognised. Subtype 1 shows a gene mutation mapped to *ATP8B1* on chromosome 18 (as in PFIC-1) and subtype 2 has a mutation in the *ABCB11* gene (also the target in PFIC-2).[142] Affected patients have multiple attacks of jaundice and itching, often starting in childhood or early adult life.[132,134,143] Histologically, canalicular cholestasis is seen in attacks, usually unaccompanied by any substantial degree of inflammation (**Fig. 13.21**). Between attacks the liver returns to normal and there is no fibrosis or progression to cirrhosis. A clinical continuum between BRIC and PFIC is suggested in some cases.[144]

Additional congenital or familial cholestatic syndromes are described,[145] including Norwegian cholestasis, North American Indian cholestasis,[30,137] Navajo neurohepatopathy[2] and recurrent cholestasis in the Faeroe Islands.[146]

Cirrhosis in childhood

Children are susceptible to many of the causal cirrhotic agents affecting adults, including hepatitis virus infections. As already noted, several inherited metabolic disorders lead to cirrhosis, and the possibility of Wilson's disease should always be considered in a child with chronic liver disease. Cirrhosis in young women should raise the question of autoimmune hepatitis, either type I (with anti-actin antibodies) or type II (anti-liver–kidney microsomal antibodies)[147] (**see Ch. 9**). Rare familial forms of cirrhosis have been described.[148] Not infrequently, the aetiology of some forms of childhood cirrhosis is obscure, as for example in the cerebral degenerative disorder Alper's disease[149] in which

Figure 13.22 Indian childhood cirrhosis.

Many liver cells are swollen (centre), and surrounded by fibrosis and mononuclear cells. Mallory bodies are present within some hepatocytes (arrow). Regenerating hepatocytes are organised into small clusters. (Post-mortem liver, H&E.)

microvesicular fat is also present. Cryptogenic cirrhosis due to keratin mutations[150] is another consideration (**see Ch. 10**).

Indian childhood cirrhosis, a disease of high mortality affecting young Indian children (and occasionally reported from outside the Indian subcontinent[151–157]), greatly declined in incidence after the mid-1990s, when brass- and copper-containing vessels used for milk-feeding were identified as sources of copper contamination.[158] The major features include hepatocellular swelling at an early stage followed by ballooning, Mallory body formation and necrosis. Focal accumulations of neutrophils and pericellular fibrosis resemble steatohepatitis, but there is little or no fatty change (**Fig. 13.22**). Large amounts of copper and copper-associated protein accumulate in affected hepatocytes[159,160] and chelation therapy with d-penicillamine therapy is effective in some patients.[161] The small clusters of damaged hepatocytes surrounded by fibrosis eventually evolve to a cirrhosis characterised by very small nodules ('micro-micronodular cirrhosis').

References

1 Balistreri WF, Bezerra JA, Jansen P, et al. Intrahepatic cholestasis: summary of an American Association for the Study of Liver Diseases Single-Topic Conference. *Hepatology* 2005; **42**: 222–235.

2 Vu TH, Tanji K, Holve SA, et al. Navajao neurohepatopathy: a mitochondrial DNA depletion syndrome? *Hepatology* 2001; **34**: 116–120.

3 Lee WS, Sokol RJ. Mitochondrial hepatopathies: advances in genetics and pathogenesis. *Hepatology* 2007; **45**: 1555–1565.

4 Jansen PLM, Sturm E. Genetic cholestasis, causes and consequences for hepatobiliary transport. *Liver Int* 2003; **23**: 315–322.

5 Knisely AS, Mieli-Vergani G, Whitington PF. Neonatal hemochromatosis. *Gastroenterol Clin North Am* 2003; **32**: 877–889.

6 Faa G, Liguori C, Columbano A, et al. Uneven copper distribution in the human newborn liver. *Hepatology* 1987; **7**: 838–842.

7 Faa G, Sciot R, Farci AMG, et al. Iron concentration and distribution in the newborn liver. *Liver* 1994; **14**: 193–199.

8 Bove KE, Daugherty CC, Tyson W, et al. Bile acid synthetic defects and liver disease. *Pediatr Devel Pathol* 2000; **3**: 1–16.

9 Müller-Höcker J, Muntau A, Schäfer S, et al. Depletion of mitochondrial DNA in the liver of an infant with neonatal giant cell hepatitis. *Hum Pathol* 2002; **33**: 247–253.

10 Ruchelli ED, Uri A, Dimmick JE, et al. Severe perinatal liver disease and Down syndrome: an apparent relationship. *Hum Pathol* 1991; **22**: 1274–1280.

11 Hadchouel M, Gautier M. Histopathologic study of the liver in the early cholestatic phase of alpha-1-antitrypsin deficiency. *J Pediatr* 1976; **89**: 211–215.

12 Perlmutter DH, Shepherd RW. Extrahepatic biliary atresia: a disease or a phenotype. *Hepatology* 2002; **35**: 1297–1304.

13 Gautier M, Eliot N. Extrahepatic biliary atresia. Morphological study of 98 biliary remnants. *Arch Pathol Lab Med* 1981; **105**: 397–402.

14 Chandra RS, Altman RP. Ductal remnants in extrahepatic biliary atresia: a histopathologic study with clinical correlation. *J Pediatr* 1978; **93**: 196–200.

15 Gautier M, Jehan P, Odièvre M. Histologic study of biliary fibrous remnants in 48 cases of extrahepatic biliary atresia: correlation with postoperative bile flow restoration. *J Pediatr* 1976; **89**: 704–709.

16 Haas JE. Bile duct and liver pathology in biliary atresia. *World J Surg* 1978; **2**: 561–569.

17 Kasai M, Suzuki S. A new operation for 'non-correctable' biliary atresia. *Shujitsu* 1959; **13**: 173–179.

18 Logan S, Stanton A. Screening for biliary atresia. *Lancet* 1993; **342**: 256.

19 Whitington PF, Balistreri WF. Liver transplantation in pediatrics: indications, contraindications, and pretransplant management. *J Pediatr* 1991; **118**: 169–177.

20 Chen L, Goryachev A, Sun J, et al. Altered expression of genes involved in hepatic morphogenesis and fibrogenesis are identified by cDNA microarray analysis in biliary atresia. *Hepatology* 2003; **38**: 567–576.

21 Silveira TR, Salzano FM, Howard ER, et al. Congenital structural abnormalities in biliary atresia: evidence for etiopathogenic heterogeneity and therapeutic implications. *Acta Paediatr Scand* 1991; **80**: 1192–1199.

22 Fain JS, Lewin KJ. Intrahepatic biliary cysts in congenital biliary atresia. *Arch Pathol Lab Med* 1989; **113**: 1383–1386.

23 Zhang D-Y, Sabla G, Shivakumar P, et al. Coordinate expression of regulatory genes differentiates embryonic and perinatal forms of biliary atresia. *Hepatology* 2004; **39**: 954–962.

24 Raweily EA, Gibson AAM, Burt AD. Abnormalities of intrahepatic bile ducts in extrahepatic biliary atresia. *Histopathology* 1990; **17**: 521–527.

25 Nietgen GW, Vacanti JP, Perez-Atayde AR. Intrahepatic bile duct loss in biliary atresia despite portoenterostomy: a consequence of ongoing obstruction? *Gastroenterology* 1992; **102**: 2126–2133.

26 Alagille D. Extrahepatic biliary atresia. *Hepatology* 1984; **4**: 7S–10S.

27 Jörgensen MJ. The ductal plate malformation: a study of the intrahepatic bile-duct lesion in infantile polycystic disease and congenital hepatic fibrosis. *Acta Pathol Microbiol Scand* 1977; **257**(Suppl): 1–88.

28 Brough AJ, Bernstein J. Conjugated hyperbilirubinemia in early infancy. A reassessment of liver biopsy. *Hum Pathol* 1974; **5**: 507–516.

29 Ramm GA, Nair VG, Bridle KR, et al. Contribution of hepatic parenchymal and nonparenchymal cells to hepatic fibrogenesis in biliary atresia. *Am J Pathol* 1998; **153**: 527–535.

30 Riely CA. Familial intrahepatic cholestatic syndromes. *Semin Liver Dis* 1987; **7**: 119–133.

31 Dahms BB, Petrelli M, Wyllie R, et al. Arteriohepatic dysplasia in infancy and childhood: a longitudinal study of six patients. *Hepatology* 1982; **2**: 350–358.

32 Kahn EI, Daum F, Markowitz J, et al. Arteriohepatic dysplasia. II. Hepatobiliary morphology. *Hepatology* 1983; **3**: 77–84.

33 Nijjar SS, Crosby HA, Wallace L, et al. Notch receptor expression in adult human liver: a possible role in bile duct formation and hepatic neovascularisation. *Hepatology* 2001; **34**: 1184–1192.

34 Libbrecht L, Spinner NB, Moore EC, et al. Peripheral bile duct paucity and cholestasis in the liver of a patient with Alagille syndrome. Further evidence supporting a lack of postnatal bile duct branching and elongation. *Am J Surg Pathol* 2005; **29**: 820–826.

35 Emerick KM, Rand EB, Goldmuntz E, et al. Features of Alagille syndrome in 92 patients: frequency and relation to prognosis. *Hepatology* 1999; **29**: 822–829.

36 Finegold MJ, Carpenter RJ. Obliterative cholangitis due to cytomegalovirus: a possible precursor of paucity of intrahepatic bile ducts. *Hum Pathol* 1982; **13**: 662–665.

37 Bruguera M, Llach J, Rodés J. Nonsyndromic paucity of intrahepatic bile ducts in infancy and idiopathic ductopenia in adulthood: the same syndrome? *Hepatology* 1992; **15**: 830–834.

38 Ludwig J, Wiesner RH, La Russo NF. Idiopathic adulthood ductopenia: a cause of chronic cholestatic liver disease and biliary cirrhosis. *J Hepatol* 1988; **7**: 193–199.

39 Kahn E, Daum F, Markowitz J, et al. Nonsyndromatic paucity of interlobular bile ducts: light and electron microscopic evaluation of sequential liver biopsies in early childhood. *Hepatology* 1986; **6**: 890–901.

40 Fabris L, Cadamuro M, Guido M, et al. Analysis of liver repair mechanisms in Alagille syndrome and biliary atresia reveals a role for Notch signaling. *Am J Pathol* 2007; **171**: 641–653.

41 Heathcote J, Deodhar KP, Scheuer PJ, et al. Intrahepatic cholestasis in childhood. *N Engl J Med* 1976; **295**: 801–805.

42 Leblanc A, Hadchouel M, Jehan P, et al. Obstructive jaundice in children with histiocytosis X. *Gastroenterology* 1981; **80**: 134–139.

43 Kaplan KJ, Goodman ZD, Ishak KG. Liver involvement in Langerhans' cell histiocytosis: a study of nine cases. *Mod Pathol* 1999; **12**: 370–378.

44 Gregorio GV, Portmann B, Karani J, et al. Autoimmune hepatitis/sclerosing cholangitis overlap syndrome in childhood: a 16-year prospective study. *Hepatology* 2001; **33**: 544–553.

45 Summerfield JA, Nagafuchi Y, Sherlock S, et al. Hepatobiliary fibropolycystic diseases. A clinical and histological review of 51 patients. *J Hepatol* 1986; **2**: 141–156.

46 Desmet VJ. Congenital diseases of intrahepatic bile ducts: variations on the theme 'ductal plate malformation'. *Hepatology* 1992; **16**: 1069–1083.

47 Desmet VJ. What is congenital hepatic fibrosis? *Histopathology* 1992; **20**: 465–477.

48 Desmet VJ. Pathogenesis of ductal plate abnormalities. *Mayo Clin Proc* 1998; **73**: 80–89.

49 Scott J, Shousha S, Thomas HC, et al. Bile duct carcinoma: a late complication of congenital hepatic fibrosis. Case

report and review of literature. *Am J Gastroenterol* 1980; **73**: 113–119.

50 Chaudhuri PK, Chaudhuri B, Schuler JJ, et al. Carcinoma associated with congenital cystic dilation of bile ducts. *Arch Surg* 1982; **117**: 1349–1351.

51 Honda N, Cobb C, Lechago J. Bile duct carcinoma associated with multiple von Meyenburg complexes in the liver. *Hum Pathol* 1986; **17**: 1287–1290.

52 Case records of the Massachusetts General Hospital. Case 48-1988. *N Engl J Med* 1988; **319**: 1465–1474.

53 Hodgson HJF, Davies DR, Thompson RPH. Congenital hepatic fibrosis. *J Clin Pathol* 1976; **29**: 11–16.

54 de Koning TJ, Nikkels PGJ, Dorland L, et al. Congenital hepatic fibrosis in 3 siblings with phosphomannose isomerase deficiency. *Virchows Arch* 2000; **437**: 101–105.

55 Nakanuma Y, Terada T, Ohta G, et al. Caroli's disease in congenital hepatic fibrosis and infantile polycystic disease. *Liver* 1982; **2**: 346–354.

56 Ludwig J, MacCarty RL, LaRusso NF, et al. Intrahepatic cholangiectases and large-duct obliteration in primary sclerosing cholangitis. *Hepatology* 1986; **6**: 560–568.

57 Thommesen N. Biliary hamartomas (von Meyenburg complexes) in liver needle biopsies. *Acta Pathol Microbiol Scand A* 1978; **86**: 93–99.

58 Landing BH, Wells TR, Claireaux AE. Morphometric analysis of liver lesions in cystic diseases of childhood. *Hum Pathol* 1980; **11**: 549–560.

59 Chatelain D, Chailley-Heu B, Terris B, et al. The ciliated hepatic foregut cyst, an unusual bronchiolar foregut malformation: a histological, histochemical, and immunohistochemical study of 7 cases. *Hum Pathol* 2000; **31**: 241–246.

60 Forbes A, Murray-Lyon IM. Cystic disease of the liver and biliary tract. *Gut* 1991; **32: Suppl**: S116–S122.

61 Terada T, Nakanuma Y. Congenital biliary dilatation in autosomal dominant adult polycystic disease of the liver and kidneys. *Arch Pathol Lab Med* 1988; **112**: 1113–1116.

62 Ramos A, Torres VE, Holley KE, et al. The liver in autosomal dominant polycystic kidney disease. Implications for pathogenesis. *Arch Pathol Lab Med* 1990; **114**: 180–184.

63 Scott-Jupp R, Lama M, Tanner MS. Prevalence of liver disease in cystic fibrosis. *Arch Dis Child* 1991; **66**: 698–701.

64 Nagel RA, Westaby D, Javaid A, et al. Liver disease and bileduct abnormalities in adults with cystic fibrosis. *Lancet* 1989; **ii**: 1422–1425.

65 Marino CR, Gorelick FS. Scientific advances in cystic fibrosis. *Gastroenterology* 1992; **103**: 681–693.

66 Lindblad A, Hultcrantz R, Strandvik B. Bile-duct destruction and collagen deposition: a prominent ultrastructural feature of the liver in cystic fibrosis. *Hepatology* 1992; **16**: 372–381.

67 Furuya KN, Roberts EA, Canny GJ, et al. Neonatal hepatitis syndrome with paucity of interlobular bile ducts in cystic fibrosis. *J Pediatr Gastroenterol Nutr* 1991; **12**: 127–130.

68 Isenberg JI. Cystic fibrosis: its influence on the liver, biliary tree, and bile salt metabolism. *Semin Liver Dis* 1982; **4**: 302–313.

69 Lewindon PJ, Pereira TN, Hoskins AC, et al. The role of hepatic stellate cells and transforming growth factor-beta-1 in cystic fibrosis liver disease. *Am J Pathol* 2002; **160**: 1705–1715.

70 Ishak KG. Hepatic morphology in the inherited metabolic diseases. *Semin Liver Dis* 1986; **6**: 246–258.

71 Ishak KG, Sharp HL. Metabolic errors and liver disease. In: MacSween RNM, Anthony PP, Scheuer PJ, et al., eds. Pathology of the Liver, 3rd edn. Edinburgh: Churchill Livingstone, 1994; Ch. 4: 123–218.

72 Portmann BC. Liver biopsy in the diagnosis of inherited metabolic disorders. In: Anthony PP, MacSween RNM, eds. Recent Advances in Histopathology, **Vol 14.** Edinburgh: Churchill Livingstone, 1989: 139–159.

73 Resnick JM, Whitley CB, Leonard AS, et al. Light and electron microscopic features of the liver in mucopolysaccharidosis. *Hum Pathol* 1994; **25**: 276–286.

74 Phillips MJ, Poucell S, Patterson J, et al., eds. The Liver. An Atlas and Text of Ultrastructural Pathology. New York: Raven Press, 1987.

75 Resnick JM, Krivit W, Snover DC, et al. Pathology of the liver in mucopolysaccharidosis: light and electron microscopic assessment before and after bone marrow transplantation. *Bone Marrow Transplant* 1992; **10**: 273–280.

76 Smanik EJ, Tavill AS, Jacobs GH, et al. Orthotopic liver transplantation in two adults with Niemann–Pick and Gaucher's diseases: implications for the treatment of inherited metabolic disease. *Hepatology* 1993; **17**: 42–49.

77 McAdams AJ, Hug G, Bove KE. Glycogen storage disease, types I to X: criteria for morphologic diagnosis. *Hum Pathol* 1974; **5**: 463–487.

78 Itoh S, Ishida Y, Matsuo S. Mallory bodies in a patient with type Ia glycogen storage disease. *Gastroenterology* 1987; **92**: 520–523.

79 Howell RR, Stevenson RE, Ben-Menachem Y, et al. Hepatic adenomata with type 1 glycogen storage disease. *JAMA* 1976; **236**: 1481–1484.

80 Coire CI, Qizilbash AH, Castelli MF. Hepatic adenomata in type Ia glycogen storage disease. *Arch Pathol Lab Med* 1987; **111**: 166–169.

81 Limmer J, Fleig WE, Leupold D, et al. Hepatocellular carcinoma in type I glycogen storage disease. *Hepatology* 1988; **8**: 531–537.

82 Markowitz AJ, Chen Y-T, Muenzer J, et al. A man with type III glycogenosis associated with cirrhosis and portal hypertension. *Gastroenterology* 1993; **105**: 1882–1885.

83 Bannayan GA, Dean WJ, Howell RR. Type IV glycogen-storage disease. Light-microscopic, electron-microscopic, and enzymatic study. *Am J Clin Pathol* 1976; **66**: 702–709.

84 Vázquez JJ. Ground glass hepatocytes: light and electron microscopy. Characterization of the different types. *Histol Histopathol* 1990; **5**: 379–386.

85 Jack CIA, Evans CC. Three cases of alpha-1-antitrypsin deficiency in the elderly. *Postgrad Med J* 1991; **67**: 840–842.

86 Rakela J, Goldschmiedt M, Ludwig J. Late manifestation of chronic liver disease in adults with alpha-1-antitrypsin deficiency. *Dig Dis Sci* 1987; **32**: 1358–1362.

87 Deutsch J, Becker H, Auböck L. Histopathological features of liver disease in alpha-1-antitrypsin deficiency. *Acta Paediatr* 1994; **393**(Suppl): 8–12.

88 Fairbanks KD, Tavill AS. Liver disease in alpha-1-antitrypsin deficiency: a review. *Am J Gastroenterol* 2008; **103**: 2136–2141.

89 Perlmutter DH. The cellular basis for liver injury in α_1-antitrypsin deficiency. *Hepatology* 1991; **13**: 172–185.

90 Aldonyte R, Jamsson L, Ljungberg O, et al. Polymerized α_1-antitrypsin is present on lung vascular endothelium. New insights into the biological significance of α_1-antitrypsin polymerization. *Histopathology* 2004; **45**: 587–592.

91 Carrell RW, Lomas DA. Alpha-1-antitrypsin deficiency – a model for conformational diseases. *N Engl J Med* 2002; **346**: 45–53.

92 Callea F, Fevery J, De Groote J, et al. Detection of Pi Z phenotype individuals by alpha-1-antitrypsin (AAT) immunohistochemistry in paraffin-embedded liver tissue specimens. *J Hepatol* 1986; **2**: 389–401.

93 Theaker JM, Fleming KA. Alpha-1-antitrypsin and the liver: a routine immunohistological screen. *J Clin Pathol* 1986; **39**: 58–62.

94 Qizilbash A, Young-Pong O. Alpha 1 antitrypsin liver disease differential diagnosis of PAS-positive, diastase-resistant globules in liver cells. *Am J Clin Pathol* 1983; **79**: 697–702.

95 Hay CR, Preston FE, Triger DR, et al. Progressive liver disease in haemophilia: an understated problem? *Lancet* 1985; **1**: 1495–1498.

96 Geller SA, Nichols WS, Dycaico MJ, et al. Histopathology of α_1-antitrypsin liver disease in a transgenic mouse model. *Hepatology* 1990; **12**: 40–47.

97 Talbot IC, Mowat AP. Liver disease in infancy: histological features and relationship to alpha-antitrypsin phenotype. *J Clin Pathol* 1975; **28**: 559–563.

98 Odièvre M, Martin JP, Hadchouel M, et al. Alpha1-antitrypsin deficiency and liver disease in children: phenotypes, manifestations, and prognosis. *Pediatrics* 1976; **57**: 226–231.

99 Propst T, Propst A, Dietze O, et al. High prevalence of viral infection in adults with homozygous and heterozygous alpha-1-antitrypsin deficiency and chronic liver disease. *Ann Intern Med* 1992; **117**: 641–645.

100 Palmer PE, Wolfe HJ. Alpha-antitrypsin deposition in primary hepatic carcinomas. *Arch Pathol Lab Med* 1976; **100**: 232–236.

101 Reintoft I, Hagerstrand I. Demonstration of alpha 1-antitrypsin in hepatomas. *Arch Pathol Lab Med* 1979; **103**: 495–498.

102 Eriksson S, Carlson J, Velez R. Risk of cirrhosis and primary liver cancer in alpha 1-antitrypsin deficiency. *N Engl J Med* 1986; **314**: 736–739.

103 Graziadei IW, Joseph JJ, Wiesner RH, et al. Increased risk of chronic liver failure in adults with heterozygous α_1-antitrypsin deficiency. *Hepatology* 1998; **28**: 1058–1063.

104 Pittschieler K. Liver disease and heterozygous alpha-1-antitrypsin deficiency. *Acta Paediatr Scand* 1991; **80**: 323–327.

105 Marwick TH, Cooney PT, Kerlin P. Cirrhosis and hepatocellular carcinoma in a patient with heterozygous (MZ) alpha-1-antitrypsin deficiency. *Pathology* 1985; **17**: 649–652.

106 Reid CL, Wiener GJ, Cox DW, et al. Diffuse hepatocellular dysplasia and carcinoma associated with the Mmalton variant of α_1-antitrypsin. *Gastroenterology* 1987; **93**: 181–187.

107 Callea F, Brisigotti M, Fabbretti G, et al. Hepatic endoplasmic reticulum storage diseases. *Liver* 1992; **12**: 357–362.

108 Lindmark B, Eriksson S. Partial deficiency of α_1-antichymotrypsin is associated with chronic cryptogenic liver disease. *Scand J Gastroenterol* 1991; **26**: 508–512.

109 Rubbia-Brandt L, Neerman-Arbez M, Rougemont A-L, et al. Fibrinogen gamma 375 Arg->trp mutation (fibrinogen Aguadilla) causes hereditary hypofibrinogenemia, hepatic endoplasmic reticulum storage disease and cirrhosis. *Am J Surg Pathol* 2006; **30**: 906–911.

110 James SP, Stromeyer FW, Chang C, et al. Liver abnormalities in patients with Gaucher's disease. *Gastroenterology* 1981; **80**: 126–133.

111 Long RG, Lake BD, Pettit JE, et al. Adult Niemann–Pick disease: its relationship to the syndrome of the sea-blue histiocyte. *Am J Med* 1977; **62**: 627–635.

112 Tassoni JP, Fawaz KA, Johnston DE. Cirrhosis and portal hypertension in a patient with adult Niemann–Pick disease. *Gastroenterology* 1991; **100**: 567–569.

113 Lake BD, Patrick AD. Wolman's disease: deficiency of E600-resistant acid esterase activity with storage of lipids in lysosomes. *J Pediatr* 1970; **76**: 262–266.

114 Beaudet AL, Ferry GD, Nichols BL Jr, et al. Cholesterol ester storage disease: clinical, biochemical, and pathological studies. *J Pediatr* 1977; **90**: 910–914.

115 Applebaum MN, Thaler MM. Reversibility of extensive liver damage in galactosemia. *Gastroenterology* 1975; **69**: 496–502.

116 Mieles LA, Esquivel COO, Van Thiel DH, et al. Liver transplantation for tyrosinemia: a review of 10 cases from the University of Pittsburgh. *Dig Dis Sci* 1990; **35**: 153–157.

117 Lichtenstein GR, Kaiser LR, Tuchman M, et al. Fatal hyperammonemia following orthotopic lung transplantation. *Gastroenterology* 1997; **112**: 236–240.

118 Badizadegan K, Perez-Atayde AR. Focal glycogenosis of the liver in disorders of ureagenesis: its occurrence and diagnostic significance. *Hepatology* 1997; **26**: 365–373.

119 Kilpatrick-Smith L, Hale DE, Douglas SD. Progress in Reye syndrome: epidemiology, biochemical mechanisms and animal models. *Dig Dis Sci* 1989; **7**: 135–146.

120 Lichtenstein PK, Heubi JE, Daugherty CC, et al. Grade I Reye's syndrome. A frequent cause of vomiting and liver dysfunction after varicella and upper-respiratory-tract infection. *N Engl J Med* 1983; **309**: 133–139.

121 Mowat AP. Reye's syndrome: 20 years on. *BMJ Clin Res* 1983; **286**: 1999–2001.

122 Brown RE, Ishak KG. Hepatic zonal degeneration and necrosis in Reye's syndrome. *Arch Pathol Lab Med* 1976; **100**: 123–126.

123 Kimura S, Kobayashi T, Tanaka Y, et al. Liver histopathology in clinical Reye syndrome. *Brain Dev* 1991; **13**: 95–100.

124 Tonsgard JH. Effect of Reye's syndrome serum on the ultrastructure of isolated liver mitochondria. *Lab Invest* 1989; **60**: 568–573.

125 Mandel H, Hartman C, Berkowitz D, et al. The hepatic mitochondrial DNA depletion syndrome: ultrastructural changes in liver biopsies. *Hepatology* 2001; **34**: 776–784.

126 Balistreri WF, Bove KE. Hepatobiliary consequences of parenteral alimentation. In: Popper H, Schaffner F, eds. Progress in Liver Diseases, **Vol IX**. Philadelphia, PA: WB Saunders, 1990: 567–602.

127 Quigley EMM, Marsh MN, Shaffer JL, et al. Hepatobiliary complications of total parenteral nutrition. *Gastroenterology* 1993; **104**: 286–301.

128 Cohen C, Olsen MM. Pediatric total parenteral nutrition. Liver histopathology. *Arch Pathol Lab Med* 1981; **105**: 152–156.

129 Mullick FG, Moran CA, Ishak KG. Total parenteral nutrition: a histopathologic analysis of the liver changes in 20 children. *Mod Pathol* 1994; **7**: 190–194.

130 Bosma PJ. Inherited disorders of bilirubin metabolism. *J Hepatol* 2003; **38**: 107–117.

131 Berthelot P, Dhumeaux D. New insights into the classification and mechanisms of hereditary, chronic, non-haemolytic hyperbilirubinaemias. *Gut* 1978; **19**: 474–480.

132 Traunder M, Meier PJ, Boyer JL. Molecular pathogenesis of cholestasis. *N Engl J Med* 1998; **339**: 1217–1227.

133 Knisely AS, Strautnieks SS, Meier Y, et al. Hepatocellular carcinoma in ten children under five years of age with bile salt export pump deficiency. *Hepatology* 2006; **44**: 478–486.

134 Oude Elferink RPJ, Van Berge Henegouwen GP. Cracking the genetic code for benign recurrent and progressive familial intrahepatic cholestasis. *J Hepatol* 1998; **29**: 317–320.

135 Müller M, Jansen PLM. The secretory function of the liver: new aspects of hepatobiliary transport. *J Hepatol* 1998; **28**: 344–354.

136 Bull LN, Carolton VEH, Stricker NL, et al. Genetic and morphological findings in progressive familial intrahepatic cholestasis (Byler disease [PFIC-1] and Byler syndrome): evidence for heterogeneity. *Hepatology* 1997; **26**: 155–164.

137 Desmet VJ. Cholestasis: extrahepatic obstruction and secondary biliary cirrhosis. In: MacSween RNM, Anthony PP, Scheuer PJ, et al., eds. Pathology of the Liver, 3rd edn. Edinburgh: Churchill Livingstone, 1994; Ch. 11: 425–476.

138 Scheimann AO, Strautnieks SS, Knisely AS, et al. Mutations in bile salt export pump (*ABCB11*) in two children with progressive familial intrahepatic cholestasis and cholangiocarcinoma. *J Pediatr* 2007; **150**: 556–559.

139 Lykavieris P, van Mil S, Cresteil D, et al. Progressive familial intrahepatic cholestasis type 1 and extrahepatic features: no catch-up of stature growth, exacerbation of diarrhea, and appearance of liver steatosis after liver transplantation. *J Hepatol* 2003; **39**: 447–452.

140 Shneider BL. Liver transplantation for progressive familial intrahepatic cholestasis: the evolving role of genotyping. *Liver Transplant* 2009; **15**: 565–566.

141 Miyagawa-Hayashino A, Egaqa H, Yorifuji T, et al. Allograft steatohepatitis in progressive familial intrahepatic cholestasis type 1 after living donor liver transplantation. *Liver Transplant* 2009; **15**: 610–618.

142 van Mil SWC, Van Der Woerd WL, Van Der Brugge G, et al. Benign recurrent intrahepatic cholestasis type 2 is caused by mutations in ABCB11. *Gastroenterology* 2004; **127**: 379–384.

143 Beaudoin M, Feldmann G, Erlinger S, et al. Benign recurrent cholestasis. *Digestion* 1973; **9**: 49–65.

144 van Ooteghem NAM, Klomp LWJ, van Berge-Henegouwen GP, et al. Benign recurrent intrahepatic cholestasis progressing to progressive familial intrahepatic cholestasis: low GGT cholestasis is a clinical continuum. *J Hepatol* 2002; **36**: 439–443.

145 Jansen PLM, Müller M, Sturm E. Genes and cholestasis. *Hepatology* 2001; **34**: 1067–1074.

146 Tygstrup N, Steig BA, Juijn JA, et al. Recurrent familial intrahepatic cholestasis in the Faeroe Islands. Phenotypic heterogeneity but genetic homogeneity. *Hepatology* 1999; **29**: 506–508.

147 Johnson PJ, McFarlane IG, Eddleston ALWF. The natural course and heterogeneity of autoimmune-type chronic active hepatitis. *Semin Liver Dis* 1991; **11**: 187–196.

148 Barnett JL, Appelman HD, Moseley RH. A familial form of incomplete septal cirrhosis. *Gastroenterology* 1992; **102**: 674–678.

149 Narkewicz MR, Sokol RJ, Beckwith B, et al. Liver involvement in Alpers disease. *J Pediatr* 1991; **119**: 260–267.

150 Ku N-O, Gish R, Wright TL, et al. Keratin 8 mutations in patients with cryptogenic liver disease. *N Engl J Med* 2001; **344**: 1580–1587.

151 Klass HJ, Kelly JK, Warnes TW. Indian childhood cirrhosis in the United Kingdom. *Gut* 1980; **21**: 344–350.

152 Lefkowitch JH, Honig CL, King ME, et al. Hepatic copper overload and features of Indian childhood cirrhosis in an American sibship. *N Engl J Med* 1982; **307**: 271–277.

153 Müller-Höcker J, Meyer U, Wiebecke B, et al. Copper storage disease of the liver and chronic dietary copper intoxication in two further German infants mimicking Indian childhood cirrhosis. *Pathol Res Pract* 1988; **183**: 39–45.

154 Adamson M, Reiner B, Olson JL, et al. Indian childhood cirrhosis in an American child. *Gastroenterology* 1992; **102**: 1771–1777.

155 Aljajeh IA, Mughal S, Al-Tahou B, et al. Indian childhood cirrhosis-like liver disease in an Arab child. A brief report. *Virchows Arch* 1994; **424**: 225–227.

156 Baker A, Gormally S, Saxena R, et al. Copper-associated liver disease in childhood. *J Hepatol* 1995; **23**: 538–543.

157 Müller T, Feichtinger H, Berger H, et al. Endemic Tyrolean infantile cirrhosis: an ecogenetic disorder. *Lancet* 1996; **347**: 877–880.

158 Tanner MS, Kantarjian AH, Bhave SA, et al. Early introduction of copper-contaminated animal mild feeds as a possible cause of Indian childhood cirrhosis. *Lancet* 1983; **2**: 992–995.

159 Popper H, Goldfischer S, Sternlieb I, et al. Cytoplasmic copper and its toxic effects. Studies in Indian childhood cirrhosis. *Lancet* 1979; **1**: 1205–1208.

160 Tanner MS, Portmann B, Mowat AP, et al. Increased hepatic copper concentration in Indian childhood cirrhosis. *Lancet* 1979; **1**: 1203–1205.

161 Bhusnurmath SR, Walia BNS, Singh S, et al. Sequential histopathologic alterations in Indian childhood cirrhosis treated with d-penicillamine. *Hum Pathol* 1991; **22**: 653–658.

General reading

Chandra RS, Stocker JT. The liver, gallbladder, and biliary tract. In: Stocker JT, Dehner LP, eds. Pediatric Pathology. Philadelphia, PA: JB Lippincott, 1992: 703–790.

Elferink RPJO, Paulusma CC, Groen AK. Hepatocanalicular transport defects: pathophysiologic mechanisms of rare diseases. *Gastroenterology* 2006; **130**: 908–925.

Feingold MJ. Common diagnostic problems in pediatric liver pathology. *Clin Liver Dis* 2002; **6**: 421–454.

Hansen K, Horslen S. Metabolic liver disease in children. *Liver Transpl* 2008; **14**: 391–411.

Ishak KG. Inherited metabolic diseases of the liver. *Clin Liver Dis* 2002; **6**: 455–480.

Kelly DA (ed). Diseases of the Liver and Biliary System in Children. 3rd edn. Chichester, West Sussex, UK: Wiley-Blackwell, 2008.

Portmann BC, Roberts EA. Developmental abnormalities and liver disease in childhood. In: Burt AD, Portmann BC, Ferrell LD, eds. MacSween's Pathology of the Liver, 5th edn. Edinburgh: Churchill Livingstone/Elsevier, 2007: 147–198.

Portmann BC, Thompson RJ, Roberts EA, Paterson AC. Genetic and metabolic liver disease. In: Burt AD, Portmann BC, Ferrell LD, eds. MacSween's Pathology of the Liver, 5th edn. Edinburgh: Churchill Livingstone/Elsevier, 2007: 199–326.

Disturbances of Copper and Iron Metabolism

Wilson's disease (hepatolenticular degeneration)

Wilson's disease is an autosomal recessive disorder due to mutations in the gene *ATP7B* for copper-transporting ATPase located in the *trans*-Golgi network of the liver.[1] It is uncommon but important and treatable. Normal hepatic copper transport[2] is disrupted owing to various ATP7B mutations,[3] leading to the accumulation of copper in hepatocytes and liver disease. The large number and diverse mutations identified currently precludes simple genetic testing,[4] in contrast to hereditary haemochromatosis (discussed later). Liver biopsy is important for histological diagnosis and monitoring.[4a]

Chemical quantitation of copper concentration in the biopsy sample helps to establish the diagnosis and is sometimes used for determination of the genetic status of a patient's siblings.[5,6] Copper determination can be made from specimens obtained by routine liver biopsy or retrieved from paraffin blocks, without special copper-free solutions or instruments.[7] Homozygous individuals have increased liver copper levels from an early age but do not develop symptoms of liver disease in the first few years of life. Increased liver copper levels precede the development of histological abnormalities. Hepatic copper levels are typically greater than 4 µmol/g dry weight (>250 µg/g dry weight).[7]

Histological lesions develop before the disease is clinically apparent. In the early, pre-cirrhotic phase there is fatty change,[6] sometimes with the formation of fat granulomas.[5] Slender fibrous septa extend from portal tracts (**Fig. 14.1**). There may be unusually abundant lipofuscin pigment in hepatocytes and glycogen vacuolation of hepatocyte nuclei, but neither feature is easy to evaluate; both are found in normal individuals, and nuclear vacuolation is particularly common in the young. Lipofuscin granules may be larger and less regular in outline than normal.[8] Inflammation is absent or mild in the early stages. Kupffer cells are sometimes enlarged and may stain for iron as a result of haemolysis. Electron microscopy helps in the diagnosis of both early and late disease because of characteristic changes in mitochondria and lysosomes (**see Ch. 17**).

In some patients a phase of chronic hepatitis develops next that is difficult to distinguish histologically from chronic viral hepatitis. Stains for copper and copper-associated protein may be helpful, as discussed below. Cirrhosis develops in untreated patients, with or without a recognisable preceding phase of chronic hepatitis. A common though not invariable pattern is of active cirrhosis with fatty change, ballooned hepatocytes, focally dense eosinophilic cytoplasm and glycogen vacuolation of nuclei (**Fig. 14.2**). Cholestasis may be present. Hepatocytes often contain Mallory bodies and these are sometimes very

©2010 Elsevier Ltd
DOI: 10.1016/B978-0-7020-3410-7.00020-4

**Figure 14.1
Wilson's disease.**
At this early stage slender septa extend from portal tracts (P) but acinar architecture is intact. There is steatosis, just visible in this reticulin preparation. (Wedge biopsy, reticulin.)

**Figure 14.2
Wilson's disease.**
Active cirrhosis with liver-cell swelling, steatosis (arrowheads) and nuclear vacuolation (arrow). (Wedge biopsy, H&E.)

abundant. They are associated with an infiltrate rich in neutrophils, as in steatohepatitis (**Fig. 14.3**). Partial fibrous occlusion of efferent veins has been reported.[8] Hepatocellular carcinoma is a rare sequel of cirrhosis in Wilson's disease.[9,10]

Fulminant hepatic failure may be the first manifestation of Wilson's disease and is a major indication for liver transplantation.[11] The presence of haemolysis in a young individual with acute liver failure should therefore prompt consideration of Wilson's disease.[12] Cirrhosis is usually already present in such cases[13,14] in contradistinction to acute liver failure, owing to viral or drug hepatitis where recent massive necrosis is evident. The

Figure 14.3
Wilson's disease.
Numerous Mallory bodies (arrowheads) are seen within hepatocytes. (Post-mortem liver, H&E.)

cirrhotic nodules are frequently small and separated by septa containing abundant ductular structures and variable chronic inflammatory cells (**Fig. 14.4**). The death of hepatocytes in the fulminant disease occurs by both apoptosis and necrosis,[15] resulting in new zones of confluent necrosis superimposed on the underlying cirrhotic architecture. Cholestasis is often striking and hepatocytes may contain large- or small-droplet fat. The presence of much stainable copper and/or copper-associated protein in hepatocytes and Kupffer cells distinguishes Wilson's disease from other causes of fulminant hepatic failure.

Staining for copper and copper-associated protein plays a part in the diagnosis of Wilson's disease, though staining results (as well as the copper concentration) can vary considerably throughout the liver.[16] Failure to stain in either case is common at some stages of the disease and does not therefore exclude the diagnosis. Conversely, both copper and copper-associated protein are found in other liver diseases, usually as a result of failure to secrete copper into the bile. Thus, in a child with liver disease strong staining for copper might reflect loss of bile ducts rather than Wilson's disease. Other copper storage disorders have been described, including Indian childhood cirrhosis (**see Ch. 13, Fig. 13.22**), which is also occasionally seen elsewhere in the world.[17–19] Furthermore, neonatal liver is normally rich in copper.[20]

In the early phases of Wilson's disease, liver copper levels are high, but the copper is difficult to demonstrate histochemically. This is because it is diffusely distributed in hepatocytes and not concentrated in lysosomes. Sensitive histochemical methods (e.g. Timm's silver method or rhodanine) may show faint cytoplasmic staining. Later in the course of the disease copper begins to accumulate in liver-cell lysosomes and is then more easily stained. Once cirrhosis has developed, the distribution of copper is typically uneven, some nodules staining strongly while others are negative (**Fig. 14.5**). Staining for copper and copper–protein may be dissociated, although in most cases both are positive.[21,22] Timm's silver stain appears to be the most sensitive staining method for demonstrating copper in this disease.[23]

Because of the great variety of histological lesions in the liver, Wilson's disease can easily be mistaken for other liver disorders. Clinicians and pathologists should consider

Figure 14.4 Fulminant liver failure in Wilson's disease.

Fulminant hepatitis in Wilson's disease usually develops on a background of already developed cirrhosis, as seen in this case. **A:** Cirrhotic nodules (N) are surrounded by inflamed fibrous septa with numerous bile ductular structures. The acute illness is related to progressive hepatocyte necrosis, inflammation and ductular reaction at the septal–parenchymal interface as seen in the upper right field. **B:** Severe bile canalicular and hepatocellular cholestasis with both small- and large-droplet steatosis are present. (Explant liver, H&E.)

Figure 14.4, cont'd
C: Copper-binding protein is present in both periportal hepatocytes and sinusoidal Kupffer cells. (Explant liver, Victoria blue.)

Figure 14.5
Wilson's disease. The upper nodule is strongly positive for copper, stained orange-red. The lower nodule is completely negative. (Wedge biopsy, rhodanine.)

Wilson's disease in the differential diagnosis of hepatocellular disease especially in the young, but also at all ages, including (uncommonly) older-aged individuals.[24] The disease can be arrested by treatment and its development prevented in siblings. The penalties for missing the diagnosis are therefore very great.

Iron overload

Siderosis

Siderosis (or haemosiderosis) means the presence of demonstrable iron in tissues, irrespective of cause. The main forms of iron in hepatocytes are ferritin, haemosiderin and haem.[25] Stainable iron is mainly haemosiderin which is principally located in lysosomes and is seen as granules concentrated towards the biliary poles of the cells. Ferritin gives rise to more diffuse staining, imparting a bluish hue to the liver-cell cytoplasm on iron staining. Hepatocellular siderosis almost always shows a diminishing gradient of intensity from the periphery of lobules towards the central (efferent) veins. It is most severe in periportal regions (acinar zones 1) near small portal tracts, and least severe in centrilobular regions (acinar zones 3). The normal adult liver is usually negative on iron staining or at best shows minimal siderosis.[26] This is also true of the neonatal liver, although some cases may show mild periportal liver-cell siderosis (residual iron storage from the active period of hepatic haemopoiesis of the third trimester).[27]

Since iron stains of liver tissue are expected to be negative in most instances, a positive stain requires explanation. In this regard, two major categories of hepatic iron storage disease need to be considered, designated as **primary and secondary iron overload disorders**[28] (**Table 14.1**). The *primary disorders* are predominantly forms of hereditary haemochromatosis in which genetic mutations alter iron homeostasis in the gastrointestinal tract and liver. The *secondary disorders* are acquired conditions in which increased iron in the liver is due to exogenous sources of iron, abnormal erythrocyte destruction or changes in iron absorption and distribution related to underlying liver disease. The pathologist may be able to suggest the reason for the siderosis, based on the distribution of the stainable iron. For example, in most of the primary iron overload disorders, such as classic *HFE*-related haemochromatosis, the excess iron is mainly hepatocellular. In thalassaemia both hepatocytes and macrophages are positive, while exogenous iron overload leads to Kupffer-cell storage in the first instance. Various types of underlying liver disease are also associated with siderosis. Cirrhotic livers of varied aetiology may contain much iron,[29–31] even within macroregenerative nodules.[32] In viral hepatitis and alcoholic liver disease small amounts of stainable iron are often found. Siderosis in the setting of non-alcoholic fatty liver disease (**dysmetabolic hepatic iron overload**) is increasingly recognised.[33] Dense, iron-positive granules are common in endothelial cells in a variety of conditions including acute hepatitis,[34] chronic hepatitis B and C[35] and alcoholic liver disease, but their significance is not known.

Table 14.1 Primary and secondary iron overload disorders

Primary

Classic HFE-related hereditary haemochromatosis (type 1*)

Non-HFE hereditary haemochromatosis

  Juvenile hereditary haemochromatosis

    Hemojuvelin or HJV (HFE2)-related (type 2A*)

    Hepcidin or HAMP-related (type 2B*)

  Transferrin receptor 2-related haemochromatosis (type 3*)

  Ferroportin-related iron overload (type 4*)

Aceruloplasminaemia

Others

Secondary

  Transfusion

  Haemolysis

  Haemodialysis

  Dietary

  Underlying liver disease (e.g. chronic hepatitis, atty liver)

* Types 1–4 are classified as forms of hereditary haemochromatosis in the OMIM (Online Mendelian Inheritance in Man) database.[44]

The siderotic liver should be evaluated for the **distribution of stainable iron** among the various cell types, the **grade of siderosis**, the **presence of any related tissue damage** (fibrosis, cirrhosis, necrosis or even hepatocellular carcinoma) and **coexisting liver disease of other aetiology**. Various numerical methods of assessing the degree of siderosis (discussed below) are also helpful in evaluating causation and the effectiveness of therapeutic iron removal.

Numerical assessment of tissue iron

Many different systems have been devised for the quantification of iron in tissue sections.[36] **Histological grading of hepatocellular iron** can be simply scored on a scale from 1 to 4, with grade 1 representing minimal deposition (recognisable only with a high-power objective), grade 4 massive deposits with obliteration of the usual lobular gradient, and grades 2 and 3 intermediate amounts. Examples are shown in various illustrations to this chapter. The alternative comprehensive grading system of Deugnier and colleagues[37] measures iron not only in hepatocytes, but also in mesenchymal cells, bile-duct epithelium, blood vessels and connective tissue, generating a score between 0 and 60. This has proved helpful in the assessment of patients with hereditary haemochromatosis.

Tissue for **measuring the iron concentration** can be taken separately at the time a specimen is obtained for histology or by fine-needle aspiration biopsy,[38] or the actual paraffin block can be analysed[39] after histological examination is complete. This has the advantage that the nature of the sample is known.[40] Once the hepatic iron concentration is determined, the hepatic iron index (HII) described by Bassett and colleagues[41] can be calculated: HII = tissue iron in μmol/g dry weight, divided by the age of the patient in years (or tissue iron in μg/g dry weight divided by [55.8 $\times$ age in years]).[40,41] Because of the progressive accumulation of iron in classic HFE-related hereditary haemochromatosis, this enables patients with the disease (who have an iron index of 1.9 or more) to be distinguished from heterozygous patients and those with siderosis from other causes. However, in some patients with cirrhosis due to alcohol or other aetiologies unrelated to hereditary haemochromatosis, secondary accumulations of large amounts of iron in the liver may result in a calculated HII of 1.9 or greater, thereby mimicking the hereditary disease.[29,30] Conversely, a small percentage of individuals with hereditary haemochromatosis may have an iron index of less than 1.9.[42] In recent years genetic analysis has diminished the importance of these calculations.

The HII has been found to correlate well with a similar index derived from histological assessment and age, using the grading system of Deugnier and colleagues described above.[43] Use of this histological iron index avoids destruction of the tissue block and can be performed when the hepatic iron concentration is not available. Computerised image analysis is another approach to measuring iron deposition which correlates well with biochemical assay.[36]

Primary iron overload disorders

Molecular genetic studies have now defined a variety of heritable disorders affecting iron handling by the gastrointestinal tract and liver.[44] Several of these are listed in **Table 14.1** and the reader is encouraged to consult the section on General reading at the end of this chapter for further details. The best understood of the primary iron overload disorders was first described in 1889 by von Recklinghausen[45] and is the disease referred to as 'hereditary haemochromatosis'. The majority of these cases are examples of what is currently known to be classic *HFE*-related hereditary haemochromatosis, which is discussed below. However, the identical picture of predominantly periportal hepatocellular iron overload can be found in patients with various combinations of the gene defects listed in **Table 14.1**. There is thus a pathological pattern of **classic haemochromatosis** with more than one possible cause.[44]

Table 14.2 Characteristic diagnostic profile in *HFE* homozygous hereditary haemochromatosis

Diagnostic modality	Typical result(s)
Serum transferrin saturation	>62% (screening threshold is >45%[46])
Serum ferritin	≥300 µg/l (men); ≥200 µg/l (women)
Hepatic iron concentration	>2200 µg/g dry weight (men);
	>1600 µg/g dry weight (women)
Hepatic iron index	≥1.9
Genetic testing	C282Y/C282Y
Liver biopsy	Hepatocellular iron ≥grade 2
	Minimal or no Kupffer-cell iron

Classic *HFE*-related hereditary haemochromatosis

This autosomal recessive disorder is associated with progressive accumulation of iron in the liver, heart, pancreas and other organs. The frequency of homozygous disease is approximately 1 person in 300,[46] while heterozygotes are found in about 1 person in 8–10.[47] Overt disease may be found in as few as 1 in 5000,[25] and even within families homozygous persons may show different rates of iron accumulation.[48] The **HFE gene**, the gene for this type of haemochromatosis, is located on the short arm of chromosome 6 at some distance from the HLA-A locus.[47,49–52] A mis-sense mutation in *HFE* known as Cys282Tyr (C282Y) has been identified which results in tyrosine substitution for cysteine at position 282 of the gene protein product.[52] The majority (80–100%) of individuals with the typical phenotype of hereditary haemochromatosis are homozygous for this mutation (designated C282Y/C282Y).[46,52] Genetic tests for C282Y can be performed on peripheral blood or on paraffin-embedded tissue.[53] Expression of the mutated HFE protein on duodenal crypt epithelium is one of several factors that have been considered important in the pathogenesis of iron overload in haemochromatosis.[54] A second mutation, His63Asp (H63D), has been identified in fewer patients with haemochromatosis, either in homozygous form or as compound heterozygotes in conjunction with C282Y or the wild-type (normal) protein.[52] Other HFE mutations such as S65C (serine to cysteine) are also reported.[55] Non-*HFE* hereditary haemochromatosis[28] and other genetic disorders associated with iron overload are discussed later.

Until recently, a comprehensive panel of **diagnostic tests** combined with liver biopsy findings could be expected to provide a firm diagnosis of hereditary haemochromatosis (**Table 14.2**). However, the availability of genetic testing for *HFE*-related and other forms of haemochromatosis now sometimes obviates the need for liver biopsy, particularly if certain criteria indicate that the likelihood of hepatic fibrosis is low[56] (i.e. the patient is less than 40 years old, ferritin is less than 1000 ng/ml, serum liver tests are normal and hepatomegaly is absent). However, when there are coexisting liver diseases such as chronic hepatitis C or alcoholism that may accelerate hepatic fibrosis in the presence of a genetic iron overload disorder[57] or there are other reasons for direct morphological assessment of liver tissue, liver biopsy continues to offer considerable information. Moreover, understanding the pathological progression of classic *HFE*-related hereditary haemochromatosis (discussed below) provides a useful comparative model of iron-related liver damage.

The first histological abnormality in homozygous *HFE*-related haemochromatosis is the appearance of stainable iron in periportal hepatocytes. This may be found incidentally in the course of investigation for other diseases. The unexplained presence of more than

Figure 14.6 Hereditary haemochromatosis. At this early stage of fibrosis lobular architecture is still intact and vascular relationships are maintained. The portal tracts (P) are expanded by fibrous tissue. (Needle biopsy, reticulin.)

very small amounts of iron in hepatocytes should always raise the possibility of early hereditary haemochromatosis. The diagnosis can then be confirmed or refuted by means of genetic testing and/or calculating the hepatic iron index, as discussed previously. Early diagnosis is most important, because cirrhosis can be prevented by appropriate treatment both in patients and in their homozygous relatives, and life expectancy returned to normal.[58] In heterozygotes, stainable liver iron is either absent or very scanty.[43]

As iron stores increase, fibrosis begins to expand the portal tracts and slender septa extend from these to give a pattern of fibrosis resembling holly leaves (**Fig. 14.6**). The enlarged tracts contain iron-rich macrophages and a ductular reaction, but usually show little or no inflammatory infiltration. Iron may be seen in the ductular structures and in the epithelium of interlobular ducts in small amounts; larger quantities are not found until a later stage, when parenchymal siderosis is severe. It is a challenging paradox that in early haemochromatosis most of the iron is in hepatocytes but there is little or no evidence of liver-cell damage, liver-cell function remains virtually unimpaired, and the progressive lesion is portal in location. However, with increasing iron overload foci of sideronecrosis[37] are found, comprising eosinophilic or lytic necrosis of iron-laden hepatocytes, often in close association with clusters of macrophages. The ratio of non-hepatocytic to hepatocytic iron, as assessed histologically, rises progressively. The ultrastructural progression of iron overload has also been examined.[59]

In fully developed hereditary haemochromatosis the lobular gradient of iron staining is obliterated; iron in hepatocytes is now seen throughout the lobules, whereas earlier it is more abundant in periportal and mid-zonal regions.[37] Within individual hepatocytes the iron is seen to be deposited in pericanalicular granules, outlining the bile canalicular system (**Fig. 14.7**). Cirrhosis slowly develops as fibrosis and hepatocellular hyperplasia alter the normal architectural relationships. True nodule formation is, however, a late event and for a long period there is fibrosis rather than cirrhosis, with irregular islands of parenchyma demarcated by fibrous septa (**Fig. 14.8**). The pattern is somewhat like that of chronic biliary tract disease. At this stage some regression of fibrosis as a result of treatment remains possible.[60] Once cirrhosis has developed, biopsy assessment of the effect of treatment on structural changes becomes more difficult because of a tendency for increasing nodule size and compression or remodelling of septa. The onset of cirrhosis marks a fall in life expectancy and an increased risk of hepatocellular carcinoma.[58] The presence of iron-free foci may represent an early stage of malignant transformation.[61,62] Carcinoma has

**Figure 14.7
Hereditary
haemochromatosis.**
Grade 4 (maximal)
liver-cell siderosis.
Iron-rich granules in
a pericanalicular
location outline bile
canaliculi (arrow).
(Needle biopsy, Perls'
stain.)

**Figure 14.8
Hereditary
haemochromatosis.**
Fibrous septa
surround irregular
islands of liver
parenchyma.
(Wedge biopsy,
H&E.)

been recorded in non-cirrhotic patients with hereditary haemochromatosis, but is very rare.[61,63]

Effective treatment leads to a steady reduction in stainable iron. Iron encrusted onto portal collagen is usually the most resistant to removal and may be the only stainable iron remaining in the liver. Removal of iron unmasks a brown lipofuscin-like pigment in hepatocytes and connective tissue. Following liver transplantation for haemochromatosis, iron may reaccumulate in hepatocytes of the donor liver, but the rate is uncertain.[64]

Other primary iron overload disorders

Several types of **non-*HFE* haemochromatosis**[28] (**Box 14.1**) and other genetic diseases such as **aceruloplasminaemia**[65] result in hepatic iron overload, with marked hepatocellular siderosis present in the majority. However, some of these diseases show an atypical iron distribution. Both early and later stages of **ferroportin-related iron overload** feature abundant Kupffer-cell siderosis[66] (in contrast to *HFE*-related haemochromatosis). Liver-cell haemosiderin is absent or minimal in the early stage and as it progresses it is seen throughout the lobule, without the usual gradient from periportal to centrilobular regions.[28] The importance of ceruloplasmin in mediating egress of iron from cells is demonstrated in **aceruloplasminaemia** where both hepatocytes and Kupffer cells accumulate haemosiderin.[65,67] Excessive Kupffer-cell siderosis that cannot be accounted for by one of the causes of secondary iron overload (see below) should therefore also raise the suspicion of a genetic iron overload disorder.

Secondary iron overload disorders

In routine practice most siderosis is secondary and located in sinusoidal Kupffer cells (**Fig. 14.9**). Haemolysis, transfusions and haemodialysis are common causes. Identification of significant iron overload with this distribution is evidence against most genetic forms of haemochromatosis with the exception of ferroportin disease.[66] It is only when the threshold for macrophage iron storage is reached in such acquired disorders that liver-cell haemosiderin becomes evident in periportal regions (e.g. thalassaemia, sickle-cell disease).

Neonatal iron overload (neonatal haemochromatosis)

This condition of severe iron overload in stillborn or premature infants is characterised by extensive hepatocellular necrosis, giant-cell formation, siderosis, fibrosis and nodule formation.[68,69] Whether the disease is a genetic, infectious[70] or an acquired insult remains uncertain,[68] but the condition is not related to hereditary haemochromatosis of adults.

Iron overload in haematological disorders

Siderosis is found in patients with thalassaemia and, less commonly, other haematological disorders. The iron overload is partly the result of blood transfusion. In addition to the hepatocytic siderosis, portal fibrosis and septum formation seen in hereditary haemochromatosis, there is iron in macrophages from an early stage (**Fig. 14.10**) and haemopoietic cells may be present. There is often more infiltration of portal tracts, septa and sinusoids by lymphocytes than in hereditary haemochromatosis (**Fig. 14.11**). This, together with focal hepatocellular damage in some cases, is attributable to transfusion-related hepatitis, usually hepatitis C.[71,72] The pattern of fibrosis and degree of inflammation in a liver biopsy often help to determine the relative roles of iron overload and hepatitis C in the progression of the disease. Kupffer-cell siderosis is a common finding in haemolysis, haemophagocytic syndrome,[73] haemodialysis and sickle-cell disease.[74]

Liver disease of varied aetiology

Chronic viral hepatitis, alcoholic and non-alcoholic fatty liver disease and cirrhosis of diverse aetiologies unrelated to hereditary haemochromatosis[29,30] are often associated with

Figure 14.9 Secondary (acquired) iron overload.
A: Diffuse siderosis of sinusoidal Kupffer cells is present. Common causes are haemolysis, transfusions and hemodialysis. (Needle biopsy, Prussian blue iron stain.) **B:** Refractile brown haemosiderin granules are present within sinusoidal Kupffer cells. (Needle biopsy, H&E.)

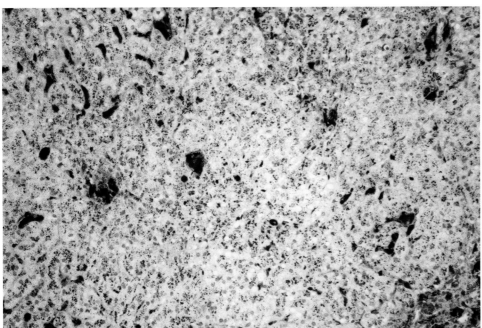

**Figure 14.10
Thalassaemia.**
In this example of secondary iron overload hepatocytes show grade 3 siderosis. The darker clumps are iron-laden macrophages. (Needle biopsy, Perls' stain.)

**Figure 14.11
Thalassaemia.**
There are iron-laden macrophages in the portal tract and in sinusoids. Haemosiderin granules are also evident in hepatocytes. The portal inflammation is probably due to transfusion-transmitted hepatitis C. (Needle biopsy, H&E.)

**Figure 14.12
Cirrhosis with
siderosis.**

This case of relatively
inactive cirrhosis due
to chronic hepatitis
C demonstrates
considerable
variability in the
degree of
hepatocellular
siderosis among the
nodules. (Explant
liver, Perls' stain.)

variable degrees of siderosis (**Fig. 14.12**). In **chronic hepatitis**, levels of serum iron and ferritin are sometimes increased as a result of release of iron from damaged hepatocytes, and iron may be seen on liver biopsy. The iron may be located in periportal hepatocytes, in Kupffer cells or in the endothelium of portal vessels.[35,75] Patchy iron-rich foci of hepatocytes in an otherwise non-siderotic biopsy may occasionally be seen.[76] In chronic hepatitis C, iron overload adversely affects therapy with interferon.[77] The severe siderosis, which can complicate **cirrhosis** due to viral hepatitis, may sometimes mimic hereditary haemochromatosis,[29,30] with marked elevations in hepatic iron concentration and hepatic iron index. Such cases require a comprehensive correlation of the histopathological features, biochemical test results, genetic analysis and other clinical data in order to clarify the aetiology of the iron overload. Biopsies from patients with **steatosis** sometimes show siderosis in periportal hepatocytes and in Kupffer cells, in which instance the possibility of **dysmetabolic hepatic iron overload (insulin resistance–iron overload/metabolic syndrome) (see Fig. 7.7)** – associated with central obesity, hypertension, hyperlipidaemia, hyperglycaemia and insulin resistance – should be considered.[33,78]

The presence of underlying liver disease is not in itself necessarily sufficient to explain the presence of hepatocellular haemosiderosis, nor does it preclude the diagnosis of a coexisting genetic iron overload disorder. An example of this is **porphyria cutanea tarda** in which siderosis is present and increased frequencies of both hepatitis C virus infection[79,80] and *HFE* gene mutations have been identified.[80] Histological siderosis in **alcoholic liver disease (Fig. 14.13)** may reflect underlying homozygous or heterozygous haemochromatosis or concomitant spur-cell haemolytic anaemia.[81] Alcohol and chronic hepatitis C are known to accelerate the progression of liver disease in patients with *HFE*-related homozygous hereditary haemochromatosis.[57,82]

Figure 14.13
Cirrhosis with siderosis.
In this fatty cirrhosis in an alcohol abuser there is grade 2 hepatocellular siderosis, the cause of which needs investigation. (Needle biopsy, Perls' stain.)

References

1   Riordan SM, Williams R. The Wilson's disease gene and phenotypic diversity. *J Hepatol* 2001; **34**: 165–171.

2   Tao TY, Gitlin JD. Hepatic copper metabolism: insights from genetic disease. *Hepatology* 2003; **37**: 1241–1247.

3   Huster D, Hoppert M, Lutsenko S, et al. Defective cellular localization of mutant ATP7B in Wilson's disease patients and hepatoma cell lines. *Gastroenterology* 2003; **124**: 335–345.

4   Schmidt HHJ. Role of genotyping in Wilson's disease. *J Hepatol* 2009; **50**: 449–452.

4a   Cope-Yokoyama S, Finegold MJ, Sturniolo GC, et al. Wilson disease: histopathological correlations with treatment on follow-up liver biopsies. *World J Gastroenterol* 2010; **16**: 1487–1494.

5   Scheinberg IH, Sternlieb I. Wilson's Disease. Major Problems in Internal Medicine XXIII. Philadelphia, PA: WB Saunders, 1984.

6   Walshe JM. Diagnosis and treatment of presymptomatic Wilson's disease. *Lancet* 1988; **ii**: 435–437.

7   Ludwig J, Moyer TP, Rakela J. The liver biopsy diagnosis of Wilson's disease. Methods in pathology. *Am J Clin Pathol* 1994; **102**: 443–446.

8   Stromeyer FW, Ishak KG. Histology of the liver in Wilson's disease: a study of 34 cases. *Am J Clin Pathol* 1980; **73**: 12–24.

9   Polio J, Enriquez RE, Chow A, et al. Hepatocellular carcinoma in Wilson's disease. Case report and review of the literature. *J Clin Gastroenterol* 1989; **11**: 220–224.

10   Cheng WSC, Govindarajan S, Redeker AG. Hepatocellular carcinoma in a case of Wilson's disease. *Liver* 1992; **12**: 42–45.

11   Schilsky ML, Scheinberg IH, Sternlieb I. Liver transplantation for Wilson's disease: indications and outcome. *Hepatology* 1994; **19**: 583–587.

12   Eleazar JA, Memeo L, Jhang JS, et al. Progenitor cell expansion: an important source of hepatocyte regeneration in chronic hepatitis. *J Hepatol* 2004; **41**: 983–991.

13   Roberts EA, Schilsky ML. Diagnosis and treatment of Wilson disease: an update. *Hepatology* 2008; **47**: 2089–2111.

14   Davies SE, Williams R, Portmann B. Hepatic morphology and histochemistry of Wilson's disease presenting as fulminant hepatic failure: a study of 11 cases. *Histopathology* 1989; **15**: 385–394.

15   Strand S, Hofmann WJ, Grambihler A, et al. Hepatic failure and liver cell damage in acute Wilson's disease involve CD95 (APO-1/Fas) mediated apoptosis. *Nat Med* 1998; **4**: 588–593.

16   Faa G, Nurchi V, Demelia L, et al. Uneven hepatic copper distribution in Wilson's disease. *J Hepatol* 1995; **22**: 303–308.

17   Müller-Höcker J, Meyer U, Wiebecke B, et al. Copper storage disease of the liver and chronic dietary copper intoxication in two further German infants mimicking Indian childhood cirrhosis. *Pathol Res Pract* 1988; **183**: 39–45.

18   Baker A, Gormally S, Saxena R, et al. Copper-associated liver disease in childhood. *J Hepatol* 1995; **23**: 538–543.

19   Müller T, Feichtinger H, Berger H, et al. Endemic Tyrolean infantile cirrhosis: an ecogenetic disorder. *Lancet* 1996; **347**: 877–880.

20 Faa G, Liguori C, Columbano A, et al. Uneven copper distribution in the human newborn liver. *Hepatology* 1987; **7**: 838–842.

21 Elmes ME, Clarkson JP, Mahy NJ, et al. Metallothionein and copper in liver disease with copper retention – a histopathological study. *J Pathol* 1989; **158**: 131–137.

22 Mulder TPJ, Janssens AR, Verspaget HW, et al. Metallothionein concentration in the liver of patients with Wilson's disease, primary biliary cirrhosis, and liver metastasis of colorectal cancer. *J Hepatol* 1992; **16**: 346–350.

23 Pilloni L, Lecca S, Van Eyken P, et al. Value of histochemical stains for copper in the diagnosis of Wilson's disease. *Histopathology* 1998; **33**: 28–33.

24 Ala A, Borjigin J, Rochwarger A, et al. Wilson disease in septuagenarian siblings: raising the bar for diagnosis. *Hepatology* 2005; **41**: 668–670.

25 Tavill AS, Sharma BK, Bacon BR. Iron and the liver: genetic hemochromatosis and other hepatic iron overload disorders. In: Popper H, Schaffner F, eds. Progress in Liver Diseases, Vol. IX. Philadelphia, PA: WB Saunders, 1990: 281–306.

26 Searle J, Leggett BA, Crawford DHG, et al. Iron storage diseases. In: MacSween RNM, Burt AD, Portmann BC, Ishak KG, Scheuer PJ, Anthony PP, eds. Pathology of the Liver, 4th edn. Edinburgh: Churchill Livingstone, 2002; Ch. 5: 257–272.

27 Faa G, Sciot R, Farci AMG, et al. Iron concentration and distribution in the newborn liver. *Liver* 1994; **14**: 193–199.

28 Pietrangelo A. Non-*HFE* hemochromatosis. *Hepatology* 2004; **39**: 21–29.

29 Deugnier Y, Turlin B, Le Quilleuc D, et al. A reappraisal of hepatic siderosis in patients with end-stage cirrhosis: practical implications for the diagnosis of hemochromatosis. *Am J Surg Pathol* 1997; **21**: 669–675.

30 Ludwig J, Hashimoto E, Porayko MK, et al. Hemosiderosis in cirrhosis: a study of 447 native livers. *Gastroenterology* 1997; **112**: 882–888.

31 Bergmann OM, Mathahs MM, Broadhurst KA, et al. Altered expression of iron regulatory genes in cirrhotic human livers: clues to the cause of hemosiderosis? *Lab Invest* 2008; **88**: 1349–1357.

32 Terada T, Nakanuma Y. Survey of iron-accumulative macroregenerative nodules in cirrhotic livers. *Hepatology* 1989; **10**: 851–854.

33 Turlin B, Mendler MH, Moirand R, et al. Histologic features of the liver in insulin resistance-associated iron overload. A study of 139 patients. *Am J Clin Pathol* 2001; **116**: 263–270.

34 Bardadin KA, Scheuer PJ. Endothelial cell changes in acute hepatitis. A light and electron microscopic study. *J Pathol* 1984; **144**: 213–220.

35 Kaji K, Nakanuma Y, Sasaki M, et al. Hemosiderin deposition in portal endothelial cells: a novel hepatic hemosiderosis frequent in chronic viral hepatitis B and C. *Hum Pathol* 1995; **26**: 1080–1085.

36 Olynyk J, Hall P, Sallie R, et al. Computerized measurement of iron in liver biopsies: a comparison with biochemical iron measurement. *Hepatology* 1990; **12**: 26–30.

37 Deugnier YM, Loréal O, Turlin B, et al. Liver pathology in genetic hemochromatosis: a review of 135 homozygous cases and their bioclinical correlations. *Gastroenterology* 1992; **102**: 2050–2059.

38 Olynyk J, Williams P, Fudge A, et al. Fine-needle aspiration biopsy for the measurement of hepatic iron concentration. *Hepatology* 1992; **15**: 502–506.

39 Olynyk JK, O'Neill R, Britton RS, et al. Determination of hepatic iron concentration in fresh and paraffin-embedded tissue: diagnostic implications. *Gastroenterology* 1994; **106**: 674–677.

40 Ludwig J, Batts KP, Moyer TP, et al. Liver biopsy diagnosis of homozygous hemochromatosis: a diagnostic algorithm. *Mayo Clin Proc* 1993; **68**: 263–267.

41 Bassett ML, Halliday JW, Powell LW. Value of hepatic iron measurements in early hemochromatosis and determination of the critical iron level associated with fibrosis. *Hepatology* 1986; **6**: 24–29.

42 Kowdley KV, Trainer TD, Saltzman JR, et al. Utility of hepatic iron index in American patients with hereditary hemochromatosis: a multicenter study. *Gastroenterology* 1997; **113**: 1270–1277.

43 Deugnier YM, Turlin B, Powell LW, et al. Differentiation between heterozygotes and homozygotes in genetic hemochromatosis by means of a histological hepatic iron index: a study of 192 cases. *Hepatology* 1993; **17**: 30–34.

44 Pietrangelo A. Hereditary hemochromatosis – a new look at an old disease. *N Engl J Med* 2004; **350**: 2383–2397.

45 von Recklinghausen FD. Hemochromatosis. *Taggeblatt Versammlung Dtsch Naturforsch Arzte Heidelberg* 1889; **62**: 324–325.

46 Powell LW, George K, McDonnell SM, et al. Diagnosis of hemochromatosis. *Ann Intern Med* 1998; **129**: 925–931.

47 Pietrangelo A. Hemochromatosis 1998: is one gene enough? *J Hepatol* 1998; **29**: 502–509.

48 Adams PC. Intrafamilial variation in hereditary hemochromatosis. *Dig Dis Sci* 1992; **37**: 361–363.

49 Riedel H-D, Stremmel W. The haemochromatosis gene. *J Hepatol* 1997; **26**: 941–944.

50 Ramrakhiani S, Bacon BR. Hemochromatosis. Advances in molecular genetics and clinical diagnosis. *J Clin Gastroenterol* 1998; **27**: 41–46.

51 Brissot P, Moirand R, Guyader D, et al. Hemochromatosis after the gene discovery: revisiting the diagnostic strategy. *J Hepatol* 1998; **28**: 14–18.

52 Bacon BR. Diagnosis and management of hemochromatosis. *Gastroenterology* 1997; **113**: 995–999.

53 Bartolo C, McAndrew PE, Sosolik RC, et al. Differential diagnosis of hereditary hemochromatosis from other liver disorders by genetic analysis. Gene mutation analysis of patients previously diagnosed with hemochromatosis by liver biopsy. *Arch Pathol Lab Med* 1998; **122**: 633–637.

54 Parkkila S, Niemelä O, Britton RS, et al. Molecular aspects of iron absorption and HFE expression. *Gastroenterology* 2001; **121**: 1489–1496.

55 Wallace DF, Walker AP, Pietrangelo A, et al. Frequency of the S65C mutation of HFE and iron overload in 309 subjects heterozygous for C282Y. *J Hepatol* 2002; **36**: 474–479.

56 Harrison SA, Bacon BR. Hereditary hemochromatosis: update for 2003. *J Hepatol* 2003; **38**: S14–S23.

57 Diwarkaran HH, Befeler AS, Britton RS, et al. Accelerated hepatic fibrosis in patients with combined hereditary hemochromatosis and chronic hepatitis C infection. *J Hepatol* 2002; **36**: 687–691.

58 Niederau C, Fischer R, Sonnenberg A, et al. Survival and causes of death in cirrhotic and in noncirrhotic patients with primary hemochromatosis. *N Engl J Med* 1985; **313**: 1256–1262.

59   Iancu TC, Deugnier Y, Halliday JW, et al. Ultrastructural sequences during liver iron overload in genetic hemochromatosis. *J Hepatol* 1997; **27**: 628–638.

60   Falize L, Guillygomarc'h A, Perrin M, et al. Reversibility of hepatic fibrosis in treated genetic hemochromatosis: a study of 36 cases. *Hepatology* 2006; **44**: 472–477.

61   Deugnier YM, Guyuder D, Crantock I, et al. Primary liver cancer in genetic hemochromatosis: a clinical, pathological, and pathogenetic study of 54 cases. *Gastroenterology* 1993; **104**: 228–234.

62   Deugnier YM, Charalambous P, Le Quilleuc D, et al. Preneoplastic significance of hepatic iron-free foci in genetic hemochromatosis: a study of 185 patients. *Hepatology* 1993; **18**: 1363–1369.

63   Fellows IW, Stewart M, Jeffcoate WJ, et al. Hepatocellular carcinoma in primary haemochromatosis in the absence of cirrhosis. *Gut* 1988; **29**: 1603–1606.

64   Farrell FJ, Nguyen M, Woodley S, et al. Outcome of liver transplantation in patients with hemochromatosis. *Hepatology* 1994; **20**: 404–410.

65   Loréal O, Turlin B, Pigeon C, et al. Aceruloplasminemia: new clinical, pathophysiological and therapeutic insights. *J Hepatol* 2002; **36**: 851–856.

66   Pietrangelo A. Hemochromatosis: an endocrine liver disease. *Hepatology* 2007; **46**: 1291–1301.

67   Kono S, Suzuki H, Takahashi K, et al. Hepatic iron overload associated with a decreased serum ceruloplasmin level in a novel clinical type of aceruloplasminemia. *Gastroenterology* 2006; **131**: 240–245.

68   Knisely AS, Mieli-Vergani G, Whitington PF. Neonatal hemochromatosis. *Gastroenterol Clin North Am* 2003; **32**: 877–889.

69   Whitington PF. Fetal and infantile hemochromatosis. *Hepatology* 2006; **43**: 654–660.

70   Kershisnik MM, Knisely AS, Sun C-CJ, et al. Cytomegalovirus infection, fetal liver disease, and neonatal hemochromatosis. *Hum Pathol* 1992; **23**: 1075–1080.

71   Wonke B, Hoffbrand AV, Brown D, et al. Antibody to hepatitis C virus in multiply transfused patients with thalassaemia major. *J Clin Pathol* 1990; **43**: 638–640.

72   Donohue SM, Wonke B, Hoffbrand AV, et al. Alpha interferon in the treatment of chronic hepatitis C infection in thalassaemia major. *Br J Haematol* 1993; **83**: 491–497.

73   de Kerguenec C, Hillaire S, Molinié V, et al. Hepatic manifestations of hemophagocytic syndrome: a study of 30 cases. *Am J Gastroenterol* 2001; **96**: 852–857.

74   Banerjee S, Owen C, Chopra S. Sickle cell hepatopathy. *Hepatology* 2001; **33**: 1021–1028.

75   Haque S, Chandra B, Gerber MA, et al. Iron overload in patients with chronic hepatitis C: a clinicopathologic study. *Hum Pathol* 1996; **27**: 1277–1281.

76   Lefkowitch JH, Yee HT, Sweeting J, et al. Iron-rich foci in chronic hepatitis. *Hum Pathol* 1998; **29**: 116–118.

77   Bonkovsky HL, Banner BF, Rothman AL. Iron and chronic viral hepatitis. *Hepatology* 1997; **25**: 759–768.

78   Deugnier Y, Brissot P, Loréal O. Iron and the liver: update 2008. *J Hepatol* 2008; **48**: S113–S123.

79   Nagy Z, Kószo F, Pár A, et al. Hemochromatosis (*HFE*) gene mutations and hepatitis C virus infection as risk factors for porphyria cutanea tarda in Hungarian patients. *Liver Int* 2004; **24**: 16–20.

80   Bonkovsky HL, Poh-Fitzpatrick M, Pimstone N, et al. Polrphyria cutanea tarda, hepatitis C and *HFE* gene mutations in North America. *Hepatology* 1998; **27**: 1661–1669.

81   Pascoe A, Kerlin P, Steadman C, et al. Spur cell anaemia and hepatic iron stores in patients with alcoholic liver disease undergoing orthotopic liver transplantation. *Gut* 1999; **45**: 301–305.

82   Fletcher LM, Dixon JL, Purdie DM, et al. Excess alcohol greatly increases the prevalence of cirrhosis in hereditary hemochromatosis. *Gastroenterology* 2002; **122**: 281–289.

General reading

Ferenci P, Caca K, Loudianos G, et al. Diagnosis and phenotypic classification of Wilson disease. *Liver Int* 2003; **23**: 139–142.

Merle U, Schaefer M, Ferenci P, et al. Clinical presentation, diagnosis and long-term outcome of Wilson's disease: a cohort study. *Gut* 2007; **56**: 115–120.

Pietrangelo A. Hereditary hemochromatosis – a new look at an old disease. *N Engl J Med* 2004; **350**: 2383–2397.

Pietrangelo A. Non-*HFE* hemochromatosis. *Hepatology* 2004; **39**: 21–29.

Pietrangelo A. Hemochromatosis: an endocrine liver disease. *Hepatology* 2007; **46**: 1291–1301.

Portmann BC, Thompson RJ, Roberts EA, Paterson AC. Genetic and metabolic liver disease. In: Burt AD, Portmann BC, Ferrell LD, eds. MacSween's Pathology of the Liver, 5th edn. Edinburgh: Churchill Livingstone/Elsevier, 2007: 199–326.

Roberts EA, Schilsky ML. A practice guideline on Wilson disease. *Gastroenterology* 2003; **37**: 1475–1492.

The Liver in Systemic Disease and Pregnancy

Introduction

Liver biopsies are often obtained to evaluate abnormalities of liver function tests in patients with known or suspected systemic disease and in the investigation of pyrexia of unknown origin.[1,2] In the latter, liver biopsy provides diagnostic information in approximately 15–30% of cases.[3] The hepatic changes associated with systemic diseases vary from obvious granulomas or steatosis (discussed in **Ch. 7**) to more subtle findings such as an increase in liver-cell mitoses. The pathologist will want to know, whenever possible, whether or not the biopsy changes are specific for a systemic disease. For example, when granulomas are present, their aetiology usually has important therapeutic implications. Liver biopsy in patients with AIDS may demonstrate suspected hepatotoxicity due to antiretroviral drugs or hepatic involvement by a micro-organism already identified elsewhere in the patient, or may disclose a new diagnosis such as lymphoma. Liver biopsy also provides tissue for culture and special stains. This chapter examines the pathology of hepatic granulomas, hepatic changes in a variety of infectious diseases, and liver involvement in gastrointestinal and haemopoietic diseases and the porphyrias.

In the unusual situation where liver dysfunction is found in pregnancy, the histopathologist may be called upon to differentiate intercurrent conditions such as viral hepatitis from several varieties of liver disease unique to pregnancy. This differential diagnosis is discussed later on in this chapter.

Granulomas

There are many causes of hepatic granulomas, including local irritants, infections, infestations and hypersensitivity to drugs. The constituents of these lesions, depending on the aetiology and inflammatory cytokines produced,[4] include large epithelioid cells, multinucleated giant cells, varied numbers of mononuclear cells and eosinophils. Hepatic granulomas can be further morphologically classified as **caseating (necrotising)**, **non-caseating**, **lipogranulomas (Ch. 7)** and **fibrin-ring granulomas**.[5–7] The causes vary in frequency from one country to another. Although the aetiology may be determined from the histological features, from special stains for micro-organisms, from culture of part of the biopsy specimen or polymerase chain reaction of the paraffin-embedded specimen,[8] or from clinical and serological data, the cause of hepatic granulomas may remain unknown in some 10–36% of cases.[9,10]

©2010 Elsevier Ltd
DOI: 10.1016/B978-0-7020-3410-7.00021-6

From a practical point of view biopsies containing granulomas fall into one of four groups:

1 The cause of the granuloma is seen under the microscope. Examples are the granulomas around schistosome ova, and the mineral oil lipogranulomas found in portal tracts or near terminal hepatic venules.
2 The cause is not seen, but other histological features and clinical circumstances make the diagnosis clear. For example, granulomas near damaged bile ducts in a patient with clinically and immunologically typical primary biliary cirrhosis are almost certainly due to this disease.
3 The cause is uncertain, but appearances favour one particular line of further investigation rather than another. For instance, sarcoidosis should be suspected when clusters of large granulomas with prominent epithelioid cells, large multinucleated giant cells and dense fibrosis are found in portal tracts.
4 The cause of the granulomas cannot be determined from the histological appearances. This is unfortunately common, and the help that the pathologist can then give to the clinician is limited.

These four circumstances can be summarised as **see the cause**, **know the cause**, **suspect the cause** and **don't know the cause**. Some of the histological guidelines for evaluating granulomas are shown in **Table 15.1**.

Granulomas are found in up to 10% of liver biopsies.[11,12] They may be sparse, and suspicion of granulomatous disease is an indication for examining step sections from different levels of a paraffin block, if no lesions are seen initially. Because identifiable granulomas are generally more than 50 μm in diameter, serial sections 5 μm thick are unnecessary unless a single granuloma is to be further investigated.

Granulomas are commonly found in the liver in **sarcoidosis** and may even recur following liver transplantation.[13] The liver is usually one of several organs involved, but occasionally extrahepatic lesions are difficult to demonstrate and chest X-ray may be normal.[14] Liver biopsy is helpful for diagnosis, especially in patients with fever and

Table 15.1 Histological features of hepatic granulomas

Aetiology	Favoured site(s)	Special features
Sarcoidosis	Portal/periportal	Clustering Hyalinisation Inclusions in giant cells May destroy bile ducts
Tuberculosis	None	Necrosis
PBC	Portal	Near damaged bile duct Lobular granulomas uncommon
Drug	None	Eosinophils Other lesions often present (hepatitis, fat, cholestasis)
Mineral oil	Portal, perivenous	Oil vacuoles
Q fever, CMV, Allopurinol, etc.	None	Fibrin-ring granuloma
CGDC	None	Brown pigment in macrophages May be necrotising
Cat-scratch disease, tularemia, yersinia	None	Purulent centre

CGDC, chronic granulomatous disease of childhood; CMV, cytomegalovirus; PBC, primary biliary cirrhosis.

**Figure 15.1
Sarcoidosis.**
A cluster of epithelioid-cell granulomas with giant cells has expanded a portal tract and surrounded a bile duct (arrow). (Needle biopsy, H&E.)

arthralgia.[15] The lesions may be found both in portal tracts and in lobules, and consist of well-defined, rounded granulomas with variable infiltration by inflammatory cells including plasma cells and eosinophils (**Fig. 15.1**). The granulomas contain reticulin fibres (**Fig. 15.2**). Multinucleated giant cells may contain inclusions of different types.[16] Central necrosis may infrequently be present, but is never as extensive as in tuberculosis. The granulomas often cluster in portal and periportal regions[17] (**Fig. 15.2**) and older lesions show dense hyalinised collagen. The fibrosis may extend to interfere with normal acinar structure, and in more severe cases may progress to cirrhosis.[16,18] A surprising degree of reactive portal and lobular inflammation may occasionally be seen in association with sarcoid granulomas, raising the question of concomitant hepatitis.[18] The lobular component consists predominantly of hyperplastic Kupffer cells; acidophil bodies are rare. The portal tracts show considerable variability in the amount of lymphocytic inflammation and the most active portal inflammation is usually near granulomas. Serological tests for viral hepatitis should be obtained if there is serious diagnostic concern. In those few patients with sarcoidosis who develop portal hypertension,[19,20] it may be related to portal and periportal fibrosis or to broad areas of replacement fibrosis,[16] nodular regenerative hyperplasia[21] or cirrhosis.[16,18] Another rare complication of sarcoidosis is a primary biliary cirrhosis-like lesion, with destruction of bile ducts and a clinical picture of chronic cholestasis.[22] Portal features suggesting biliary obstruction may also be present.[16,18] It should be noted that a diagnosis of sarcoidosis cannot be proved by histological examination of the liver alone, because very similar lesions are found in other granulomatous diseases.

In **chronic granulomatous disease of childhood,** defective neutrophil leucocyte function leads to the development of infective granulomas of different sizes, containing homogeneous eosinophilic material, necrotic debris or pus. Portal tracts are inflamed and there may be fibrosis. A brown pigment of ceroid type accumulates in portal macrophages and to a lesser extent in Kupffer cells.[23-25] Abscesses and bile-duct fibroinflammatory lesions resembling primary sclerosing cholangitis are also seen.[26] The development of non-cirrhotic portal hypertension related to nodular regenerative hyperplasia and oblitera-

**Figure 15.2
Sarcoidosis.**

The granulomas are clustered in the portal tract (P) and periportal region, a characteristic feature of sarcoidosis. They are associated with increased reticulin fibres. (Needle biopsy, reticulin.)

tive fibrosis of terminal venules and/or portal veins contributes to mortality.[27] **Common variable immunodeficiency** may be associated with portal and/or lobular epithelioid granulomas[27a] as well as with nodular regenerative hyperplasia,[27b] mild portal lymphocytic infiltrates with mild fibrosis[27c] and, rarely, primary biliary cirrhosis or autoimmune hepatitis.[27d]

A small number of patients with **chronic hepatitis C** may show non-caseating granulomas in the liver, either portal or lobular in location,[28,29] sometimes recurring after liver transplantation.[30] In one series, nearly 10% of granulomas were ascribed to this infection.[10] Their pathogenesis is unknown. In some instances, other causes such as schistosomiasis may become apparent during a thorough evaluation.[31]

Drugs and toxins should be considered in the evaluation of hepatic granulomas (**see Ch. 8**), particularly if eosinophils are prominent.[32] A diverse array of particulate materials may cause granulomas, including aluminium,[33] feldspar[34] and silicone.[35] Biopsies with granulomas should therefore be examined under polarised light for evidence of particulate material. Dense reactive fibrosis may develop in the form of **sclerohyaline nodules** in individuals exposed to silica, chromium, cobalt or magnesium, either in the workplace or by intravenous drug abuse.[36]

The **fibrin-ring granuloma** is a distinctive though non-specific[37] form described in Q fever,[37–42] Hodgkin's disease,[43] allopurinol hypersensitivity,[44] cytomegalovirus[45] and Epstein–Barr virus infections,[46] leishmaniasis,[47] toxoplasmosis,[43] hepatitis A,[48,49] giant-cell arteritis[50] and systemic lupus erythematosus.[51] This granuloma is composed of a fat vacuole surrounded by a ring of fibrin, epithelioid cells, giant cells and neutrophils (**Fig. 15.3**). Serial sections may be needed to demonstrate the typical fibrin-ring or 'doughnut' lesion.[39]

Simon and Wolff[52] described a syndrome characterised by fever, constitutional symptoms and hepatic granulomas, which does not respond to antituberculous drugs but improves on corticosteroid therapy or sometimes with methotrexate.[53] In some patients the syndrome resolves spontaneously without treatment.[54] The cause has not been established.

Figure 15.3 Q fever.
Small granulomas containing giant cells, fat vacuoles and neutrophil leucocytes are surrounded by rings of fibrin, stained red. (Needle biopsy, Martius scarlet blue.)

Viral diseases

The pathological changes in the liver resulting from virus infections other than hepatitis viruses have been reviewed by Lucas.[55] The viral haemorrhagic fevers, such as mosquito-borne **flavivirus** infection (**Dengue fever**[56]) and rodent-borne **hantavirus** infections,[57] are characterised by mid-zonal or more extensive hepatic necrosis. In **yellow fever**, acidophil bodies are typically abundant; they were first described in this disease by Councilman over a 100 years ago.[58,59]

Several viruses not normally associated with liver disease can occasionally cause liver damage. Examples include **herpes simplex virus** infection leading to irregular and randomly distributed areas of coagulative necrosis[60,61] (**Fig. 15.4**) and **adenovirus** infection.[62,63] In both infections, virus particles or antigens can be identified in hepatocytes. Paramyxovirus-like particles were described in adults with associated syncytial giant-cell hepatitis.[64] Multinucleated giant hepatocytes in liver biopsies from adults (**post-infantile giant-cell hepatitis**) may also be seen in hepatitis C virus mono-infection or co-infection with human immunodeficiency virus (HIV),[64a] human herpes virus-6A infection,[65] in autoimmune hepatitis and in other liver diseases.[66,67]

Cytomegalovirus infection

Cytomegalovirus (CMV) has been implicated in some children with neonatal hepatitis (**see Ch. 13**). Histological features include giant-cell formation as in other forms of neonatal liver damage, inflammation and cholestasis. Bile ducts are damaged and may be destroyed.[68] The CMV genome can be identified by the polymerase chain reaction in many cases.[69]

In later life, CMV infection can present as a mononucleosis-like illness, but also as hepatitis. Asymptomatic infection is common in immunocompromised patients. In these, the histological changes are often mild, but typical CMV inclusions are found in hepatocytes, bile-duct epithelium and endothelial cells (**Fig. 15.5**). Specific immunocytochemical

Figure 15.4
Herpes simplex hepatitis.
Pale, ground-glass-like intranuclear inclusions are present in a multinucleated hepatocyte (near centre) and elsewhere (arrows). An adjacent focus of necrosis with neutrophils is seen at the right of the field. (Needle biopsy, H&E.)

Figure 15.5
Cytomegalovirus hepatitis in AIDS.
Numerous cytomegalovirus inclusions (arrows) are seen within bile-duct epithelial cells. (Needle biopsy, H&E.)

staining reveals CMV antigens, even in cells without inclusions,[70] but sometimes with an abnormal granular basophilic cytoplasm.[71] Patients with CMV infection may also show aggregation of neutrophils in sinusoids, with or without evidence of CMV in neighbouring cells,[71] an important diagnostic consideration in immunocompromised patients or individuals who have received organ transplants. Larger accumulations of macrophages and lymphocytes can be seen and epithelioid-cell granulomas have been reported.[72] In immunocompetent patients, there are varying degress of focal liver-cell and bile-duct damage, portal

**Figure 15.6
Infectious
mononucleosis.**
At left, a prominent
sinusoidal 'beads-on-
a-string' pattern is
seen, consisting of
atypical lymphocytes
and hyperplastic
Kupffer cells. Atypical
lymphocytes are also
present in the portal
tract at right.
(Needle biopsy,
H&E.)

inflammation, infiltration of sinusoids with lymphoid cells and increased mitoses in hepatocytes.[73] In such patients, it may not be possible to demonstrate CMV inclusions or antigen, a situation possibly analogous to hepatitis B virus infection where inclusions and antigen may be scanty or absent during the acute attack while characteristic of the carrier state.[73]

Infectious mononucleosis

The liver is histologically abnormal in infectious mononucleosis even when there is no clinical jaundice.[74] Dense accumulations of atypical lymphocytes are found in portal tracts and sinusoids (**Fig. 15.6**). Sinusoidal aggregates must be distinguished from the more heterogeneous collections of cells found in extramedullary haemopoiesis. The infiltration also mimics that of leukaemia. Kupffer cells are enlarged. Epithelioid-cell granulomas are occasionally present.[12] Small foci of hepatocellular necrosis and acidophil bodies may be seen, but the diffuse hepatocellular damage characteristic of viral hepatitis is usually absent and extensive necrosis[75] is rare. Cholestasis is absent or mild.

Acquired immune deficiency syndrome

A spectrum of hepatobiliary lesions has been associated with AIDS and HIV-1 infection since the onset of the epidemic[76–85] (**Table 15.2**). Liver biopsy continues to play an important diagnostic role in the evaluation of abnormal liver function tests in these patients,[78,79,86] particularly in managing the potential hepatotoxicity of highly active antiretroviral therapy (HAART)[87,88] and concurrent chronic hepatitis B and/or C which may be present. Although Kupffer cells and endothelial cells[89–93] are potential target cells for HIV-1 infection, there are no specific hepatic lesions due to HIV-1, a few cases of alleged 'HIV-1 hepatitis'[94,95] notwithstanding.

Despite the reduction in morbidity and mortality due to antiretroviral therapy and prophylactic antibiotics,[96] opportunistic infections and neoplasms such as Kaposi's

Table 15.2 Hepatobiliary lesions in HIV-1 infection and AIDS

Lesion	Cause(s) or type(s)
Granulomas	Mycobacteria, fungi, drugs
Abscesses	Staphylococci, streptococci, listeria
Bacillary peliosis	*Bartonella henselae*
Biliary tract disease (AIDS cholangiopathy)	CMV, cryptosporidia, microsporidia
Neoplasms	Kaposi's sarcoma, lymphoma, smooth muscle tumours
Chronic viral hepatitis	HBV, HCV, HDV
Autoimmune hepatitis	Coexistent or following immune reconstitution
Other viral infections	CMV, herpes simplex virus, Epstein–Barr virus, adenovirus
Vascular lesions	Peliosis hepatis, sinusoidal dilatation
Drug toxicity	Sulfa agents, antiretrovirals
Miscellaneous	Steatosis, haemosiderosis, stellate cell hypertrophy, amyloidosis

sarcoma and lymphoma must still be excluded on liver biopsy. Specimens should routinely be studied with acid-fast and silver stains for detection of high-incidence pathogens such as mycobacteria and fungi. Other methods such as Gram or Warthin–Starry stains can be applied, depending on the clinical and histological indications. A portion of the biopsy should be sent for culture.

Drug-related hepatotoxicity

Antiretroviral drugs may need to be excluded as the cause of liver dysfunction in HIV-positive individuals, particularly in those with negative hepatitis virus serology. Combination therapy frequently presents the problem of distinguishing among various medications. In this instance it is helpful to consider the type of hepatic damage characteristic of the several classes of **HAART agents**.[88] The nucleoside reverse transcriptase inhibitors cause mitochondrial damage and microvesicular steatosis, while the non-nucleoside reverse transcriptase inhibitors may produce confluent necrosis. The lesions attributed to protease inhibitors are various, including bile-duct damage, hepatocyte necrosis and ballooning, Mallory body formation and perivenular fibrosis.[88] Since antiretroviral liver injury is often idiosyncratic, the Internet and other sources should be consulted for emerging descriptions of new cases.

Opportunistic infections and infestations

Opportunistic infections and infestations involving the liver and bile ducts in AIDS include *Mycobacterium avium–intracellulare* and *Mycobacterium tuberculosis* infections, cytomegalovirus infection, cryptococcosis, candidiasis, histoplasmosis, leishmaniasis,[97] malaria, cryptosporidiosis,[98] and microsporidiosis.[99–101] Mycobacterial and fungal infections frequently produce **granulomas**. *M. avium–intracellulare* results in numerous granulomas and the organisms are readily demonstrated by staining with diastase–periodic acid–Schiff (PAS) or the Ziehl–Neelsen method[102–105] (**Fig. 15.7**). Each granuloma consists of foamy

Figure 15.7
***Mycobacterium avium–intracellulare* in AIDS.**
Abundant macrophages with densely packed mycobacteria are present within a granuloma. Individual organisms are best seen in the centre of the field. (Post-mortem liver, Ziehl–Neelsen.)

histiocytes with few lymphocytes. The histiocytes often show a striated appearance on haematoxylin and eosin (H&E) staining due to the abundant packing of organisms in each cell. *M. avium–intracellulare* organisms are also well stained with Gomori methenamine silver. For screening of liver biopsies, particularly for *M. tuberculosis* which may be present in fewer numbers than *M. avium–intracellulare*, the auramine–rhodamine fluorescent method[106,107] gives excellent results. Careful examination of special stains is of particular importance, as some AIDS patients have mycobacterial infection without typical granuloma formation; scant, single mycobacteria may be present within sinusoids or portal tracts. *Pneumocystis carinii* may disseminate to the liver, producing acellular exudative masses which closely resemble the pulmonary alveolar exudates.[108]

AIDS cholangiopathy

AIDS cholangiopathy resembles sclerosing cholangitis clinically and radiographically and is due to infections of the large bile ducts by several possible pathogens, including cytomegalovirus, cryptosporidia and microsporidia.[99–101,109–111] Liver biopsy changes are those of large-duct obstruction. Cryptosporidia and microsporidia are best identified in aspirates obtained at endoscopy, duodenal biopsies, or post-mortem tissue samples of the major bile ducts.[99–101]

Peliosis hepatis

Peliosis hepatis[104,112,113] in AIDS has been postulated to be due to endothelial damage by HIV-1 infection.[93] Alternatively, **bacillary peliosis hepatis** may develop as a consequence of hepatic infection by the Gram-negative bacillus *Bartonella henselae*.[114–117] Smudge-like or granular pink-to-purple material associated with a myxoid stroma is seen within dilated vascular spaces (**Fig. 15.8**) and the Warthin–Starry stain shows clumped bacilli in these areas.

**Figure 15.8
Bacillary peliosis in
AIDS.**
The portal tract is
expanded by dilated
blood vessels (left
and right), chronic
inflammatory cells
and pink-grey
smudge-like material
(at centre) which
contains bacilli.
(Needle biopsy,
H&E.)

Lymphomas

Lymphomas involve the liver as nodular masses or portal tract infiltrates (**see Fig. 7.3**) and are high-grade large-cell, immunoblastic and Burkitt types.[118,119]

Chronic hepatitis

AIDS patients have many of the same risk factors for infection by hepatitis viruses, and serum markers of prior infection or active viral hepatitis are often present. While the liver biopsy lesions of **chronic hepatitis B, C, and delta** can vary considerably in persons infected with HIV,[120–122] it is now recognised that HIV infection may exert an adverse effect.[123–125] Fulminant hepatitis may occur[126] and in drug addicts a propensity for more severe chronic hepatitis with progression to cirrhosis has been noted.[127] Coexistent auto-immune hepatitis may need exclusion when abnormal serum liver tests are found in the HIV-infected individual[128] and rarely *de novo* autoimmune hepatitis may develop because of **immune reconstitution** after antiretroviral therapy has begun.[129]

Steatosis and other changes

Steatosis is common[130] and may be periportal (**see Fig. 7.3**). Severe macrovesicular or microvesicular fat is cause for concern because this may reflect toxicity of anti-viral medications[87,88,131,132] and can be associated with liver failure.[133] **Siderosis** of Kupffer cells is related to transfusion or viraemia-associated erythrophagocytosis. In some cases, **non-specific changes** consisting of sparse portal or acinar lymphocytic inflammation with scattered apoptotic bodies are seen, with no apparent aetiology.

Other lesions reported include **nodular regenerative hyperplasia,**[134,135] **amyloidosis**[136] and **hypertrophied perisinusoidal stellate (Ito) cells** containing numerous lipid droplets.[137] In children, **giant-cell hepatitis,**[94,138] **chronic hepatitis** of uncertain cause[139] and **primary leiomyosarcoma**[140] are described.

Rickettsial, bacterial and fungal infections

Q fever

In Q fever, due to infection with *Coxiella burnetii*, liver involvement is common although only a few patients present clinically with liver disease. Histological changes include focal necrosis, non-specific inflammation and fatty change. The most characteristic lesion is the **fibrin-ring granuloma**[37–43] **(see Fig. 15.3)**, a granulomatous lesion also seen in several other infections and in some patients taking allopurinol.[44] Atypical lesions without annular arrangement or a central clear area (but containing irregular fibrin strands) are also found, as are non-specific granulomas without fibrin. In chronic Q fever progressive fibrosis and cirrhosis have been reported.[141]

Brucellosis

In most patients with brucellosis, liver biopsy shows non-specific reactive changes comprising sinusoidal-cell hypertrophy, portal inflammation and focal necrosis. Non-necrotising granulomas, often small and located within the acini, are more commonly found in the acute phase of the infection.[142]

Typhoid fever

Liver involvement is uncommon, but most patients with 'typhoid hepatitis' are jaundiced.[143] Liver biopsy shows a mild hepatitis with marked hyperplasia of mononuclear phagocytes, and lymphocytoid cells in sinusoids.[144] Characteristic granuloma-like collections of mononuclear cells, the typhoid nodules, are described.[145] Other features include fatty change and portal inflammation.[143,146]

Cat-scratch disease

Infection by a short Gram-negative rod, *Bartonella henselae*, typically produces pyrexia and regional lymphadenopathy in children. Rarely, dissemination to the liver results in hepatic **granulomas with central stellate microabscesses** surrounded by palisaded macrophages, lymphocytes and an outer layer of fibroblasts.[147,148] The Warthin–Starry stain is used to identify the organisms.

Tuberculosis

Tuberculous lesions are present in the liver either as part of a generalised infection[149] or, less often, in the hepatobiliary form of the disease.[150] A normal chest X-ray does not exclude the diagnosis.[151] Granulomas are found randomly scattered in the parenchyma and also in the portal tracts. They range from small accumulations of macrophage-like cells to well-developed, large epithelioid-cell nodules with Langhans giant cells **(Fig. 15.9)**. Central necrosis may or may not be present, and its absence does not exclude the diagnosis. Extensive necrosis **(Fig. 15.10)** is more likely to be seen when there are widely disseminated granulomas in the liver. Mycobacteria are seen in a minority of biopsies. Acute lesions contain little reticulin, while chronic ones undergo scarring. Remaining liver tissue shows non-specific reactive features and fatty change. Patients with AIDS sometimes have mycobacterial infection without typical granulomas, or may form tuberculous abscesses.[152] In all patients in whom tuberculosis is suspected, part of the liver biopsy specimen should be cultured. Polymerase chain reaction studies may also be performed on biopsy samples.[153] Lesions similar to those of tuberculosis have been reported in patients given BCG immunotherapy.[154–157]

**Figure 15.9
Tuberculosis.**
Three parenchymal granulomas abut a portal tract. Multinucleated giant cells are visible in two of the granulomas. (Needle biopsy, H&E.)

**Figure 15.10
Tuberculosis.**
There is extensive necrosis with little residual evidence of granulomas. (Needle biopsy, H&E.)

Leprosy

In lepromatous leprosy specific granuloma-like lesions composed of foam cells are found in the liver and often contain acid-fast bacilli.[158] Organisms are also seen in Kupffer cells. Epithelioid-cell granulomas of tuberculoid type, rare in lepromatous leprosy, are found in the livers of some patients with the tuberculoid form of the disease. Either type of granuloma is seen in borderline leprosy.[159]

Spirochaetal infection

Syphilis

In congenital syphilis there is widespread fibrosis separating small groups of hepatocytes and spirochaetes are numerous. In early infections in adults, liver biopsies are normal or show non-specific changes.[160] Spirochaetes may be demonstrable histologically. In patients with secondary syphilis and jaundice or abnormal liver function tests, there is a variable degree of focal parenchymal inflammation, granuloma formation,[161] hepatocellular necrosis and portal inflammation. The portal reaction may mimic that of biliary obstruction,[162] and there may be inflammation of bile-duct epithelium as well as of the walls of small arteries and veins.[163,164] Because patients with syphilis often have other infections as well, lesions cannot always be confidently attributed to the syphilis itself.[165] The typical lesion of tertiary syphilis is the gumma, an area of necrosis surrounded by granulomatous tissue in which there is endarteritis. Healing is by fibrosis.

Leptospirosis

Most studies of the pathology of leptospirosis have dealt with autopsy material, in which disorganisation of liver-cell plates is a prominent feature. This is usually absent from liver biopsies.[166] Hepatocytes are swollen, especially in perivenular areas, and there is an increase in mitotic figures. A few acidophil bodies and fat vacuoles may be seen. Kupffer cells are prominent and there is a mild mononuclear-cell infiltrate in portal tracts. Cholestasis is common, which may persist after resolution of the other changes.[167] The diagnosis can be confirmed by demonstrating leptospiral antigen in paraffin sections by immunocytochemistry.[168]

Lyme disease

Hepatomegaly, elevated serum aminotransferase activity and biopsy features resembling viral hepatitis may be seen in patients infected with the tick-borne spirochaete *Borrelia burgdorferi*.[169] Liver-cell ballooning and numerous mitoses are accompanied by sinusoidal inflammation (hyperplastic Kupffer cells, lymphocytes, plasma cells and neutrophilic leucocytes). Rarely, necrotising granulomas with multinucleated giant cells and many eosinophils develop.[170] The organism can be identified in liver tissue by Dieterle silver stain.

Candidiasis

The most common hepatic manifestations of candidiasis in immunocompromised hosts are **microabscesses** and **granulomas**.[171,172] The more acute lesions show microabscess formation with central necrosis, visible on gross examination as 1–2 mm yellow-white nodules. Yeasts and pseudohyphae can be seen in some, but not all, cases with diastase–PAS and Gomori methenamine silver stains. The predominantly neutrophilic infiltrates are replaced by epithelioid histiocytes and granulomas as the lesions evolve, sometimes surrounded by reactive fibrosis. Candidiasis is most often diagnosed post-mortem, but should be suspected in the presence of fever, abdominal symptoms and elevated serum alkaline phosphatase activity. Systemic candidiasis has been noted as an important cause of mortality in patients with zone 3 or multilobular hepatic necrosis due to **exertional heatstroke.**[173]

Histoplasmosis

Hepatomegaly is common in disseminated histoplasmosis due to *Histoplasma capsulatum*. The disease is very occasionally seen in countries where it is not endemic.[174] The liver may rarely be the only organ clinically involved.[175] Liver biopsy shows non-specific inflammation as well as granulomas which may be mistaken for the lesions of tuberculosis.[176,177] The organisms may be scanty or abundant, and are found in Kupffer cells and granulomas. They are round or oval, 1–5 μm across, and have a capsule and central chromatin mass. Diastase–PAS and other stains for fungi can be used for their demonstration and differentiation from Leishman–Donovan bodies; the latter are PAS-negative in tissues.[178] Disseminated infection with *Histoplasma duboisii*, seen in Africa, also involves the liver. Nodular lesions contain the much larger and easily demonstrable organisms.[179]

Fibrous, calcified and even bony nodules are sometimes found in and deep to the liver capsule in long-standing histoplasmosis. The nodules, 1–3 mm in diameter, may have a necrotic core surrounded by granulomatous tissue, and the organism is demonstrable in some instances.[180]

The liver in sepsis

Hepatic changes in sepsis are the result of infection of the liver itself, of circulating toxins, of ischaemia, or of a combination of these factors. In many patients the exact cause cannot be established.

Infective lesions include **liver abscess** and **bacterial cholangitis**. Less commonly, infection produces a diffuse bacterial hepatitis in which bacterial colonisation of the liver is associated with portal inflammation.[181] Infection in areas drained by the portal venous system can give rise to **pylephlebitis (see Fig. 12.3)**. Rarely, cholangiographic and histological features resembling primary sclerosing cholangitis develop in sepsis, possibly related to ischaemic damage to large ducts.[182] Post-mortem liver sections from septic patients may show neutrophils aggregated within sinusoids and in sparse numbers dispersed throughout the connective tissue of portal tracts.

Patients with extrahepatic sepsis are often jaundiced, especially when the infection is due to Gram-negative organisms.[183] Three histological patterns have been described in such patients. The commonest is **canalicular cholestasis**, most severe in perivenular areas. This is associated with various degrees of Kupffer-cell activation, fatty change and portal inflammation, but usually little or no hepatocellular necrosis.[184]

The second pattern is one of **ductular cholestasis and inflammation.**[183,185] Bile ductular structures and canals of Hering at the margins of portal tracts are dilated and filled with bile, often in the form of dense, highly pigmented deposits, and neutrophils are seen within and around the affected ductules (**Fig. 15.11**). Perivenular cholestasis is usually present. Periportal canalicular bile is also sometimes present. These changes are not seen in uncomplicated bile-duct obstruction. They are common in the terminal stages of fatal acute or chronic liver disease complicated by sepsis. Damage to bile-duct epithelium has been reported[186] but in most instances the interlobular bile ducts are not affected. Patients with the ductular cholestasis pattern have disproportionately elevated serum bilirubin levels compared with alkaline phosphatase and aminotransferases.[187] Because of its dire implications, this biopsy finding should be communicated rapidly to the clinician and sepsis should be investigated.

**Figure 15.11
Bile ductular
cholestasis in
sepsis.**
Proliferated bile
ductules at the edge
of the portal tract
contain inspissated
bile. The patient
died of septicaemia.
(Post-mortem liver,
H&E.)

The third pattern is **non-bacterial cholangitis**, seen in the **toxic shock syndrome**.[188] The histological features are similar to those of bacterial cholangitis, but the biliary tree is anatomically normal and the lesion is attributed to a circulating staphylococcal toxin rather than to bacteraemia. In many patients, but not all, the underlying lesion is a staphylococcal vaginitis associated with the use of tampons.

Parasitic diseases

Toxoplasmosis

Toxoplasma gondii is occasionally responsible for neonatal liver injury. In adults, hepatic changes include extensive lymphocytic infiltration of sinusoids, evidence of mild liver-cell damage and granuloma formation.[12,189] Trophozoites may be seen within necrotic hepatocytes and can be identified by specific immunocytochemical methods.[190,191]

Malaria

In non-immune patients with malaria there is hypertrophy of Kupffer cells and these contain malarial pigment (haemozoin) in the form of fine, dark brown or black pigment granules (**Fig. 15.12**). In acute malaria due to *Plasmodium falciparum* they also contain erythrocytes, parasites and iron. Malarial pigment closely resembles schistosomal pigment. It often gives pin-point birefringence and, like formalin pigment, is soluble in alcoholic picric acid. This distinguishes it from carbon, with which it may be confused.[192] Other black pigment in Kupffer cells, portal tract macrophages or granulomas can be seen after gold salt therapy or following knee or hip replacement with titanium-containing prostheses.[193] Following an attack of malaria the pigment clears from the acini but can be found in portal macrophages.

**Figure 15.12
Malaria.**
Kupffer cells contain abundant dark granules of malarial pigment. (Needle biopsy, H&E.)

The **tropical splenomegaly syndrome (hyper-reactive malarial splenomegaly)** probably represents an abnormal immune response of the patient to the malarial parasite.[194] Large numbers of small T-lymphocytes are seen in dilated hepatic sinusoids (**Fig. 15.13**). Kupffer cells are enlarged but hepatocytes remain normal. Malarial pigment is scanty or absent. The differential histological diagnosis is from leukaemia, hepatitis C virus infection, infectious mononucleosis, cytomegalovirus infection and toxoplasmosis.

Visceral leishmaniasis (kala-azar)

Infection by *Leishmania donovani* produces striking hypertrophy of Kupffer cells and portal macrophages. These cells contain variable, sometimes very large numbers of Leishman–Donovan bodies, easily visible in H&E-stained sections (**Fig. 15.14**). The PAS stain after diastase digestion is negative, in contrast to the positive staining obtained with *Histoplasma*. In some patients the liver contains epithelioid-cell granulomas, which heal by fibrosis.[12,195]

Amoebiasis

In patients with liver abscesses due to *Entamoeba histolytica*,[196] the amoebae may be found at the margins of the lesion or, less often, within the necrotic debris. They may also be seen in the adjacent liver tissue. They are most easily demonstrated by the PAS or Giemsa methods. Organisms may be identified in fine-needle aspiration biopsy specimens (**Fig. 15.15**).

Schistosomiasis

Liver lesions are usually caused by *Schistosoma mansoni* or *S. japonicum*, and less commonly by other species.[197] In acute schistosomiasis due to *S. mansoni* the portal tracts are

Figure 15.13 Tropical splenomegaly syndrome (hyper-reactive malarial splenomegaly). There are groups of lymphocytes in the sinusoids. Kupffer cells are enlarged. Hepatocytes appear normal. (Needle biopsy, H&E.)

Figure 15.14 Kala-azar. There are many Leishman–Donovan bodies within several hepatocytes, just large enough to give the cells a stippled appearance at this magnification. (Post-mortem liver, H&E.)

infiltrated by eosinophils, lymphocytes and macrophages. Kupffer cells are enlarged and there is focal hepatocellular necrosis. Granulomas around ova are rare.[198]

More commonly schistosomiasis is chronic. Ova, initially containing live miracidia, are trapped in portal tracts where they excite a granulomatous reaction. This is composed of epithelioid cells, multinucleated giant cells, eosinophils and lymphocytes (**Fig. 15.16**). Healing is by fibrosis. When ova are scanty and granulomas are no longer seen, step sections may need to be searched. Ziehl–Neelsen staining is then helpful, because the ova of

Figure 15.15
Amoebic abscess.
A trophozoite of *Entamoeba histolytica* is present in this fine-needle aspiration biopsy sample, with a round nucleus above several cytoplasmic glycogen vacuoles. Adjacent cells are neutrophilic leucocytes. (Papanicolaou.) (Illustration kindly provided by Dr Alastair Deery, London, UK.)

Figure 15.16
Schistosomiasis.
An ovum (arrow) surrounded by giant cells is seen at the centre of a granuloma. The infiltrate is rich in eosinophil leucocytes. (Needle biopsy, H&E.)

species other than *S. haematobium* are acid-fast.[199] Schistosomal pigment, found in portal tracts in some patients with chronic or past schistosomiasis, is a fine, dark granular material closely resembling malarial pigment.

There are lesions in portal-vein branches of all sizes.[198] The smallest contain ova and granulomas. Angiomatoids, wide irregular thin-walled vascular channels, are characteristically found in fibrotic and enlarged portal tracts. Medium-sized veins show intimal

Figure 15.17 Schistosomiasis. Serpiginous septa contain many small blood vessels in this example of 'pipestem' fibrosis. (Wedge biopsy, H&E.)

thickening which may be eccentric and polypoid, and in large veins there are thrombi and adult worms. In the course of portal scarring, isolated smooth muscle cells may become separated from the portal-vein wall and entrapped in fibrous tissue, a helpful diagnostic feature.[200] Diffuse hyaline thickening and tortuosity of veins with surrounding fibrosis constitute 'clay pipestem fibrosis' in which hepatic artery branches and bile ducts are preserved[200] (**Fig. 15.17**).

Lobular changes are usually slight, but sinusoidal lining cells are prominent and there is an increase in fibre within the space of Disse.[201,202] Portal tract lymphocytic infiltrates and piecemeal necrosis are likely to reflect the presence of chronic hepatitis, as hepatitis B virus infection is increased in patients with hepatosplenic schistosomiasis,[203,204] as is hepatitis C.

Liver flukes

Invasion of the biliary tree by the trematodes *Clonorchis sinensis* (the Chinese liver fluke), *Opisthorchis viverrini* and *O. felineus* is followed by proliferation of duct-like structures around the large bile ducts. The ductal epithelium may undergo goblet-cell metaplasia.[205] Smaller ducts are surrounded by an eosinophil-rich infiltrate. Complications include bile-duct obstruction, infection, portal fibrosis and hypertension, and bile-duct carcinoma.[206] Infestation may present several years after the patient has left an endemic area.[207]

The liver fluke *Fasciola hepatica* enters the liver from the peritoneal cavity and reaches the biliary tree some weeks later. White nodules are seen on the liver surface at the points of entry and may be mistaken for tumour. Migration tracks extend into the liver. Histologically, capsular and subcapsular lesions are composed of serpiginous areas of necrosis containing eosinophils and Charcot–Leyden crystals and bordered by palisaded histiocytes[208] (**Fig. 15.18**). Elsewhere in the liver, portal tracts are infiltrated with eosinophils. The biliary phase of the infestation is marked by cholangitis with rather less bile-duct hyperplasia than in *Clonorchis* or *Opisthorchis* infections, and both arterial and venous

Figure 15.18 Fascioliasis. Part of a nodule near the surface of the liver. A central area of necrosis (N) filled with leucocytes is bordered by palisaded histiocytes (H). (Wedge biopsy, H&E.)

thrombosis. Features of bile-duct obstruction, periductal fibrosis, and an ovum within a granuloma have also been reported.[209]

Ascariasis

Focal areas of necrosis with infiltration by eosinophils and neutrophils are seen in the migratory phase, when larvae travel to the lungs via the liver. Adult worms may enter the biliary tree from the duodenum, giving rise to bile-duct obstruction, cholangitis and abscess formation.[199]

Larval diseases

In several parasitic diseases with larval stages, including infestation by *Toxocara*, the larvae may reach the liver and give rise to eosinophil-rich abscesses or granulomas. Larvae are sometimes seen within these lesions.[12] White capsular and subcapsular liver nodules composed of mature fibrous tissue with calcification and few infiltrating cells surround larval remnants in long-standing disease due to *Toxocara* or to arthropod larvae.[210]

Gastrointestinal disorders and the liver

Patients with **coeliac disease** sometimes have elevated serum aminotransferases with non-specific acinar or portal mononuclear inflammation, fatty liver or infrequently chronic hepatitis, cirrhosis and hepatocellular carcinoma.[211] Occasionally, coeliac disease is associated with primary biliary cirrhosis or, rarely, with autoimmune hepatitis, primary sclerosing cholangitis or autoimmune cholangitis.[211,212] In **Whipple's disease** the characteristic foamy PAS-positive macrophages may be found in the liver[213] and epithelioid-cell granulomas have been reported.[214] Granulomas, associated with a heavy infiltration by eosinophils, have also been described in **eosinophilic gastroenteritis**.[215]

Chronic inflammatory bowel disease

The spectrum of liver lesions is generally similar in ulcerative colitis and Crohn's disease. In Crohn's disease, serious hepatic complications such as sclerosing cholangitis are much less common and there may be granulomas in the liver[216] or amyloid deposition.[217] Gallstones are more common in patients with Crohn's disease than in the general population. In both Crohn's disease and ulcerative colitis, malnutrition, anaemia and toxaemia can lead to steatosis.[218]

A minority of patients with ulcerative colitis has persistent abnormalities of liver function tests.[219] Careful examination including cholangiography shows that most of these patients have primary sclerosing cholangitis (**see Ch. 5**). Bile-duct carcinoma, sometimes accompanied by diffuse dysplasia of biliary epithelium[220,221] (**see Fig. 5.18**), is increased in patients with ulcerative colitis, probably reflecting underlying sclerosing cholangitis.[222,223] Portal inflammatory lesions with or without periductal fibrosis in ulcerative colitis have occasioned use of the term 'pericholangitis'. However, patients with such portal inflammation have largely been shown to have typical primary sclerosing cholangitis[224] or its small-duct variant.[225] Furthermore, some examples of so-called pericholangitis probably represent a non-specific inflammatory response to the colitis. The term pericholangitis should therefore be discarded.[225] While liver biopsies from patients with ulcerative colitis may show features of chronic hepatitis, this may be due to intercurrent viral hepatitis (e.g. following blood transfusion). However, it should be noted that interface hepatitis is also common in primary sclerosing cholangitis. From a practical point of view it therefore seems wise to consider the possibility of sclerosing cholangitis in all patients with ulcerative colitis and chronic liver disease.

Haematological disorders and the liver

One of the most common findings in liver biopsies from patients with haematological disorders is diffuse **Kupffer-cell siderosis**, usually reflecting prior transfusion (**Ch. 14**). In **reactive haemophagocytic syndrome**[226,227] diffuse Kupffer-cell hyperplasia with siderosis and phagocytosis of erythrocytes may be seen in patients with systemic infections, disseminated carcinoma, leukaemia and lymphoma. Kupffer-cell erythrophagocytosis in **macrophage activation syndrome** (MAS) triggered by infection, malignancy or collagen vascular disease[228] is accompanied by portal and parenchymal CD8-positive T-lymphocytes which may cause a clinical and histopathological hepatitis, the latter featuring prominent apoptotic bodies and, rarely, bile-duct damage or destruction.[229,230] Phagocytosed red blood cells are well demonstrated on chromotrope–aniline blue stain and the histiocytes stain much less intensely on diastase–PAS than those engaged in necrotising processes such as viral hepatitis. Hepatic involvement by leukaemias and lymphomas is discussed in **Chapter 11**, the effects of thrombosis and sickle-cell disease in **Chapter 12**, and graft-versus-host disease following bone marrow transplantation in **Chapter 16**.

Haemophilia

Hepatitis viruses are readily transmitted in blood products, and hepatitis is therefore common in patients with haemophilia.[231–234] Hepatitis C virus and possibly other putative non-A, non-E hepatitis viruses are the most important agents involved, but markers of infection with hepatitis B virus are also present in some patients. Liver histopathology is most often that of a mild chronic hepatitis;[234] cirrhosis is infrequent. The complications of infection by HIV-1 and AIDS have been seen in some haemophiliacs who received blood products contaminated with HIV-1 prior to mandated screening for the virus which was initiated in the 1980s.

Figure 15.19 Extramedullary haemopoiesis. Clumps of haemopoietic cells are seen in the sinusoids, including a megakaryocyte at the bottom of the field. (Needle biopsy, H&E.)

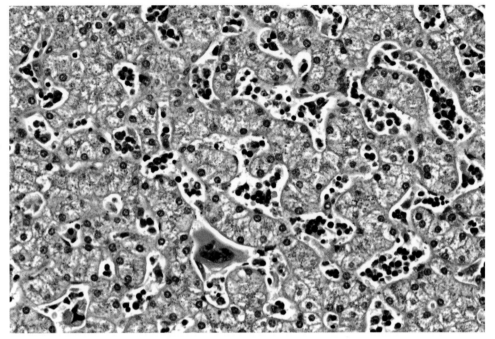

Extramedullary haemopoiesis

Haemopoiesis in the liver sinusoids is normal in fetal and neonatal life. In adults it is seen mainly in the myeloproliferative disorders and when tumours invade bone marrow. Foci of haemopoiesis may also be seen in the congested liver of patients with cardiac failure,[235] in massive hepatic necrosis,[236] in transplant livers with zone 3 necrosis[237] or in the rare situation of graft-versus-host disease in liver transplant recipients.[238] The sinusoids and spaces of Disse of the enlarged liver contain discrete clumps of haemopoietic cells (**Fig. 15.19**), and there are similar cells in portal tracts. Features which distinguish haemopoiesis from the infiltrates of leukaemias, infectious mononucleosis, other infections and the tropical splenomegaly syndrome are the variety of cells in the aggregates and the presence of recognisable marrow cells such as normoblasts and eosinophil myelocytes. Megakaryocytes are commonly seen (**Fig. 15.19**) and are sometimes the only marrow elements found. Owing to the restraints of space, these cells are more elongated than in a section or smear of bone marrow. In the liver of neonates or stillborn infants with **Down's syndrome**, megakaryocytes may be the predominant form of extramedullary haemopoiesis[239,240] and perisinusoidal fibrosis may also be present.[241]

The liver in rheumatoid, immune-complex and collagen diseases

Liver pathology is uncommon in this group of diseases, but when present is most often steatosis.[242] **Nodular regenerative hyperplasia** is also seen in many connective tissue diseases.[243,244] The presence of multisystem disordered immunity in these conditions may be reflected in some cases by associated immune damage to bile ducts (**primary biliary cirrhosis**) or in the form of hepatic vasculitis.[244]

Polyarteritis nodosa in small hepatic arteries can lead to infarction. Immune complexes containing hepatitis B surface antigen are sometimes demonstrable in vessel walls in this disease.[245] Both hepatitis B and C virus antigen–antibody complexes have been implicated in the pathogenesis of essential (type II) mixed cryoglobulinaemia.[246–249] In the polymyalgia rheumatica-giant-cell arteritis syndrome the liver may contain granulomas.[250,251] Other findings reported include fatty change, venous congestion, non-specific hepatitis and prominent stellate cells.[252,253]

Patients with rheumatoid arthritis often have abnormal liver function tests, but liver biopsy more often shows non-specific changes or normal liver than definitive liver disease.[254–256] Amyloidosis or necrotising arteritis may be found, and rheumatoid nodules in the liver such as those typically found in subcutaneous tissue have been reported.[257] In Felty's syndrome[258] (rheumatoid arthritis, leucopenia and splenomegaly), the nodular lesions may be attributable to arteritis involving small intrahepatic vessels.[259]

Scleroderma and the CRST syndrome (calcinosis, Raynaud's phenomenon, sclerodactyly and telangiectasia) may be associated with primary biliary cirrhosis.[260,261] Giant, dense mitochondria on electron microscopy, with normal liver or non-specific changes on light microscopy, have been described in patients with systemic sclerosis.[262]

Most patients with systemic lupus erythematosus (SLE) do not have significant liver pathology but chronic hepatitis, cirrhosis and hepatic granulomas have been reported.[263,264] Abnormal liver function tests may be present without serious lesions.[265,266] Other changes described in SLE include steatosis,[267] cholestasis, nodular regenerative hyperplasia, and necrotising arteritis involving arteries of 100–400 μm diameter.[264] An unusual case of malacoplakia involving the liver in a steroid-treated patient with SLE and Gram-negative bacterial infection showed aggregates of histiocytes with typical Michaelis–Gutmann bodies.[268] Although there appears to be no close relationship between systemic lupus and autoimmune ('lupoid') hepatitis, SLE with autoimmune hepatitis or with primary biliary cirrhosis may coexist.[267] The case of a patient with chronic hepatitis and mixed connective tissue disease has been reported.[269]

Amyloidosis and light chain deposition

The liver is commonly involved in systemic amyloidosis. 'Primary' (AL) and reactive (AA) amyloidosis cannot definitively be distinguished by the pattern of liver involvement,[270,271] although sinusoidal deposition in AL and vascular involvement in AA are consistent patterns reported in several studies.[270,272] Histological distinction is made by the resistance of AL amyloid to potassium permanganate before Congo red staining[273] and by immunohistochemistry for immunoglobulin light chains, AA protein, transthyretin and other proteins.[271,274,275] In most patients the amyloid is deposited in portal arteries (Figs 15.20, 15.21) or diffusely in the perisinusoidal space of Disse (Fig. 15.22). The two patterns are often combined. The perisinusoidal deposits compress both the sinusoids and the liver-cell plates, occasionally leading to portal hypertension or to cholestasis.[276–278] Rarely, AL or AA amyloid may be in the form of globular deposits[279] in the space of Disse (Fig. 15.23), within or surrounding portal arteries and veins or terminal venules, or within hepatocytes. Globular amyloid may be histologically contiguous with sinusoidal (linear) amyloid and thus be the precursor of the latter type.[280]

Amorphous perisinusoidal and portal deposits that are somewhat like amyloid are seen when the liver is involved in light chain deposit disease.[281] Immunoglobulin light chains, usually kappa, can be identified immunochemically. The characteristic green birefringence of amyloid after Congo red staining is absent. Occasionally, amyloid and light chain deposits are found in the same patient.[282,283]

Figure 15.20
Amyloidosis.
The artery at right within this portal tract is thickened by amyloid deposit. (Needle biopsy, H&E.)

Figure 15.21
Amyloidosis.
Arterial amyloid deposits in this large-calibre portal tract are highlighted by Congo red staining. (Wedge biopsy, Congo red.)

**Figure 15.22
Amyloidosis.**
Amyloid has been laid down in the space of Disse. Liver-cell plates have undergone atrophy and sinusoids are narrowed. Cholestasis, an unusual complication of hepatic amyloidosis, is seen at upper right. (Explant liver, H&E.)

**Figure 15.23
Globular amyloid.**
There are rounded deposits of amyloid (A) in the space of Disse. (Needle biopsy, Congo red.)

Figure 15.24 Erythropoietic protoporphyria. Dense brown protoporphyrin deposits are seen within sinusoids. (Needle biopsy, H&E.)

The liver in the porphyrias

Liver lesions are found in **porphyria cutanea tarda** (PCT) and **protoporphyria**.[284] Red porphyrin fluorescence can be demonstrated in both diseases using unfixed liver tissue.

In **porphyria cutanea tarda**, hepatocytes contain needle-shaped birefringent porphyrin crystals, sufficiently water-soluble to make their demonstration difficult or impossible in routinely prepared paraffin sections. They can be seen in unstained paraffin sections, with a ferric ferricyanide reduction stain[285] and in H&E-stained sections prepared with minimal exposure to water.[286] Fatty change and hepatocellular siderosis are common[287] and intra-acinar clumps of iron- and ceroid-containing macrophages, fat droplets and inflammatory cells may also be present.[288] The role of HFE mutations in PCT varies geographically.[289–291] Alcohol contributes to the pathogenesis of PCT and biopsies should be critically examined for alcohol-related injury. More importantly, **chronic hepatitis** and **cirrhosis** are common in patients with PCT and the majority have hepatitis C virus infection.[292–295] The prevalence of chronic hepatitis C in this population is approximately 50%,[296,297] which may also explain the development of **hepatocellular carcinoma**.[284]

In **protoporphyria** (erythropoietic or erythrohepatic protoporphyria) dense, dark brown deposits of poorly soluble protoporphyrin accumulate in the liver (**Fig. 15.24**). These give a diagnostic red birefringence under polarised light, with a characteristic dark maltese cross centrally.[298] There may be serious liver damage, with cholestasis, perisinusoidal and perivenular fibrosis and cirrhosis developing in some patients.[299,300]

Non-specific reactive changes

A variety of changes including portal and lobular inflammation, fat accumulation and Kupffer-cell hypertrophy is seen in extrahepatic conditions, especially febrile, inflammatory or widespread neoplastic diseases. Focal hepatocellular necroses may be found in the parenchyma. The distinction of these reactive changes from a mild form of chronic hepatitis or from residual acute hepatitis requires clinical information. The latter may sometimes be suspected from a predominantly perivenular location of inflammation and liver-cell loss. Reactive changes near space-occupying lesions such as metastatic tumours are discussed in **Chapter 1 (see Fig. 1.5)**.

The liver in pregnancy

In normal pregnancy there are no specific light microscopic findings in the liver. Electron microscopic changes reported in late pregnancy include giant mitochondria with para-crystalline inclusions, increase in the number of peroxisomes and proliferation of smooth endoplasmic reticulum.[301]

Liver disease in pregnancy is rare and falls into three categories:[302]

1 **Liver disease unique to pregnancy**. The four conditions included in this category[303] are **acute fatty liver of pregnancy** (AFLP), **pre-eclampsia/eclampsia**, the **HELLP syndrome (haemolysis, elevated liver enzymes and low platelets)** and **intrahepatic cholestasis of pregnancy** (ICP).
2 **Intercurrent liver disease during pregnancy**. Viral hepatitis and cholelithiasis are examples. Hepatocellular carcinoma, including the fibrolamellar variety,[304] occurs rarely. **Viral hepatitis** is the most common form of liver disease encountered in pregnancy.
3 **Pre-existing liver disease in the pregnant patient**. Chronic hepatitis B viral infection and autoimmune hepatitis with or without cirrhosis are examples.

Jaundice and elevated serum aminotransferases are important aspects of the clinical presentation of liver disease in pregnancy. The following discussion is limited to those diseases unique to pregnancy.

Acute fatty liver of pregnancy

This uncommon and serious complication of pregnancy develops in the last weeks of gestation[305–307] and in certain cases is due to gene mutations affecting mitochondrial fatty acid oxidation enzymes.[308,309] Steatosis involves the greater part of each acinus, usually leaving a thin and incomplete rim of normal hepatocytes around the portal tracts.[310,311] The fat is mainly in the form of fine droplets, as in Reye's syndrome and other examples of microvesicular steatosis.[312] Large fat vacuoles of the kind seen in alcoholic liver disease are scanty, and the cause of the hepatocellular swelling and pallor may not be readily apparent on examination of paraffin sections (**Fig. 15.25**). PAS and trichrome stains are sometimes more helpful than H&E for identifying the small fat vacuoles. Fat staining of frozen sections makes the diagnosis clear, and a piece of the biopsy specimen should therefore be kept for frozen sectioning in patients with unexplained jaundice in late pregnancy. Inflammatory cells, mostly lymphocytes, are prominent in some examples and may lead to confusion with acute viral hepatitis,[313] in which microvesicular steatosis is not seen. In more severe examples of AFLP there is loss of hepatocytes leading to approximation of portal tracts. Fibrin deposits are occasionally demonstrable in hepatic sinusoids. One series showed cholestasis, extramedullary haemopoiesis and giant mitochondria[311] in some patients. With rare exception,[314] AFLP does not recur in subsequent pregnancies.

Pre-eclampsia/eclampsia

Hypertension, proteinuria, peripheral oedema and occasional coagulation abnormalities in pregnancy constitute pre-eclampsia, or eclampsia if convulsions and hyper-reflexia are also present. Liver involvement is unusual, but may be manifested by elevated levels of

**Figure 15.25
Acute fatty liver of pregnancy.**
Swollen pale-staining hepatocytes are seen around a terminal hepatic venule (V). The edge of a portal tract with a mild lymphocytic infiltrate is seen at the upper left corner. No large fat vacuoles are seen. (Post-mortem liver, H&E.)

**Figure 15.26
Pre-eclampsia/ eclampsia.**
Fibrin is seen within the periportal sinusoids at lower right. (Needle biopsy, H&E.)

serum aminotransferases and/or alkaline phosphatase. The incidence of pre-eclampsia is increased in patients with acute fatty liver.[313] The liver in pre-eclampsia shows fibrin thrombi in portal vessels and periportal sinusoids (**Fig. 15.26**) associated with necrosis and haemorrhage in more severe cases.[315,316] The identity of the fibrin can be established by phosphotungstic acid–haematoxylin (PTAH) staining or immunofluorescence.[317] These changes are not seen in all patients. Infarction, haematoma and rupture of the liver[318] are complications.

HELLP syndrome

This syndrome is exceedingly uncommon in pregnancy[305,319] and is seen in 20% of patients with severe pre-eclampsia.[303] Liver biopsy changes range from non-specific portal inflammation and glycogenated hepatocyte nuclei[305,320–322] to the periportal fibrin and necrosis seen in pre-eclampsia.[303] One study demonstrated a relationship between maternal AFLP and HELLP syndrome and a mitochondrial fatty acid β-oxidation disorder with 3-hydroxyacyl-CoA dehydrogenase deficiency in their offspring.[323] Two of the children in the study had severe fatty change, necrosis and early nodules at autopsy.

Intrahepatic cholestasis of pregnancy

Pruritus, with or without cholestatic jaundice, may develop in late pregnancy and recur in subsequent pregnancies. It regresses after delivery. Liver biopsy shows little apart from canalicular cholestasis, most severe in perivenular areas.[315] Minor hepatocellular changes and inflammation are attributable to the cholestasis itself. Portal inflammation is absent or mild. No histological abnormalities are detectable between pregnancies, but the jaundice has been shown to return on administration of oral contraceptives.[324] Concomitant ICP and AFLP have been reported.[325] Some 15% of cases are accounted for by mutations in the multidrug resistance 3 (MDR3) bile transport gene.[326–329]

References

1 Bravo AA, Sheth SG, Chopra S. Liver biopsy. N Engl J Med 2001; 344: 495–500.

2 Burt AD. Liver pathology associated with diseases of other organs or systems. In: Burt AD, Portmann BC, Ferrell LD, eds. Pathology of the Liver, 5th edn. Edinburgh: Churchill Livingstone/Elsevier, 2007: Ch. 17: 881–932.

3 Holtz T, Moseley RH, Scheiman JM. Liver biopsy in fever of unknown origin. A reappraisal. J Clin Gastroenterol 1993; 17: 29–32.

4 Sandor M, Weinstock JV, Wynn TA. Granulomas in schistosome and mycobacterial infections: a model of local immune responses. Trends Immunol 2003; 24: 44–52.

5 Lefkowitch JH. Hepatic granulomas. J Hepatol 1999; 30: 40–45.

6 Ferrell LD. Hepatic granulomas: a morphologic approach to diagnosis. Surg Pathol 1990; 3: 87–106.

7 Denk H, Scheuer PJ, Baptista A, et al. Guidelines for the diagnosis and interpretation of hepatic granulomas. Histopathology 1994; 25: 209–218.

8 Drebber U, Kasper H-U, Ratering J, et al. Hepatic granulomas: histological and molecular pathological approach to differential diagnosis – a study of 442 cases. Liver Int 2008; 28: 828–834.

9 Fauci AS, Wolff SM. Granulomatous hepatitis. In: Popper H, Schaffner F, eds. Progress in Liver Diseases, Vol V. New York: Grune & Stratton, 1976; Ch. 36: 609–621.

10 Gaya DR, Thorburn KA, Oien KA, et al. Hepatic granulomas: a 10 year single centre experience. J Clin Pathol 2003; 56: 850–853.

11 Guckian JC, Perry JE. Granulomatous hepatitis: an analysis of 63 cases and review of the literature. Ann Intern Med 1966; 65: 1081–1100.

12 Ishak KG. Granulomas of the liver. In: Ioachim HL, ed. Pathology of Granulomas. New York: Raven Press, 1983: 307–370.

13 Hunt J, Gordon FD, Jenkins RL, et al. Sarcoidosis with selective involvement of a second liver allograft: report of a case and review of the literature. Mod Pathol 1999; 12: 325–328.

14 Israel HL, Margolis ML, Rose LJ. Hepatic granulomatosis and sarcoidosis. Further observations. Dig Dis Sci 1984; 29: 353–356.

15 Hercules HD, Bethlem NM. Value of liver biopsy in sarcoidosis. Arch Pathol Lab Med 1984; 108: 831–834.

16 Ishak KG. Sarcoidosis of the liver and bile ducts. Mayo Clin Proc 1998; 73: 467–472.

17 Epstein MS, Devaney KO, Goodman ZD, et al. Liver disease in sarcoidosis. Hepatology 1990; 12: 839A.

18 Devaney K, Goodman ZD, Epstein MS, et al. Hepatic sarcoidosis. Clinicopathologic features in 100 patients. Am J Surg Pathol 1993; 17: 1272–1280.

19 Maddrey WC, Johns CJ, Boitnott JK, et al. Sarcoidosis and chronic hepatic disease: a clinical and pathologic study of 20 patients. Medicine 1970; 49: 375–395.

20 Tekeste H, Latour F, Levitt RE. Portal hypertension complicating sarcoid liver disease: case report and review of the literature. Am J Gastroenterol 1984; 79: 389–396.

21 Moreno-Merlo F, Wanless IR, Shimamatsu K, et al. The role of granulomatous phlebitis and thrombosis in the pathogenesis of cirrhosis and portal hypertension in sarcoidosis. Hepatology 1997; 26: 554–560.

22 Rudzki C, Ishak KG, Zimmerman HJ. Chronic intrahepatic cholestasis of sarcoidosis. Am J Med 1975; 59: 373–387.

23 Bridges RA, Berendes H, Good RA. A fatal granulomatous disease of childhood. Am J Dis Child 1959; 97: 387–408.

24 Ishak KG, Sharp HL. Metabolic errors and liver disease. In: MacSween RNM, Anthony PP, Scheuer PJ, et al., eds. Pathology of the Liver, 3rd edn. Edinburgh: Churchill Livingstone, 1994; Ch. 4: 123–218.

25 Nakhleh RE, Glock M, Snover DC. Hepatic pathology of chronic granulomatous disease of childhood. *Arch Pathol Lab Med* 1992; **116:** 71–75.

26 Hussain N, Feld JJ, Kleiner DE, et al. Hepatic abnormalities in patients with chronic granulomatous disease. *Hepatology* 2007; **45:** 675–683.

27 Feld JJ, Hussain N, Wright EC, et al. Hepatic involvement and portal hypertension predict mortality in chronic granulomatous disease. *Gastroenterology* 2008; **134:** 1917–1926.

27a Ardeniz O, Cunningham-Rundles C. Granulomatous disease in common variable immunodeficiency. *Clin Immunol* 2009; **133:** 198–207.

27b Malamut G, Ziol M, Suarez F, et al. Nodular regenerative hyperplasia: the main liver disease in patients with primary hypogammaglobulinemia and hepatic abnormalities. *J Hepatol* 2008; **48:** 74–82.

27c Daniels JA, Torbenson M, Vivekanandan P, Anders RA, Boitnott JK. Hepatitis in common variable immunodeficiency. *Hum Pathol* 2009; **40:** 484–488.

27d Fukushima K, Ueno Y, Kanegane H, et al. A case of severe recurrent hepatitis with common variable immunodeficiency. *Hepatol Res* 2008; **38:** 415–420.

28 Emile JF, Sebagh M, Ferray C, et al. The presence of epithelioid granulomas in hepatitis C virus-related cirrhosis. *Hum Pathol* 1993; **24:** 1095–1097.

29 Barceno R, Sanroman AL, Del Campo S, et al. Posttransplant liver granulomatosis associated with hepatitis C? *Transplantation* 1998; **65:** 1494–1495.

30 Vakiani E, Hunt KK, Mazziotta RM, et al. Hepatitis C-associated granulomas after liver transplantation: morphologic spectrum and clinical implications. *Am J Clin Pathol* 2007; **127:** 128–134.

31 Goldin RD, Levine TS, Foster GR, et al. Granulomas and hepatitis C. *Histopathology* 1996; **28:** 265–267.

32 McMaster KR, Hennigar GR. Drug-induced granulomatous hepatitis. *Lab Invest* 1981; **44:** 61–73.

33 Kurumaya H, Kono N, Nakanuma Y, et al. Hepatic granulomata in long-term hemodialysis patients with hyperaluminumemia. *Arch Pathol Lab Med* 1989; **113:** 1132–1134.

34 Ballestri M, Baraldi A, Gatti AM, et al. Liver and kidney foreign bodies granulomatosis in a patient with malocclusion, bruxism and worn dental prostheses. *Gastroenterology* 2001; **121:** 1234–1238.

35 Leong ASY, Disney APS, Gove DW. Spallation and migration of silicone from blood-pump tubing in patients on hemodialysis. *N Engl J Med* 1982; **306:** 135–140.

36 Yao-Chang L, Tomashefski J, McMahon JT, et al. Mineral-associated hepatic injury: a report of seven cases with X-ray microanalysis. *Hum Pathol* 1991; **22:** 1120–1127.

37 Tjwa M, De Hertogh G, Neuville B, et al. Hepatic fibrin-ring granulomas in granulomatous hepatitis: report of four cases and review of the literature. *Acta Clin Belg* 2001; **56:** 341–348.

38 Bernstein M, Edmondson HA, Barbour BH. The liver lesion in Q-fever. Clinical and pathologic features. *Arch Intern Med* 1965; **116:** 491–498.

39 Pellegrin M, Delsol G, Auvergnat JC, et al. Granulomatous hepatitis in Q fever. *Hum Pathol* 1980; **11:** 51–57.

40 Hofmann CE, Heaton JW Jr. Q fever hepatitis: clinical manifestations and pathological findings. *Gastroenterology* 1982; **83:** 474–479.

41 Qizilbash AH. The pathology of Q fever as seen on liver biopsy. *Arch Pathol Lab Med* 1983; **107:** 364–367.

42 Srigley JR, Vellend H, Palmer N, et al. Q-fever. The liver and bone marrow pathology. *Am J Surg Pathol* 1985; **9:** 752–758.

43 Marazuela M, Moreno A, Yebra M, et al. Hepatic fibrin-ring granulomas. A clinicopathologic study of 23 patients. *Hum Pathol* 1991; **22:** 607–613.

44 Vanderstigel M, Zafrani ES, Lejonc JL, et al. Allopurinol hypersensitivity syndrome as a cause of hepatic fibrin-ring granulomas. *Gastroenterology* 1986; **90:** 188–190.

45 Lobdell DH. 'Ring' granulomas in cytomegalovirus hepatitis. *Arch Pathol Lab Med* 1987; **111:** 881–882.

46 Nenert M, Mavier P, Dubuc N, et al. Epstein–Barr virus infection and hepatic fibrin-ring granulomas. *Hum Pathol* 1988; **19:** 608–610.

47 Moreno A, Marazuela M, Yebra M, et al. Hepatic fibrin-ring granulomas in visceral leishmaniasis. *Gastroenterology* 1988; **95:** 1123–1126.

48 Ponz E, García-Pagán JC, Bruguera M, et al. Hepatic fibrin-ring granulomas in a patient with hepatitis A. *Gastroenterology* 1991; **100:** 268–270.

49 Ruel M, Sevestre H, Henry-Biabaud E, et al. Fibrin ring granulomas in hepatitis A. *Dig Dis Sci* 1992; **37:** 1915–1917.

50 De Bayser L, Roblot P, Ramassamy A, et al. Hepatic fibrin-ring granulomas in giant cell arteritis. *Gastroenterology* 1993; **105:** 272–273.

51 Murphy E, Griffiths MR, Hunter JA, et al. Fibrin-ring granulomas: a non-specific reaction to liver injury? *Histopathology* 1991; **19:** 91–93.

52 Simon HB, Wolff SM. Granulomatous hepatitis and prolonged fever of unknown origin: a study of 13 patients. *Medicine* 1973; **52:** 1–21.

53 Knox TA, Kaplan MM, Gelfand JA, et al. Methotrexate treatment of idiopathic granulomatous hepatitis. *Ann Intern Med* 1995; **122:** 592–595.

54 Zoutman DE, Ralph ED, Frei JV. Granulomatous hepatitis and fever of unknown origin. An 11-year experience of 23 cases with three years' follow-up. *J Clin Gastroenterol* 1991; **13:** 69–75.

55. Lucas SB. Other viral and infectious diseases and HIV-related liver disease. In: Burt AD, Portmann BC, Ferrell LD, eds. MacSween's Pathology of the Liver, 5th edn. Edinburgh: Churchill Livingstone/Elsevier, 2007; Ch. 9: 443–492.

56 Huerre MR, Lan NT, Marianneau P, et al. Liver histopathology and biological correlates in five cases of fatal dengue fever in Vietnamese children. *Virchows Arch* 2001; **438:** 107–115.

57 Elisaf M, Stefanaki S, Repanti M, et al. Liver involvement in hemorrhagic fever with renal syndrome. *J Clin Gastroenterol* 1993; **17:** 33–37.

58 Klotz O, Belt TH. The pathology of the liver in yellow fever. *Am J Pathol* 1930; **6:** 663–689.

59 Vieira WT, Gayotto LC, de Lima CP, et al. Histopathology of the human liver in yellow fever with special emphasis on the diagnostic role of the Councilman body. *Histopathology* 1983; **7:** 195–208.

60 Goodman ZD, Ishak KG, Sesterhenn IA. Herpes simplex hepatitis in apparently immunocompetent adults. *Am J Clin Pathol* 1986; **85**: 694–699.

61 Jacques SM, Qureshi F. Herpes simplex virus hepatitis in pregnancy: a clinicopathologic study of three cases. *Hum Pathol* 1992; **23**: 183–187.

62 Carmichael GP Jr, Zahradnik JM, Moyer GH, et al. Adenovirus hepatitis in an immunosuppressed adult patient. *Am J Clin Pathol* 1979; **71**: 352–355.

63 Varki NM, Bhuta S, Drake T, et al. Adenovirus hepatitis in two successive liver transplants in a child. *Arch Pathol Lab Med* 1990; **114**: 106–109.

64 Phillips MJ, Glendis LM, Paucell S, et al. Syncytial giant-cell hepatitis. Sporadic hepatitis with distinctive pathologic features, a severe clinical course, and paramyxoviral features. *N Engl J Med* 1991; **324**: 455–460.

64a Micchelli STL, Thomas D, Boitnott JK, et al. Hepatic giant cells in hepatitis C virus (HCV) mono-infection and HCV/HIV co-infection. *J Clin Pathol* 2008; **61**: 1058–1061.

65 Potenza L, Luppi M, Barozzi P, et al. HHV-6A in syncytial giant-cell hepatitis. *N Engl J Med* 2008; **359**: 593–602.

66 Devaney K, Goodman ZD, Ishak KG. Postinfantile giant-cell transformation in hepatitis. *Hepatology* 1992; **16**: 327–333.

67 Lau J, Koukoulis G, Mieli-Vergani G, et al. Syncytial giant-cell hepatitis – a specific disease entity? *J Hepatol* 1992; **15**: 216–219.

68 Finegold MJ, Carpenter RJ. Obliterative cholangitis due to cytomegalovirus: a possible precursor of paucity of intrahepatic bile ducts. *Hum Pathol* 1982; **13**: 662–665.

69 Chang M-H, Huang H-H, Huang E-S, et al. Polymerase chain reaction to detect human cytomegalovirus in livers of infants with neonatal hepatitis. *Gastroenterology* 1992; **103**: 1022–1025.

70 Theise ND, Conn M, Thung SN. Localization of cytomegalovirus antigens in liver allografts over time. *Hum Pathol* 1993; **24**: 103–108.

71 Vanstapel MJ, Desmet VJ. Cytomegalovirus hepatitis: a histological and immunohistochemical study. *Appl Pathol* 1983; **1**: 41–49.

72 Clarke J, Craig RM, Saffro R, et al. Cytomegalovirus granulomatous hepatitis. *Am J Med* 1979; **66**: 264–269.

73 Snover DC, Horwitz CA. Liver disease in cytomegalovirus mononucleosis: a light microscopical and immunoperoxidase study of six cases. *Hepatology* 1984; **4**: 408–412.

74 Kilpatrick ZM. Structural and functional abnormalities of liver in infectious mononucleosis. *Arch Intern Med* 1966; **117**: 47–53.

75 Chang MY, Campbell WG Jr. Fatal infectious mononucleosis. Association with liver necrosis and herpes-like virus particles. *Arch Pathol* 1975; **99**: 185–191.

76 Lebovics E, Thung SN, Schaffner F, et al. The liver in the acquired immunodeficiency syndrome: a clinical and histologic study. *Hepatology* 1985; **5**: 293–298.

77 Glasgow BJ, Anders K, Layfield LJ, et al. Clinical and pathologic findings of the liver in the acquired immune deficiency syndrome (AIDS). *Am J Clin Pathol* 1985; **83**: 582–588.

78 Dworkin BM, Stahl RE, Giardina MA, et al. The liver in acquired immune deficiency syndrome: emphasis on patients with intravenous drug abuse. *Am J Gastroenterol* 1987; **82**: 231–236.

79 Schneiderman DJ, Arenson DM, Cello JP, et al. Hepatic disease in patients with the acquired immune deficiency syndrome (AIDS). *Hepatology* 1987; **7**: 925–930.

80 Lebovics E, Dworkin BM, Heier SK, et al. The hepatobiliary manifestations of human immunodeficiency virus infection. *Am J Gastroenterol* 1988; **83**: 1–7.

81 Wilkins MJ, Lindley R, Dourakis SP, et al. Surgical pathology of the liver in HIV infection. *Histopathology* 1991; **18**: 459–464.

82 Stone VE, Bounds BC, Muse VV, Ferry JA. Case 29-2009: an 81-year-old man with weight loss, odynophagic, and failure to thrive. *N Engl J Med* 2009; **361**: 1189–1198.

83 Bach N, Theise ND, Schaffner F. Hepatic histopathology in the acquired immunodeficiency syndrome. *Semin Liver Dis* 1992; **12**: 205–212.

84 Lefkowitch JH. The liver in AIDS. *Semin Liver Dis* 1997; **17**: 335–344.

85 Lefkowitch JH. Pathology of AIDS-related liver disease. *Dig Dis* 1994; **12**: 321–330.

86 Forsmark CE. AIDS and the gastrointestinal tract. *Postgrad Med* 1993; **93**: 143–152.

87 Clark SJ, Creighton S, Portmann B, et al. Acute liver failure associate with antiretroviral treatment for HIV: a report of six cases. *J Hepatol* 2002; **36**: 295–301.

88 Spengler U, Lichterfeld M, Rockstroh JK. Antiretroviral drug toxicity – a challenge for the hepatologist? *J Hepatol* 2002; **36**: 283–294.

89 Scoazec JY, Feldmann G. Both macrophages and endothelial cells of the human hepatic sinusoid express the CD4 molecule, a receptor for the human immunodeficiency virus. *Hepatology* 1990; **12**: 505–510.

90 Housset C, Lamas E, Courgnaud V, et al. Presence of HIV-1 in human parenchymal and non-parenchymal liver cells in vivo. *J Hepatol* 1993; **19**: 252–258.

91 Steffan A-M, Lafon M-E, Gendrault J-L, et al. Primary cultures of endothelial cells from the human liver sinusoid are permissive for human immunodeficiency virus type 1. *Proc Natl Acad Sci USA* 1992; **89**: 1582–1586.

92 Housset C, Boucher O, Girard PM, et al. Immunohistochemical evidence for human immunodeficiency virus-1 infection of liver Kupffer cells. *Hum Pathol* 1990; **21**: 404–408.

93 Lafon M-E, Kirn A. Human immunodeficiency virus infection of the liver. *Semin Liver Dis* 1992; **12**: 197–204.

94 Witzleben CL, Marshall GS, Wenner W, et al. HIV as a cause of giant cell hepatitis. *Hum Pathol* 1988; **19**: 603–605.

95 Molina J-M, Welker Y, Ferchal F, et al. Hepatitis associated with primary HIV infection. *Gastroenterology* 1992; **102**: 739–746.

96 Palella FJ, Delaney KM, Moorman AC, et al. Declining morbidity and mortality among patients with advanced human immunodeficiency virus infection. *N Engl J Med* 1998; **338**: 853–860.

97 Hofman V, Marty P, Perrin C, et al. The histological spectrum of visceral leishmaniasis caused by Leishmania infantum MON-1 in acquired immune deficiency syndrome. *Hum Pathol* 2000; **31**: 75–84.

98 Kahn DG, Garfinkle JM, Klonoff DC, et al. Cryptosporidial and cytomegaloviral hepatitis and cholecystitis. *Arch Pathol Lab Med* 1987; **111**: 879–881.

99 Beaugerie L, Teilhac M-F, Deluol A-M, et al. Cholangiopathy associated with Microsporidia infection of the common bile duct mucosa in a patient with HIV infection. *Ann Intern Med* 1992; **117**: 401–402.

100 Pol S, Romana C, Richard S, et al. *Enterocytozoon bieneusi* infection in acquired-immunodeficiency syndrome-related sclerosing cholangitis. *Gastroenterology* 1992; **102**: 1778–1781.

101 Pol S, Romana CA, Richard S, et al. Microsporidia infection in patients with the human immunodeficiency virus and unexplained cholangitis. *N Engl J Med* 1993; **328**: 95–99.

102 Greene JB, Sidhu GS, Lewin S, et al. Mycobacterium avium-intracellulare: a cause of disseminated life-threatening infection in homosexuals and drug abusers. *Ann Intern Med* 1982; **97**: 539–546.

103 Orenstein MS, Tavitian A, Yonk B, et al. Granulomatous involvement of the liver in patients with AIDS. *Gut* 1985; **26**: 1220–1225.

104 Gordon SC, Reddy KR, Gould EE, et al. The spectrum of liver disease in the acquired immunodeficiency syndrome. *J Hepatol* 1986; **2**: 475–484.

105 Nakanuma Y, Liew CT, Peters RL, et al. Pathologic features of the liver in acquired immune deficiency syndrome (AIDS). *Liver* 1986; **6**: 158–166.

106 Stevens A. Micro-organisms. In: Bancroft JD, Stevens A, eds. Theory and Practice of Histological Techniques, 2nd edn. Edinburgh: Churchill Livingstone, 1982; Ch. 15: 278–296.

107 Kuper SWA, May JR. Detection of acid-fast-organisms in tissue sections by fluorescence microscopy. *J Pathol Bacteriol* 1960; **79**: 59–68.

108 Poblete RB, Rodriguez K, Foust RT, et al. *Pneumocystis carinii* hepatitis in the acquired immunodeficiency syndrome (AIDS). *Ann Intern Med* 1989; **110**: 737–738.

109 Margulis SJ, Honig CL, Soave R, et al. Biliary tract obstruction in the acquired immunodeficiency syndrome [published erratum appears in *Ann Intern Med* 1986 Oct; **105**(4): 634]. *Ann Intern Med* 1986; **105**: 207–210.

110 Cello J. Human immunodeficiency virus-associated biliary tract disease. *Semin Liver Dis* 1992; **12**: 213–218.

111 Bouche H, Housset C, Dumont J-L, et al. AIDS-related cholangitis: diagnostic features and course in 15 patients. *J Hepatol* 1993; **17**: 34–39.

112 Czapar CA, Weldon-Linne CM, Moore DM, et al. Peliosis hepatis in the acquired immunodeficiency syndrome. *Arch Pathol Lab Med* 1986; **110**: 611–613.

113 Boylston AW, Cook HT, Francis ND, et al. Biopsy pathology of acquired immune deficiency syndrome (AIDS). *J Clin Pathol* 1987; **40**: 1–8.

114 Perkocha LA, Geaghan SM, Yen TSB, et al. Clinical and pathological features of bacillary peliosis hepatis in association with human immunodeficiency virus infection. *N Engl J Med* 1990; **323**: 1581–1586.

115 Garcia-Tsao G, Panzini L, Yoselevitz M, et al. Bacillary peliosis hepatis as a cause of acute anemia in a patient with the acquired immunodeficiency syndrome. *Gastroenterology* 1992; **102**: 1065–1070.

116 Tappero JW, Koehler JE, Berger TG, et al. Bacillary angiomatosis and bacillary splenitis in immunocompetent adults. *Ann Intern Med* 1993; **118**: 363–365.

117 Koehler JE, Sanchez MA, Garrido CS, et al. Molecular epidemiology of bartonella infections in patients with bacillary angiomatosis–peliosis. *N Engl J Med* 1997; **337**: 1876–1883.

118 Caccamo D, Pervez NK, Marchevsky A. Primary lymphoma of the liver in the acquired immunodeficiency syndrome. *Arch Pathol Lab Med* 1986; **110**: 553–555.

119 Beral V, Peterman T, Berkelman R, et al. AIDS-associated non-Hodgkin lymphoma. *Lancet* 1991; **337**: 805–809.

120 Newell A, Francis N, Nelson M. Hepatitis and HIV: interrelationship and interactions. *Br J Clin Pract* 1995; **49**: 247–251.

121 Horvath J, Raffanti SP. Clinical aspects of the interactions between human immunodeficiency virus and the hepatotropic viruses. *Clin Infect Dis* 1994; **18**: 339–347.

122 Petrovic LM. HIV/HCV co-infection: histopathologic findings, natural history, fibrosis, and impact of antiretroviral treatment: a review article. *Liver Int* 2007; **27**: 598–606.

123 Colin J-F, Cazals-Hatem D, Loriot MA, et al. Influence of human immunodeficiency virus infection on chronic hepatitis B in homosexual men. *Hepatology* 1999; **29**: 1306–1310.

124 Collier J, Heathcote J. Hepatitis C viral infection in the immunosuppressed patient. *Hepatology* 1998; **27**: 1–6.

125 Di Martino V, Rufat P, Boyer N, et al. The influence of human immunodeficiency virus coinfection on chronic hepatitis C in injection drug users: a long-term retrospective cohort study. *Hepatology* 2001; **34**: 1193–1199.

126 Lichtenstein DR, Makadon HJ, Chopra S. Fulminant hepatitis B and delta virus coinfection in AIDS. *Am J Gastroenterol* 1992; **87**: 1643–1647.

127 Housset C, Pol S, Carnot F, et al. Interactions between human immunodeficiency virus-1, hepatitis delta virus and hepatitis B virus infections in 260 chronic carriers of hepatitis B virus. *Hepatology* 1992; **15**: 578–583.

128 Puius YA, Dove LM, Brust DG, et al. Three cases of autoimmune hepatitis in HIV-infected patients. *J Clin Gastroenterol* 2008; **42**: 424–429.

129 O'Leary JG, Zachary K, Misdraji J, et al. De novo autoimmune hepatitis during immune reconstitution in an HIV-infected patient receiving highly active antiretroviral therapy. *Clin Infect Dis* 2008; **46**: e12–e14.

130 Crum-Cianflone N, Dilay A, Collins G, et al. Nonalcoholic fatty liver disease among HIV-infected persons. *J AIDS* 2009; **50**: 464–473.

131 Bissuel F, Bruneel F, Habersetzer F, et al. Fulminant hepatitis with severe lactate acidosis in HIV-infected patients on didanosine therapy. *J Int Med* 1994; **235**: 367–372.

132 Olano JP, Borucki MJ, Wen JW, et al. Massive hepatic steatosis and lactic acidosis in a patient with AIDS who was receiving zidovudine. *Clin Infect Dis* 1995; **21**: 973–976.

133 Freiman JP, Helfert KE, Hamrell MR, et al. Hepatomegaly with severe steatosis in HIV-seropositive patients. *AIDS* 1993; **7**: 379–385.

134 Tateo M, Sebagh M, Bralet M-P, et al. A new indication for liver transplantation: nodular regenerative hyperplasia in human immunodeficiency virus-infected patients. *Liver Transplant* 2008; **14**: 1194–1198.

135 Mallet V, Blanchard P, Verkarre V, et al. Nodular regenerative hyperplasia is a new cause of chronic liver disease in HIV-infected patients. *AIDS* 2007; **21**: 187–192.

136 Osick LA, Lee T-P, Pedemonte MB, et al. Hepatic amyloidosis in intravenous drug abusers and AIDS patients. *J Hepatol* 1993; **19**: 79–84.

137 Kossaifi T, Dupon M, Le Bail B, et al. Perisinusoidal cell hypertrophy in a patient with acquired immunodeficiency syndrome. *Arch Pathol Lab Med* 1990; **114**: 876–879.

138 Kahn E, Greco A, Daum F, et al. Hepatic pathology in pediatric acquired immunodeficiency syndrome. *Hum Pathol* 1991; **22**: 1111–1119.

139 Duffy LF, Daum F, Kahn E, et al. Hepatitis in children with acquired immune deficiency syndrome. Histopathologic and immunocytologic features. *Gastroenterology* 1986; **90**: 173–181.

140 Ross JS, Del Rosario A, Bui HX, et al. Primary hepatic leiomyosarcoma in a child with the acquired immunodeficiency syndrome. *Hum Pathol* 1992; **23**: 69–72.

141 Turck WP, Howitt G, Turnberg LA, et al. Chronic Q fever. *Q J Med* 1976; **45**: 193–217.

142 Cervantes F, Bruguera M, Carbonell J, et al. Liver disease in brucellosis. A clinical and pathological study of 40 cases. *Postgrad Med J* 1982; **58**: 346–350.

143 Khosla SN. Typhoid hepatitis. *Postgrad Med J* 1990; **66**: 923–925.

144 De Brito T, Trench Vieira W, D'Agostino Dias M. Jaundice in typhoid hepatitis: a light and electron microscopy study based on liver biopsies. *Acta Hepatol Gastroenterol* 1977; **24**: 426–433.

145 Nasrallah SM, Nassar VH. Enteric fever: a clinicopathological study of 104 cases. *Am J Gastroenterol* 1978; **69**: 63–69.

146 Pais P. A hepatitis like picture in typhoid fever. *Br Med J Clin Res* 1984; **289**: 225–226.

147 Lamps LW, Gray GF, Scott MA. The histologic spectrum of hepatic cat scratch disease. A series of six cases with confirmed Bartonella henselae infection. *Am J Surg Pathol* 1996; **20**: 1253–1259.

148 Thudi KR, Kreikemeier JT, Phillips NJ, et al. Cat scratch disease causing hepatic masses after liver transplant. *Liver Int* 2007; **27**: 145–148.

149 Asada Y, Hayashi T, Sumiyoshi A, et al. Miliary tuberculosis presenting as fever and jaundice with hepatic failure. *Hum Pathol* 1991; **22**: 92–94.

150 Alvarez SZ, Carpio R. Hepatobiliary tuberculosis. *Dig Dis Sci* 1983; **28**: 193–200.

151 Essop AR, Posen JA, Hodkinson JH, et al. Tuberculosis hepatitis: a clinical review of 96 cases. *Q J Med* 1984; **53**: 465–477.

152 Pottipati AR, Dave PB, Gumaste V, et al. Tuberculous abscess of the liver in acquired immunodeficiency syndrome. *J Clin Gastroenterol* 1991; **13**: 549–553.

153 Alcantra-Payawal DE, Matsumura M, Shiratori Y, et al. Direct detection of Mycobacterium tuberculosis using polymerase chain reaction assay among patients with hepatic granuloma. *J Hepatol* 1997; **27**: 620–627.

154 Hunt JS, Silverstein MJ, Sparks FC, et al. Granulomatous hepatitis: a complication of BCG immunotherapy. *Lancet* 1973; **2**: 820–821.

155 Bodurtha A, Kim YH, Laucius JF, et al. Hepatic granulomas and other hepatic lesions associated with BCG immunotherapy for cancer. *Am J Clin Pathol* 1974; **61**: 747–752.

156 Proctor DD, Chopra S, Rubenstein SC, et al. Mycobacteremia and granulomatous hepatitis following initial intravesical bacillus Calmette–Guérin instillation for bladder carcinoma. *Am J Gastroenterol* 1993; **88**: 1112–1115.

157 Case records of the Massachusetts General Hospital. Case 29-1998. *N Engl J Med* 1998; **339**: 831–837.

158 Karat AB, Job CK, Rao PS. Liver in leprosy: histological and biochemical findings. *BMJ* 1971; **1**: 307–310.

159 Chen TS, Drutz DJ, Whelan GE. Hepatic granulomas in leprosy. Their relation to bacteremia. *Arch Pathol Lab Med* 1976; **100**: 182–185.

160 Terry SI, Hanchard B, Brooks SE, et al. Prevalence of liver abnormality in early syphilis. *Br J Vener Dis* 1984; **60**: 83–86.

161 Murray FE, O'Loughlin S, Dervan P, et al. Granulomatous hepatitis in secondary syphilis. *Irish J Med Sci* 1990; **159**: 53–54.

162 Sobel HJ, Wolf EH. Liver involvement in early syphilis. *Arch Pathol* 1972; **93**: 565–568.

163 Fehér J, Somogyi T, Timmer M, et al. Early syphilitic hepatitis. *Lancet* 1975; **2**: 896–899.

164 Romeu J, Rybak B, Dave P, et al. Spirochetal vasculitis and bile ductular damage in early hepatic syphilis. *Am J Gastroenterol* 1980; **74**: 352–354.

165 Veeravahu M. Diagnosis of liver involvement in early syphilis. A critical review. *Arch Intern Med* 1985; **145**: 132–134.

166 De Brito T, Machado MM, Montans SD, et al. Liver biopsy in human leptospirosis: a light and electron microscopy study. *Virchows Arch Pathol Anat Physiol* 1967; **342**: 61–69.

167 De Brito T, Penna DO, Hoshino S, et al. Cholestasis in human leptospirosis: a clinical, histochemical, biochemical and electron microscopy study based on liver biopsies. *Beitr Pathol* 1970; **140**: 345–361.

168 Ferreira Alves VA, Vianna MR, Yasuda PH, et al. Detection of leptospiral antigen in the human liver and kidney using an immunoperoxidase staining procedure. *J Pathol* 1987; **151**: 125–131.

169 Goellner MH, Agger WA, Burgess JH, et al. Hepatitis due to recurrent Lyme disease. *Ann Intern Med* 1988; **108**: 707–708.

170 Zanchi A, Gingold AR, Theise ND, et al. Necrotizing granulomatous hepatitis as an unusual manifestation of Lyme disease. *Dig Dis Sci* 2007; **52**: 2629–2632.

171 Thaler M, Pastakia B, Shawker TH, et al. Hepatic candidiasis in cancer patients: the evolving picture of the syndrome. *Ann Intern Med* 1988; **108**: 88–100.

172 Lewis JH, Patel HR, Zimmerman HJ. The spectrum of hepatic candidiasis. *Hepatology* 1982; **2**: 479–487.

173 Hassanein T, Perper JA, Tepperman L, et al. Liver failure occurring as a component of exertional heatstroke. *Gastroenterology* 1991; **100**: 1442–1447.

174 Jariwalla A, Tulloch BR, Fox H, et al. Disseminated histoplasmosis in an English patient with diabetes mellitus. *BMJ* 1977; **1**: 1002–1004.

175 Lanza FL, Nelson RS, Somayaji BN. Acute granulomatous hepatitis due to histoplasmosis. *Gastroenterology* 1970; **58**: 392–396.

176 Smith JW, Utz JP. Progressive disseminated histoplasmosis. A prospective study of 26 patients. *Ann Intern Med* 1972; **76**: 557–565.

177 Edmondson RP, Eykyn S, Davies DR, et al. Disseminated histoplasmosis successfully treated with amphotericin B. *J Clin Pathol* 1974; **27**: 308–310.

178 Ridley DS. The laboratory diagnosis of tropical diseases with special reference to Britain: a review. [Review.] *J Clin Pathol* 1974; **27**: 435–444.

179 Williams AO, Lawson EA, Lucas AO. African histoplasmosis due to *Histoplasma duboisii*. *Arch Pathol* 1971; **92**: 306–318.

180 Okudaira M, Straub M, Schwarz J. The etiology of discrete splenic and hepatic calcifications in an endemic area of histoplasmosis. *Am J Pathol* 1961; **39**: 599–611.

181 Weinstein L. Bacterial hepatitis: a case report on an unrecognized cause of fever of unknown origin. *N Engl J Med* 1978; **299**: 1052–1054.

182 Engler S, Elsing C, Flechtenmacher C, et al. Progressive sclerosing cholangitis after shock: a new variant of vanishing bile duct disorders. *Gut* 2003; **52**: 688–693.

183 Banks JG, Foulis AK, Ledingham IM, et al. Liver function in septic shock. *J Clin Pathol* 1982; **35**: 1249–1252.

184 Zimmerman HJ, Fang M, Utili R, et al. Jaundice due to bacterial infection. *Gastroenterology* 1979; **77**: 362–374.

185 Lefkowitch JH. Bile ductular cholestasis: an ominous histopathologic sign related to sepsis and 'cholangitis lenta'. *Hum Pathol* 1982; **13**: 19–24.

186 Vyberg M, Poulsen H. Abnormal bile duct epithelium accompanying septicaemia. *Virchows Arch [A]* 1984; **402**: 451–458.

187 Riely CA, Dean PJ, Park AL, et al. A distinct syndrome of liver disease with multisystem organ failure associated with bile ductular cholestasis. *Hepatology* 1989; **10**: 739A.

188 Ishak KG, Rogers WA. Cryptogenic acute cholangitis – association with toxic shock syndrome. *Am J Clin Pathol* 1981; **76**: 619–626.

189 Weitberg AB, Alper JC, Diamond I, et al. Acute granulomatous hepatitis in the course of acquired toxoplasmosis. *N Engl J Med* 1979; **300**: 1093–1096.

190 Andres TL, Dorman SA, Winn W Jr, et al. Immunohistochemical demonstration of Toxoplasma gondii. *Am J Clin Pathol* 1981; **75**: 431–434.

191 Conley FK, Jenkins KA, Remington JS. *Toxoplasma gondii* infection of the central nervous system. Use of the peroxidase–antiperoxidase method to demonstrate toxoplasma in formalin fixed, paraffin embedded tissue sections. *Hum Pathol* 1981; **12**: 690–698.

192 Pounder DJ. Malarial pigment and hepatic anthracosis [letter]. *Am J Surg Pathol* 1983; **7**: 501–502.

193 Brenard R, Dumortier P, Del Natale M, et al. Black pigments in the liver related to gold and titaniium deposits. A report of four cases. *Liver Int* 2007; **27**: 408–413.

194 Editorial: tropical splenomegaly syndrome. *Lancet* 1976; **i**: 1058–1059.

195 Daneshbod K. Visceral leishmaniasis (kala-azar) in Iran: a pathologic and electron microscopic study. *Am J Clin Pathol* 1972; **57**: 156–166.

196 Maltz G, Knauer CM. Amebic liver abscess: a 15-year experience. *Am J Gastroenterol* 1991; **86**: 704–710.

197 Dunn MA, Kamel R. Hepatic schistosomiasis. [Review.] *Hepatology* 1981; **1**: 653–661.

198 Andrade ZA. Hepatic schistosomiasis. Morphological aspects. In: Popper H, Schaffner F, eds. Progress in Liver Diseases, Vol. II. New York: Grune & Stratton, 1965; **Ch. 16**: 228–242.

199 Lucas SB. Other viral and infectious diseases. In: MacSween RNM, Anthony PP, Scheuer PJ, et al., eds.

Pathology of the Liver, 3rd edn. Edinburgh: Churchill Livingstone, 1994; **Ch. 7**: 269–316.

200 Andrade ZA, Peixoto E, Guerret S, et al. Hepatic connective tissue changes in hepatosplenic schistosomiasis. *Hum Pathol* 1992; **23**: 566–573.

201 Canto AL, Sesso A, De Brito T. Human chronic Mansonian schistosomiasis-cell proliferation and fibre formation in the hepatic sinusoidal wall: a morphometric, light and electron-microscopy study. *J Pathol* 1977; **123**: 35–44.

202 Grimaud JA, Borojevic R. Chronic human schistosomiasis mansoni. Pathology of the Disse's space. *Lab Invest* 1977; **36**: 268–273.

203 Lyra LG, Reboucas G, Andrade ZA. Hepatitis B surface antigen carrier state in hepatosplenic schistosomiasis. *Gastroenterology* 1976; **71**: 641–645.

204 Nash TE, Cheever AW, Ottesen EA, et al. Schistosome infections in humans: perspectives and recent findings. *Ann Intern Med* 1982; **97**: 740–754.

205 Sun T. Pathology and immunology of *Clonorchis sinensis* infection in the liver. *Ann Clin Lab Sci* 1984; **14**: 208–215.

206 Ona FV, Dytoc JNT. Clonorchis-associated cholangiocarcinoma: a report of two cases with unusual manifestations. *Gastroenterology* 1991; **101**: 831–839.

207 Hartley JP, Douglas AP. A case of clonorchiasis in England. *BMJ* 1975; **3**: 575.

208 Acosta-Ferreira W, Vercelli-Retta J, Falconi LM. *Fasciola hepatica* human infection. Histopathological study of sixteen cases. *Virchows Arch [A]* 1979; **383**: 319–327.

209 Jones EA, Kay JM, Milligan HP, et al. Massive infection with *Fasciola hepatica* in man. *Am J Med* 1977; **63**: 836–842.

210 Drury RAB. Larval granulomata in the liver. *Gut* 1962; **3**: 289–294.

211 Rubio-Tapia A, Murray JA. The liver in celiac disease. *Hepatology* 2007; **46**: 1650–1658.

212 Gogos CA, Nikolopoulou V, Zolota V, et al. Autoimmune cholangitis in a patient with celiac disease: a case report and review of the literature. *J Hepatol* 1999; **30**: 321–324.

213 MacSween RNM, Burt AD. Liver pathology associated with diseases of other organs. In: MacSween RNM, Anthony PP, Scheuer PJ, et al., eds. Pathology of the Liver, 3rd edn. Edinburgh: Churchill Livingstone, 1994; **Ch. 17**: 713–764.

214 Saint-Marc Girardin MF, Zafrani ES, Chaumette MT, et al. Hepatic granulomas in Whipple's disease. *Gastroenterology* 1984; **86**: 753–756.

215 Everett GD, Mitros FA. Eosinophilic gastroenteritis with hepatic eosinophilic granulomas. Report of a case with 30-year follow-up. *Am J Gastroenterol* 1980; **74**: 519–521.

216 Eade MN, Cooke WT, Brooke BN, et al. Liver disease in Crohn's colitis. A study of 21 consecutive patients having colectomy. *Ann Intern Med* 1971; **74**: 518–528.

217 Shorvon PJ. Amyloidosis and inflammatory bowel disease. *Am J Dig Dis* 1977; **22**: 209–213.

218 Quigley EMM, Zetterman RK. Hepatobiliary complications of malabsorption and malnutrition. *Semin Liver Dis* 1988; **8**: 218–228.

219 Shepherd HA, Selby WS, Chapman RW, et al. Ulcerative colitis and persistent liver dysfunction. *Q J Med* 1983; **52**: 503–513.

220 Haworth AC, Manley PN, Groll A, et al. Bile duct carcinoma and biliary tract dysplasia in chronic ulcerative colitis. *Arch Pathol Lab Med* 1989; **113**: 434–436.

221 Fleming KA, Boberg KM, Glaumann H, et al. Biliary dysplasia as a marker of cholangiocarcinoma in primary sclerosing cholangitis. *J Hepatol* 2001; **34**: 360–365.

222 Wee A, Ludwig J, Coffey RJ Jr, et al. Hepatobiliary carcinoma associated with primary sclerosing cholangitis and chronic ulcerative colitis. *Hum Pathol* 1985; **16**: 719–726.

223 Mir-Madjlessi SH, Farmer RG, Sivak MV Jr. Bile duct carcinoma in patients with ulcerative colitis. Relationship to sclerosing cholangitis: report of six cases and review of the literature. [Review.] *Dig Dis Sci* 1987; **32**: 145–154.

224 Blackstone MO, Nemchausky BA. Cholangiographic abnormalities in ulcerative colitis associated pericholangitis which resemble sclerosing cholangitis. *Am J Dig Dis* 1978; **23**: 579–585.

225 Wee A, Ludwig J. Pericholangitis in chronic ulcerative colitis: primary sclerosing cholangitis of the small bile ducts? *Ann Intern Med* 1985; **102**: 581–587.

226 Tsui WMS, Wong KF, Tse CCH. Liver changes in reactive haemophagocytic syndrome. *Liver* 1992; **12**: 363–367.

227 de Kerguenec C, Hillaire S, Molinié V, et al. Hepatic manifestations of hemophagocytic syndrome: a study of 30 cases. *Am J Gastroenterol* 2001; **96**: 852–857.

228 Tristano AG. Macrophage activation syndrome: a frequent but under-diagnosed complication associated with rheumatic diseases. *Med Sci Monit* 2008; **14**: RA27–RA36.

229 Billiau AD, Roskams T, Van Damme-Lombaerts R, et al. Macrophage activation syndrome: characteristic findings on liver biopsy illustrating the key role of activated IFN-α-producing lymphocytes and IL-6- and TNF-α-producing macrophages. *Blood* 2005; **105**: 1648–1651.

230 Bihl F, Emmenegger U, Reichen J, et al. Macrophage activating syndrome is associated with lobular hepatitis and severe bile duct injury with cholestasis. *J Hepatol* 2006; **44**: 1208–1212.

231 Aledort LM, Levine PH, Hilgartner M, et al. A study of liver biopsies and liver disease among hemophiliacs. *Blood* 1985; **66**: 367–372.

232 Colombo M, Mannucci PM, Carnelli V, et al. Transmission of non-A, non-B hepatitis by heat-treated factor VIII concentrate. *Lancet* 1985; **ii**: 1–4.

233 Hay CR, Preston FE, Triger DR, et al. Progressive liver disease in haemophilia: an understated problem? *Lancet* 1985; **1**: 1495–1498.

234 Bianchi L, Desmet VJ, Popper H, et al. Histologic patterns of liver disease in hemophiliacs, with special reference to morphologic characteristics of non-A, non-B hepatitis. *Semin Liver Dis* 1987; **7**: 203–209.

235 Lefkowitch JH, Mendez L. Morphologic features of hepatic injury in cardiac disease and shock. *J Hepatol* 1986; **2**: 313–327.

236 Craig CEH, Quaglia A, Dhillon AP. Extramedullary haematopoiesis in massive hepatic necrosis. *Histopathology* 2004; **45**: 518–525.

237 Ludwig J, Gross JB, Perkins JD, et al. Persistent centrilobular necroses in hepatic allografts. *Hum Pathol* 1990; **21**: 656–661.

238 Collins RH, Anastasi J, Terstappen LWMM, et al. Brief report: donor-derived long-term multilineage hematopoiesis in a liver-transplant recipient. *N Engl J Med* 1993; **328**: 762–765.

239 Gilson TP, Bendon RW. Megakaryocytosis of the liver in a trisomy 21 stillbirth. *Arch Pathol Lab Med* 1993; **117**: 738–739.

240 Ruchelli ED, Uri A, Dimmick JE, et al. Severe perinatal liver disease and Down syndrome: an apparent relationship. *Hum Pathol* 1991; **22**: 1274–1280.

241 Arai H, Ishida A, Nakajima W, et al. Immunohistochemical study on transforming growth factor-beta 1 expression in liver fibrosis of Down's syndrome with transient abnormal myelopoiesis. *Hum Pathol* 1999; **30**: 474–476.

242 Youssef WI, Tavill AS. Connective tissue diseases and the liver. *J Clin Gastroenterol* 2002; **35**: 345–349.

243 Keshavarzian A, Rentsch R, Hodgson HJF. Clinical implications of liver biopsy findings in collagen–vascular disorders. *J Clin Gastroenterol* 1993; **17**: 219–226.

244 Matsumoto T, Kobayashi S, Shimizu H, et al. The liver in collagen diseases: pathologic study of 160 cases with particular reference to hepatic arteritis, primary biliary cirrhosis, autoimmune hepatitis and nodular regenerative hyperplasia of the liver. *Liver* 2000; **20**: 366–373.

245 Gocke DJ, Hsu K, Morgan C, et al. Association between polyarteritis and Australia antigen. *Lancet* 1970; **2**: 1149–1153.

246 Levo Y, Gorevic PD, Kassab HJ, et al. Liver involvement in the syndrome of mixed cryoglobulinemia. *Ann Intern Med* 1977; **87**: 287–292.

247 Misiani R, Bellavita P, Fenili D, et al. Hepatitis C virus infection in patients with essential mixed cryoglobulinemia. *Ann Intern Med* 1992; **117**: 573–577.

248 Agnello V, Chung RT, Kaplan LM. A role for hepatitis C virus infection in type II cryoglobulinemia. *N Engl J Med* 1992; **327**: 1490–1495.

249 Peña LR, Nand S, De Maria N, et al. Hepatitis C virus infection and lymphoproliferative disorders. *Dig Dis Sci* 2000; **45**: 1854–1860.

250 Long R, James O. Polymyalgia rheumatica and liver disease. *Lancet* 1974; **1**: 77–79.

251 Litwack KD, Bohan A, Silverman L. Granulomatous liver disease and giant cell arteritis. Case report and literature review. *J Rheumatol* 1977; **4**: 307–312.

252 Gossmann HH, Dolle W, Korb G, et al. Liver changes in giant-cell arteritis: temporal arteritis and rheumatic polymyalgia (author's transl.). [German.] *Deutsche Med Wochenschr* 1979; **104**: 1199–1202.

253 Leong AS, Alp MH. Hepatocellular disease in the giant-cell arteritis/polymyalgia rheumatica syndrome. *Ann Rheum Dis* 1981; **40**: 92–95.

254 Rao R, Pfenniger K, Boni A. Liver function tests and liver biopsies in patients with rheumatoid arthritis. *Ann Rheum Dis* 1975; **34**: 198–199.

255 Mills PR, MacSween RN, Dick WC, et al. Liver disease in rheumatoid arthritis. *Scottish Med J* 1980; **25**: 18–22.

256 Mills PR, Sturrock RD. Clinical associations between arthritis and liver disease. [Review.] *Ann Rheum Dis* 1982; **41**: 295–307.

257 Smits JG, Kooijman CD. Rheumatoid nodules in liver [letter]. *Histopathology* 1986; **10**: 1211–1213.

258 Thorne C, Urowitz MB, Wanless I, et al. Liver disease in Felty's syndrome. *Am J Med* 1982; **73**: 35–40.

259 Reynolds WJ, Wanless IR. Nodular regenerative hyperplasia of the liver in a patient with rheumatoid vasculitis: a morphometric study suggesting a role for hepatic arteritis in the pathogenesis. *J Rheumatol* 1984; **11**: 838–842.

260 Murray-Lyon IM, Thompson RP, Ansell ID, et al. Scleroderma and primary biliary cirrhosis. *BMJ* 1970; **1**: 258–259.

261 Reynolds TB, Denison EK, Frankl HD, et al. Primary biliary cirrhosis with scleroderma, Raynaud's phenomenon and telangiectasia. New syndrome. *Am J Med* 1971; **50**: 302–312.

262 Feldmann G, Maurice M, Husson JM, et al. Hepatocyte giant mitochondria: an almost constant lesion in systemic scleroderma. *Virchows Arch [A]* 1977; **374**: 215–227.

263 Runyon BA, LaBrecque DR, Anuras S. The spectrum of liver disease in systemic lupus erythematosus. Report of 33 histologically-proved cases and review of the literature. *Am J Med* 1980; **69**: 187–194.

264 Matsumoto T, Yoshimine T, Shimouchi K, et al. The liver in systemic lupus erythematosus: pathologic analysis of 52 cases and review of Japanese autopsy registry data. *Hum Pathol* 1992; **23**: 1151–1158.

265 Gibson T, Myers AR. Subclinical liver disease in systemic lupus erythematosus. *J Rheumatol* 1981; **8**: 752–759.

266 Miller MH, Urowitz MB, Gladman DD, et al. The liver in systemic lupus erythematosus. *Q J Med* 1984; **53**: 401–409.

267 Chowdhary VR, Crowson CS, Poterucha JJ, et al. Liver involvement in systemic lupus erythematosus: case review of 40 patients. *J Rheumatol* 2008; **35**: 1–6.

268 Robertson SJ, Higgins RB, Powell C. Malacoplakia of liver: a case report. *Hum Pathol* 1991; **22**: 1294–1295.

269 Marshall JB, Ravendhran N, Sharp GC. Liver disease in mixed connective tissue disease. *Arch Intern Med* 1983; **143**: 1817–1818.

270 Chopra S, Rubinow A, Koff RS, et al. Hepatic amyloidosis. A histopathologic analysis of primary (AL) and secondary (AA) forms. *Am J Pathol* 1984; **115**: 186–193.

271 Buck FS, Koss MN. Hepatic amyloidosis: morphologic differences between systemic AL and AA types. *Hum Pathol* 1991; **22**: 904–907.

272 Looi L-M, Sumithran E. Morphologic differences in the pattern of liver infiltration between systemic AL and AA amyloidosis. *Hum Pathol* 1988; **19**: 732–735.

273 Wright JR, Calkins E, Humphrey RL. Potassium permanganate reaction in amyloidosis. A histologic method to assist in differentiating forms of this disease. *Lab Invest* 1977; **36**: 274–281.

274 Shirahama T, Skinner M, Cohen AS. Immunocytochemical identification of amyloid in formalin-fixed paraffin sections. *Histochemistry* 1981; **72**: 161–171.

275 Falk RH, Comenzo RL, Skinner M. The systemic amyloidoses. *N Engl J Med* 1997; **337**: 898–909.

276 Rubinow A, Koff RS, Cohen AS. Severe intrahepatic cholestasis in primary amyloidosis: a report of four cases and a review of the literature. *Am J Med* 1978; **64**: 937–946.

277 Finkelstein SD, Fornasier VL, Pruzanski W. Intrahepatic cholestasis with predominant pericentral deposition in systemic amyloidosis. *Hum Pathol* 1981; **12**: 470–472.

278 Case records of the Massachusetts General Hospital. Case 50-1987. *N Engl J Med* 1987; **317**: 1520–1531.

279 Agaram N, Shia J, Klimstra DS, et al. Globular hepatic amyloid: a diagnostic peculiarity that bears clinical significance. *Hum Pathol* 2005; **36**: 845–849.

280 Makhlouf HR, Goodman ZD. Globular hepatic amyloid: an early stage in the pathway of amyloid formation. A study of 20 new cases. *Am J Surg Pathol* 2007; **31**: 1615–1621.

281 Droz D, Noel LH, Carnot F, et al. Liver involvement in nonamyloid light chain deposits disease. *Lab Invest* 1984; **50**: 683–689.

282 Kirkpatrick CJ, Curry A, Galle J, et al. Systemic kappa light chain deposition and amyloidosis in multiple myeloma: novel morphological observations. *Histopathology* 1986; **10**: 1065–1076.

283 Smith NM, Malcolm AJ. Simultaneous AL-type amyloid and light chain deposit disease in a liver biopsy: a case report. *Histopathology* 1986; **10**: 1057–1064.

284 Bruguera M. Liver involvement in porphyria. *Semin Dermatol* 1986; **5**: 178–185.

285 Fakan F, Chlumská A. Demonstration of needle-shaped hepatic inclusions in porphyria cutanea tarda using the ferric ferricyanide reduction test. *Virchows Arch [A]* 1987; **411**: 365–368.

286 Cortés JM, Oliva H, Paradinas FJ, et al. The pathology of the liver in porphyria cutanea tarda. *Histopathology* 1980; **4**: 471–485.

287 Campo E, Bruguera M, Rodés J. Are there diagnostic histologic features of porphyria cutanea tarda in liver biopsy specimens? *Liver* 1990; **10**: 185–190.

288 Lefkowitch JH, Grossman ME. Hepatic pathology in porphyria cutanea tarda. *Liver* 1983; **3**: 19–29.

289 Nagy Z, Kószo F, Pár A, et al. Hemochromatosis (*HFE*) gene mutations and hepatitis C virus infection as risk factors for porphyria cutanea tarda in Hungarian patients. *Liver Int* 2004; **24**: 16–20.

290 Bonkovsky HL, Poh-Fitzpatrick M, Pimstone N, et al. Porphyria cutanea tarda, hepatitis C and *HFE* gene mutations in North America. *Hepatology* 1998; **27**: 1661–1669.

291 Bulaj ZJ, Phillips JD, Ajioka RS, et al. Hemochromatosis genes and other factors contributing to the pathogenesis of porphyria cutanea tarda. *Blood* 2000; **95**: 1565–1571.

292 Fargion S, Piperno A, Cappellini MD, et al. Hepatitis C virus and porphyria cutanea tarda: evidence of a strong association. *Hepatology* 1992; **16**: 1322–1326.

293 Herrero C, Vicente A, Bruguera M, et al. Is hepatitis C virus infection a trigger of porphyria cutanea tarda? *Lancet* 1993; **341**: 788–789.

294 DeCastro M, Sánchez J, Herrera JF, et al. Hepatitis C virus antibodies and liver disease in patients with porphyria cutanea tarda. *Hepatology* 1993; **17**: 551–557.

295 Bonkovsky H, Poh-Fitzpatrick M, Tattrie C, et al. Porphyria cutanea tarda and hepatitis C in the USA. *Hepatology* 1996; **24**: 486A.

296 Gisbert JP, García-Buey L, Pajares JM, et al. Prevalence of hepatitis C virus infection in porphyria cutanea tarda: systematic review and meta-analysis. *J Hepatol* 2003; **39**: 620–627.

297 Fargion S, Fracanzani AL. Prevalence of hepatitis C virus infection in porphyria cutanea tarda. *J Hepatol* 2003; **39**: 635–638.

298 Klatskin G, Bloomer JR. Birefringence of hepatic pigment deposits in erythropoietic protoporphyria. Specificity of polarization microscopy in the identification of hepatic protoporphyrin deposits. *Gastroenterology* 1974; **67**: 294–302.

299 Bloomer JR, Phillips MJ, Davidson DL, et al. Hepatic disease in erythropoietic protoporphyria. *Am J Med* 1975; **58**: 869–882.

300 Bonkovsky HL, Schned AR. Fatal liver failure in protoporphyria. Synergism between ethanol excess and the genetic defect. *Gastroenterology* 1986; **90**: 191–201.

301 Pérez V, Gorodisch S, Casavilla F, et al. Ultrastructure of human liver at the end of normal pregnancy. *Am J Obstet Gynecol* 1971; **110**: 428–431.

302 Hay JE. Liver disease in pregnancy. *Hepatology* 2008; **47**: 1067–1076.

303 Riely CA. Liver disease in the pregnant patient. *Am J Gastroenterol* 1999; **94**: 1728–1732.

304 Kroll D, Mazor M, Zirkin H, et al. Fibrolamellar carcinoma of the liver in pregnancy. A case report. *J Reprod Med* 1991; **36**: 823–827.

305 Schorr-Lesnick B, Lebovics E, Dworkin B, et al. Liver diseases unique to pregnancy. *Am J Gastroenterol* 1991; **86**: 659–670.

306 Samuels P, Cohen AW. Pregnancies complicated by liver disease and liver dysfunction. *Obstet Gynecol Clin North Am* 1992; **19**: 745–763.

307 Kaplan MM. Acute fatty liver of pregnancy. *N Engl J Med* 1985; **313**: 367–370.

308 Sibai BM. Imitators of severe preeclampsia. *Obstet Gynecol* 2007; **109**: 956–966.

309 Ibdah JA. Acute fatty liver of pregnancy: an update on pathogenesis and clinical implications. *World J Gastroenterol* 2006; **46**: 7397–7404.

310 Burroughs AK, Seong NH, Dojcinov DM, et al. Idiopathic acute fatty liver of pregnancy in 12 patients. *Q J Med* 1982; **51**: 481–497.

311 Rolfes DB, Ishak KG. Acute fatty liver of pregnancy: a clinicopathologic study of 35 cases. *Hepatology* 1985; **5**: 1149–1158.

312 Sherlock S. Acute fatty liver of pregnancy and the microvesicular fat diseases. *Gut* 1983; **24**: 265–269.

313 Riely CA. Acute fatty liver of pregnancy. *Semin Liver Dis* 1987; **7**: 47–54.

314 Schoeman MN, Batey RG, Wilcken B. Recurrent acute fatty liver of pregnancy associated with a fatty-acid oxidation defect in the offspring. *Gastroenterology* 1991; **100**: 544–548.

315 Rolfes DB, Ishak KG. Liver disease in toxemia of pregnancy. *Am J Gastroenterol* 1986; **81**: 1138–1144.

316 Rolfes DB, Ishak KG. Liver disease in pregnancy. [Review.] *Histopathology* 1986; **10**: 555–570.

317 Arias F, Mancilla-Jimenez R. Hepatic fibrinogen deposits in pre-eclampsia. Immunofluorescent evidence. *N Engl J Med* 1976; **295**: 578–582.

318 Cheung H, Hamzah H. Liver rupture in pregnancy: a typical case? *Singapore Med J* 1992; **33**: 89–91.

319 Schorr-Lesnick B, Dworkin B, Rosenthal WS. Hemolysis, elevated liver enzymes, and low platelets in pregnancy (HELLP syndrome). A case report and literature review. *Dig Dis Sci* 1991; **36**: 1649–1652.

320 Weinstein L. Syndrome of hemolysis, elevated liver enzymes, and low platelet count: a severe consequence of hypertension in pregnancy. *Am J Obstet Gynecol* 1982; **142**: 159–167.

321 Weinstein L. Preeclampsia/eclampsia with hemolysis, elevated liver enzymes, and thrombocytopenia. *Obstet Gynecol* 1985; **66**: 657–660.

322 Baca L, Gibbons RB. The HELLP syndrome: a serious complication of pregnancy with hemolysis, elevated levels of liver enzymes, and low platelet count. *Am J Med* 1988; **85**: 590–591.

323 Ibdah JA, Bennett MJ, Rinaldo P, et al. A fetal fatty-acid oxidation disorder as a cause of liver disease in pregnant women. *N Engl J Med* 1999; **340**: 1723–1731.

324 Adlercreutz H, Tenhunen R. Some aspects of the interaction between natural and synthetic female sex hormones and the liver. [Review.] *Am J Med* 1970; **49**: 630–648.

325 Vanjak D, Moreau R, Roche-Sicot J, et al. Intrahepatic cholestasis of pregnancy and acute fatty liver of pregnancy. An unusual but favorable association? *Gastroenterology* 1991; **100**: 1123–1125.

326 Dixon PH, Weerasekera N, Linton KJ, et al. Heterozygous *MDR3* missense mutation associated with intrahepatic cholestasis of pregnancy: evidence for a defect in protein trafficking. *Hum Mol Genet* 2000; **9**: 1209–1217.

327 Schneider G, Paus TC, Kullak-Ublick GA, et al. Linkage between a new splicing site mutation in the MDR3 alias ABCB4 gene and intrahepatic cholestasis of pregnancy. *Hepatology* 2007; **45**: 150–158.

328 Keitel V, Vogt C, Häussinger D, et al. Combined mutations of canalicular transporter proteins cause severe intrahepatic cholestasis of pregnancy. *Gastroenterology* 2006; **131**: 624–629.

329 Floreani A, Carderi I, Paternoster D, et al. Intrahepatic cholestasis of pregnancy: three novel MDR3 gene mutations. *Aliment Pharmacol Ther* 2006; **23**: 1649–1653.

General reading

Burt AD. Liver pathology associated with diseases of other organs or systems. In: Burt AD, Portmann BC, Ferrell LD, eds. Pathology of the Liver, 5th edn. Edinburgh: Churchill Livingstone/Elsevier, 2007: 881–932.

Ferrell LD. Hepatic granulomas: a morphologic approach to diagnosis. *Surg Pathol* 1990; **3**: 87–106.

Gaya DR, Thorburn KA, Oien KA, Morris AJ, Stanley AJ. Hepatic granulomas: a 10 year single center experience. *J Clin Pathol* 2003; **56**: 850–853.

Lucas SB. Other viral and infectious diseases and HIV-related liver disease. In: Burt AD, Portmann BC, Ferrell LD, eds.

Pathology of the Liver, 5th edn. Edinburgh: Churchill Livingstone/Elsevier, 2007: 443–492.

Sandor M, Weinstock JV, Wynn TA. Granulomas in schistosome and mycobacterial infections: a model of local immune responses. *Trends Immunol* 2003; **24**: 44–52.

Sartin JS, Walker RC. Granulomatous hepatitis: a retrospective review of 88 cases at the Mayo Clinic. *Mayo Clin Proc* 1991; **66**: 914–918.

CHAPTER

The Liver in Organ Transplantation

16

Introduction

The pathologist is often asked to examine liver biopsies obtained to evaluate liver dysfunction in transplant patients, including recipients of liver, renal and bone marrow grafts. For liver transplantation, liver biopsy remains the diagnostic 'gold standard' when jaundice and allograft dysfunction develop, since biochemical tests do not adequately discriminate between rejection and other conditions that may develop in the allograft.[1] Moreover, even when serum liver function tests are normal, histological abnormalities (including rejection lesions) may be present.[2,3] At the time of harvesting or engraftment, the donor liver may also require assessment, sometimes by frozen section, for lesions that may determine whether or not the graft can be used, and that can affect the postoperative course and appearance of subsequent post-transplantation biopsies. This chapter reviews the histopathological features of liver transplant rejection and other conditions affecting the allograft. The concluding sections discuss liver disease in recipients of renal and bone marrow transplants.

Liver transplantation

Assessment of the donor liver

The source of the donor allograft is an important consideration when evaluating liver biopsies obtained prior to transplantation, after graft revascularisation or at later times. Biopsies from potential living donors in apparent good health may disclose conditions such as steatohepatitis or primary biliary cirrhosis, which disqualifies their candidacy.[4] Living donor left or right lobe grafts, if small in relation to the recipient's size, may show cholestasis or congestion associated with ascites, prolonged coagulation parameters and impaired metabolic function immediately after transplantation (**small-for-size syndrome**[5]) due to problems in venous drainage[6] and portal hyperperfusion.[5] Postoperative portal tract biliary obstructive changes may also be present due to ischaemia or mechanical obstruction of the large bile ducts associated with this type of procedure.[7] Cadaveric livers are subject to preservation (ischaemia/reperfusion) injury[8] after harvesting and transport to the site of surgery, which in early baseline biopsies is evident as variable degrees of perivenular necrosis, liver-cell ballooning and/or apoptosis. The increased risk of postoperative biliary strictures and bile leaks with 'donation after cardiac death' grafts[9] should be kept in mind if cholestasis and features of biliary obstruction are seen in a post-trans-

©2010 Elsevier Ltd
DOI: 10.1016/B978-0-7020-3410-7.00022-8

plantation biopsy. If an allograft is used from a donor with known chronic hepatitis B or C ('extended donor criteria'), a baseline biopsy warrants careful attention to the grade and stage of the chronic hepatitis (**see Ch. 9**) for later comparison with subsequent biopsies. Allograft biopsies obtained soon after transplantation sometimes disclose an unsuspected condition in the donor such as α_1-antitrypsin deficiency, iron overload or amyloidosis.[10]

Frozen section of potential donor livers may be requested to exclude pre-existing disease. Pathologists providing frozen section coverage should be aware of three common reasons that frozen sections are requested: (1) *to determine whether steatosis is present*, and its degree; (2) *to exclude changes of chronic hepatitis* if the donor is known to be positive for antibodies to hepatitis B core antigen but negative for surface antigen (i.e. possible occult hepatitis B), or is positive for hepatitis C virus; and (3) *to evaluate a mass* found in the donor liver. Concern about a substantially **fatty liver** is based on the increased incidence of **primary graft dysfunction** or **non-function** when this is present.[11] The degree of macrovesicular (large droplet) fatty change should be categorised according to the percentage of parenchymal involvement as either absent, mild (<30%), moderate (30–60%) or marked (>60%).[12,13] Transplant surgeons have considered the last category unsuitable for use because of the high risk of primary dysfunction or non-function associated with severe steatosis.[11,13] Microvesicular (small droplet) fat is held not to be a contraindication, however,[14] but should also be graded and merits discussion with the transplant team if substantial. Diffuse portal mononuclear inflammatory cell infiltrates in donors with markers of hepatitis B or C viral infection support the presence of **chronic hepatitis**. The significance of this finding needs to be considered by the transplant team. With regard to **mass lesions** in the donor liver, demonstration of a malignant or metastatic tumour is an obvious contraindication to its use. However, the features of benign lesions such as focal nodular hyperplasia (**see Ch. 11**) are important to recognise since they are often encountered in this setting.

The liver allograft biopsy: general considerations

Needle liver biopsies are obtained as part of a liver transplantation protocol or because of clinical deterioration.[15] Discussion with the clinical team and careful review of pertinent radiographic, biochemical and microbiological findings are critical to biopsy interpretation and institution of appropriate therapy. Serial biopsies may be necessary to resolve difficult diagnostic problems.

There are many causes of allograft injury in addition to rejection (**Table 16.1**) and these should be considered in the context of the time elapsed since transplantation[16] (**Fig. 16.1**). For several weeks following transplantation, **functional cholestasis** may be present and must, if possible, be distinguished from the cholestasis of acute rejection, bile-duct obstruction, hepatitis, drug toxicity and sepsis. Bile is present within hepatocytes and canaliculi. This impairment of bile flow can be explained by exposure of the donor liver to cold ischaemia and reperfusion injury ('preservation injury') with resultant damage to liver-cell organelles.[17] Liver-cell death due to preservation injury actually shows features of both necrosis and apoptosis ('necrapoptosis').[18] Early postoperative cholestasis may also be due to a 'small-for-size' graft.[19] Cholestasis may be accompanied by **hepatocellular ballooning** in perivenular regions (**Fig. 16.2**) or in a diffuse distribution.[20,21] In the absence of frank perivenular necrosis, ballooning does not confer an unfavourable prognosis.[20] Hypoperfusion liver damage in the perioperative period may result in necrosis in periportal or perivenular regions and sometimes an irregular subcapsular band of infarction.[22] If the donor liver is fatty, rupture of hepatocytes affected by preservation injury may rarely cause sinusoidal engorgement by lipid vacuoles (**lipopeliosis**)[23] (**Fig. 16.3**).

In evaluating post-transplant biopsies, special attention should be paid to the portal tracts, the major sites of rejection lesions. The type of cellular infiltrate, the bile ducts, portal-vein branches and hepatic arterioles are examined to distinguish rejection from other conditions with portal tract pathology, particularly **bile-duct obstruction**, **recurrent** viral hepatitis, **drug toxicity** and immunosuppression-related **lymphoproliferative disease** (see Differential diagnosis in transplant biopsies). The perivenular region also requires inspection for possible preservation injury, cholestasis or inflammation, and for necroinflammation which may accompany portal tract lesions in more severe cases of acute rejection.[24] The lobular parenchyma shows few alterations in rejection apart from cholestasis and the occasional apoptotic bodies and scattered liver-cell mitoses which develop as the allograft equilibrates to the appropriate size for the recipient. As a result, in cases where confusion arises in the interpretation of portal changes, it is important to carefully evaluate the lobular parenchyma for evidence of intercurrent diseases such as viral or drug hepatitis. *The pathologist should always bear in mind that a given biopsy may show superimposed features attributable to several different post-transplantation complications.*

Graft rejection

The histopathological lesions of liver allograft rejection have been well characterised[25-29] and are classified as **humoral rejection, acute (cellular) rejection** and **chronic (ductopenic) rejection**, as recommended by an international working party which met in 1994.[24] Acute and chronic rejection are the most common forms seen in clinical practice.

Humoral rejection

Humoral rejection (antibody-mediated or hyperacute rejection) is rare after liver transplantation, developing in patients with pre-formed antibodies or subsequently formed antibodies to a donor liver that is incompatible with ABO blood groups. Microvascular damage evolves

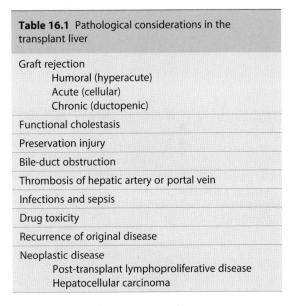

Table 16.1 Pathological considerations in the transplant liver

Graft rejection
Humoral (hyperacute)
Acute (cellular)
Chronic (ductopenic)
Functional cholestasis
Preservation injury
Bile-duct obstruction
Thrombosis of hepatic artery or portal vein
Infections and sepsis
Drug toxicity
Recurrence of original disease
Neoplastic disease
Post-transplant lymphoproliferative disease
Hepatocellular carcinoma

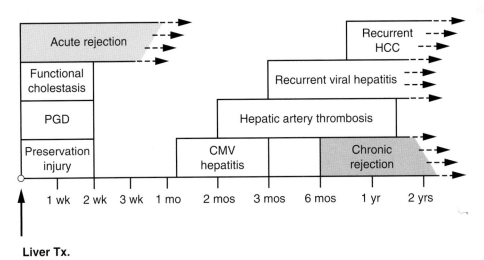

Liver Tx.

Figure 16.1 Timeline of pathologic lesions after liver transplantation.
Common post-transplantation problems are shown correlated with the approximate time frame in which they develop. Hatched arrows indicate the potential for the condition to develop at a later time. CMV, cytomegalovirus; HCC, hepatocellular carcinoma; PGD, primary graft dysfunction, Tx, transplantation.

**Figure 16.2
Liver-cell
ballooning after
transplantation.**
A liver biopsy
obtained in week 2
following transplant
shows ballooning of
hepatocytes in a
perivenular area.
Intracellular
cholestasis is visible.
(Needle biopsy, H&E.)

**Figure 16.3
Lipopeliosis.**
The enlarged empty
spaces in this
perivenular region
represent ruptured
and coalescent lipid
vacuoles within
sinusoids. This
developed due to
necrosis and rupture
of steatotic
hepatocytes
following allograft
preservation injury. A
Kupffer-cell foreign
body reaction
engulfing the lipid is
present (arrow).
(Needle biopsy, H&E.)

over the first few hours after transplantation, consisting of sinusoidal infiltrates of neutrophilic leucocytes, fibrin and red blood cells associated with focal haemorrhages. This progresses to portal and periportal oedema with coagulative and haemorrhagic necrosis over the next few days[30] (**Fig. 16.4**). Immunofluorescent studies show linear deposits of IgG or IgM, complement fractions C1q, C3 and C4 and fibrinogen in arterial walls.[24,31] The graft may remain stable in some patients for the first few days, however, possibly because of Kupffer-cell protection against the effects of circulating antibodies.[32] Graft

Figure 16.4 Humoral rejection after ABO-incompatible liver transplantation.
Mild residual portal tract oedema and focal periportal liver-cell necrosis (short arrows) remain present in this postoperative day 19 biopsy. Periportal ductular reaction with neutrophils (long arrows) has also developed. Mild lymphocytic infiltrates reflect a component of acute rejection. (Needle biopsy, H&E.) (Photomicrograph kindly provided by Dr Hironori Haga, Hokkaido University, Sapporo, Japan.)

failure within 2–4 weeks is associated with a progressive and marked rise in serum amino-transferase activity. The liver appears mottled and cyanotic at gross examination. Recipients of ABO-unmatched livers may also develop **graft-versus-host haemolysis**, associated with erythrophagocytosis and **Kupffer-cell siderosis**.[33]

Acute (cellular) rejection

Acute (cellular) rejection, the most common form of rejection, is a cell-mediated immune injury directed at bile-duct epithelium and the endothelium of portal-vein branches and terminal hepatic venules. This usually occurs within the first month to 6 weeks after transplantation,[34] but may be seen later if immunosuppression is lowered or discontinued. The characteristic histological **triad** of cellular rejection includes **portal inflammation, bile-duct damage** and **endotheliitis (endothelialitis)**. Endotheliitis is not present in all cases. The portal inflammatory lesion is typically heterogeneous, with lymphocytes predominating among plasma cells, neutrophils and, occasionally, large lymphoid cells, some in mitosis (**Fig. 16.5**). Eosinophils are often abundant (**Fig. 16.6**), which is a very helpful diagnostic sign that acute rejection is present.[35,36] Bile ducts are surrounded and infiltrated by immune cells and damage to their epithelium takes the form of variation in nuclear size, vacuolation of cytoplasm, regions of cell stratification or cell loss, and irregularity of duct outlines (**Figs 16.5–16.7**). Endotheliitis comprises attachment of lymphoid cells to the endothelium of portal-vein branches or

**Figure 16.5
Acute rejection.**
Heterogeneous portal inflammation consisting of lymphocytes, plasma cells and scattered neutrophils infiltrates the bile duct (between arrows) and the portal vein branch at top. (Needle biopsy, H&E.)

**Figure 16.6
Acute rejection.**
The portal tract infiltrate is rich in eosinophils. The portal-vein branch at bottom shows endotheliitis, with subendothelial lymphocytes and eosinophils. (Needle biopsy, H&E.)

terminal hepatic venules, variable degrees of endothelial damage, subendothelial inflammation (**Figs 16.5, 16.6**) and lifting-off of endothelial cells from the underlying vein wall (**Fig. 16.8**). Sinusoidal endotheliitis is occasionally also present. Mild focal endotheliitis is sometimes found in association with hypoperfusion damage in baseline biopsies, but extensive endotheliitis in the postoperative period is very characteristic of rejection.[25]

**Figure 16.7
Acute rejection.**
A damaged bile duct, cut twice in this portal tract, shows irregular epithelium with mild nuclear pleomorphism. Neutrophils are admixed with lymphocytes around and above the duct at left. The duct profile at right shows a mitotic figure (arrow). (Needle biopsy, H&E.) (Case kindly provided by Dr Jurgen Ludwig, Rochester, MN, USA.)

**Figure 16.8
Endotheliitis in acute rejection.**
An efferent vein shows lymphocytic infiltration of its wall. The endothelium is focally lifted off the underlying vein wall and partially destroyed. (Needle biopsy, H&E.)

Necrosis of perivenular hepatocytes, accompanied by endotheliitis of terminal hepatic venules and expansive portal inflammatory lesions involving the periportal parenchyma, is indicative of severe acute rejection.[37] **Central perivenulitis (central venulitis)** – characterised by endotheliitis of terminal venules, dropout and apoptosis of nearby hepatocytes (sometimes with focal sinusoidal congestion and dilatation) – often presages later

Table 16.2 Banff grading scheme for acute rejection*

Category	Criteria	Score
Portal inflammation	Mostly lymphocytic inflammation involving, but not noticeably expanding, a minority of the triads	1
	Expansion of most or all of the triads, by a mixed infiltrate containing lymphocytes with occasional blasts, neutrophils and eosinophils	2
	Marked expansion of most or all of the triads by a mixed infiltrate containing numerous blasts and eosinophils with inflammatory spillover into the periportal parenchyma	3
Bile-duct inflammation damage	A minority of the ducts are cuffed and infiltrated by inflammatory cells and show only mild reactive changes such as increased nucleus–cytoplasm ratio of the epithelial cells	1
	Most or all of the ducts infiltrated by inflammatory cells. More than an occasional duct shows degenerative changes such as nuclear pleomorphism, disordered polarity and cytoplasmic vacuolisation of the epithelium	2
	As above for 2, with most or all of the ducts showing degenerative changes or focal luminal disruption	3
Venous endothelial inflammation	Subendothelial lymphocytic infiltration involving some, but not the majority, of the portal and/or hepatic venules	1
	Subendothelial infiltration involving most or all of the portal and/or hepatic venules	2
	As above for 2, with moderate or severe perivenular inflammation that extends into the perivenular parenchyma and is associated with perivenular hepatocyte necrosis	3

Note: total score = sum of components. Criteria that can be used to score liver allograft biopsies with acute rejection are as defined in the World Gastroenterology Consensus Document.
*The Rejection Activity Index (RAI) is the sum of the scores for each of the three components of acute rejection. RAI ≥ 4 (mild), RAI ≥ 6 (moderate or severe).
Source: Reprinted with permission from International Panel.[37]

episodes of acute rejection and chronic ductopenic rejection.[38–40] Central perivenulitis is a common expression of rejection in paediatric allografts.[41] It is sometimes the chief manifestation of rejection, with few or no portal tract changes, as **isolated central perivenulitis**[42] in both paediatric and adult allografts, many months or longer after transplantation (see Late liver allograft dysfunction, below).

Descriptive and semi-quantitative **grading of acute rejection** can effectively be accomplished using the scoring system presented in the Banff international consensus document[37] (**Table 16.2**). Using the semi-quantitative approach of assigning a numerical score to each component of the acute rejection triad, a total **Rejection Activity Index (RAI)** can be conveyed in the biopsy report. Alternatively, a simpler global assessment of the biopsy as showing indeterminate, mild, moderate or severe changes of acute rejection can be used (**Table 16.3**). The choice of grading system, as with grading and staging for chronic hepatitis, should be made after discussion with clinicians.

Table 16.3 Descriptive terminology for acute rejection

Global assessment*	Criteria
Indeterminate	Portal inflammatory infiltrate that fails to meet the criteria for the diagnosis of acute rejection (see text)
Mild	Rejection infiltrate in a minority of the triads that is generally mild and confined within the portal spaces
Moderate	Rejection infiltrate, expanding most or all of the triads
Severe	As above for moderate, with spillover into periportal areas and moderate-to-severe perivenular inflammation that extends into the hepatic parenchyma and is associated with perivenular hepatocyte necrosis

Note: global assessment of rejection grade is made on a review of the biopsy and after the diagnosis of rejection has been established.
*Verbal description of mild, moderate or severe acute rejection could also be labelled as grades I, II and III, respectively.
Source: Reprinted with permission from International Panel.[37]

Chronic (ductopenic) rejection

Chronic (ductopenic) rejection ('vanishing bile-duct syndrome') is defined as obliterative vasculopathy and loss of bile ducts occurring 60 days or longer after transplantation.[24,43] The incidence of chronic rejection in liver transplant patients has declined to less than 5% in some series[44-46] as immunosuppression regimens have improved. In most cases, vasculopathy and ductopenia occur together, but in a minority they can be present independently.[47]

The diagnosis of chronic rejection can be problematic even for experienced hepatic pathologists,[48,49] particularly in the early stages.[24] Atrophy, nuclear pleomorphism and pyknosis of small ducts (bile-duct 'dystrophy') often precede frank ductopenia.[50] The presence of ductopenia is established when a formal count of small bile ducts and hepatic artery branches within portal tracts demonstrates loss of bile ducts from over 50% of portal tracts (**Fig. 16.9**). Progressive bile-duct loss results from a destructive cholangitis, which in most cases stems from bouts of acute rejection that are not controlled by immunosuppression. Cytokeratin immunostaining may help identify remnants of bile-duct epithelium.[28] Portal tract hepatic arterioles may also be lost.[43] Over time, portal inflammation becomes sparse and bile ducts disappear from the majority of portal tracts, usually without a ductular reaction[43] (**Fig. 16.9**). Episodes of acute rejection with increased inflammation and endotheliitis may develop superimposed on changes of chronic rejection. The pathology report in chronic rejection should therefore include consideration of the following points:[43] (1) whether acute rejection is present; (2) the degree of bile-duct loss in portal tracts; (3) the presence of perivenular necrosis or fibrosis; and (4) the degree of hepatic arteriole loss in relation to the total number of portal tracts.

The presence of obliterative vasculopathy (rejection arteriopathy) may be more difficult to demonstrate on needle biopsies, since the characteristic subintimal accumulations of foamy histiocytes and myointimal cells predominantly affect the large-calibre arteries of the liver hilum[47,51] (**Fig. 16.10**). However, foam-cell lesions can sometimes be demonstrated in medium-sized portal arterioles present in biopsies and occasionally in portal veins and sinusoids (**Fig. 16.11**). The presence of arteriopathy in most cases must be inferred when perivenular ischaemic necrosis and fibrosis are seen in liver biopsies obtained in the appropriate time frame of chronic rejection. Demonstration of perivenular necrosis in repeated biopsies indicates a poor prognosis.[52] Mismatch of recipient and

Figure 16.9 Chronic (ductopenic) rejection.
An hepatic artery branch (arrow) is present in the portal tract but the corresponding interlobular bile duct has disappeared as a result of rejection. A sparse lymphocytic infiltrate remains. (Explanted donor liver, H&E.) (Case kindly provided by Dr Jurgen Ludwig, Rochester, MN, USA.)

Figure 16.10 Rejection arteriopathy.
A hilar artery from a transplant liver removed because of rejection shows an accumulation of subintimal foam cells. (Explanted donor liver, H&E.) (Case kindly provided by Dr Jurgen Ludwig, Rochester, MN, USA.)

donor histocompatibility antigens, activation of the complement membrane attack complex and persistent cytomegalovirus infection in the allograft have been invoked in the pathogenesis of bile-duct loss and arteriopathy.[28,53–57]

Chronic rejection usually leads to irreversible graft failure, although some patients may recover.[28,58] The late stage characteristically shows marked cholestasis and bile-duct loss,

**Figure 16.11
Sinusoidal foam
cells in transplant
rejection.**
Months after
transplantation,
foam cells may
be deposited in
large-calibre arteries
and also within
hepatic sinusoids.
(Needle biopsy, H&E.)

portal and periportal fibrosis, perivenular fibrosis and variable numbers of bridging fibrous septa linking portal tracts or central veins to portal tracts. Cirrhosis develops after liver transplantation in only a minority of patients and is typically due to recurrent or acquired viral hepatitis, rather than chronic rejection[59] (see Recurrent disease).

Other causes of graft dysfunction

Infection

Cytomegalovirus (CMV) is a common pathogen in liver allografts, most cases of CMV hepatitis occurring 4–8 weeks after transplant.[60] Typical intranuclear and cytoplasmic CMV inclusions (**see Ch. 15**) can be found in hepatocytes, bile-duct epithelium (**see Fig. 15.5**) and endothelial cells. CMV infection should be suspected when small **microabscess**-like foci of necrosis with an infiltrate of neutrophils are present (**Fig. 16.12**). Smaller collections of parenchymal neutrophils ('**mini-microabscesses**') are occasionally seen in patients without CMV infection, apparently without adverse effects on the graft.[61] CMV infection may also lead to formation of epithelioid granulomas. Immunohistochemical staining for CMV antigens is a sensitive method of demonstrating occult infection.[62]

    Epstein–Barr virus infection should be considered if portal tracts and sinusoids contain a preponderance of atypical lymphocytes and immunoblasts.[63–65] The possibility that as yet unidentified hepatitis viruses may cause post-transplantation liver dysfunction has been considered.[66]

    Infection by **Gram-negative bacilli** may produce hepatocellular and canalicular cholestasis or, with sepsis, the more unusual picture of inspissated bile in periportal bile ductules ('bile ductular cholestasis') (**see Ch. 15 and Fig. 15.11**). Cholestasis due to infection and/or sepsis must be distinguished from that seen in bile-duct obstruction and rejection. Assessment of portal tract changes as well as results of microbiological studies are important in making these distinctions. Culture and special stains of liver biopsy specimens that show microabscesses or granulomas are the best means of documenting **bacterial, fungal or other infections.**[67]

**Figure 16.12
Cytomegalovirus
hepatitis.**
A microabscess-like
cluster of neutrophils
surrounds a
hepatocyte with a
smudged
intranuclear
inclusion. (Needle
biopsy, H&E.)

Thrombosis

Thrombosis of the hepatic artery[68,69] or portal vein[70] (the latter particularly in children) may develop within the first few weeks or months of transplantation, leading to infarction of the liver (**see Ch. 12**). Needle biopsy specimens may not be representative owing to the irregular distribution of infarcted liver parenchyma. Thrombosis, stricture or foam-cell arteriopathy of perihilar arteries may cause necrosis, stricture or cholangiectases of perihilar bile ducts due to impaired duct perfusion.[71] Liver biopsy in such cases may show features of biliary obstruction.[71]

Drug toxicity

The therapeutic regimen for immunosuppression in liver transplant patients includes several potentially hepatotoxic agents. **Azathioprine** hepatotoxicity has been reported primarily in renal transplant patients (see Renal transplantation, below). Elevated activities of serum aminotransferases with **sinusoidal congestion** and **perivenular necrosis** have been described in liver transplant patients treated with this drug,[72] and **veno-occlusive disease** elsewhere in the graft should be suspected, even if not demonstrated in the biopsy sample. There may also be **fibrosis of terminal hepatic venules**, particularly in patients with cellular rejection and endotheliitis.[73] **Ciclosporin** may cause **cholestasis**[74] by inhibition of ATP-dependent bile-salt transport.[75,76] Although a similar mechanism of cholestasis obtains for **FK 506**, hepatotoxicity is rare, probably due to the lower dose of FK 506 required for immunosuppression.[77,78]

Recurrent disease

Many of the diseases for which liver transplantation is performed have the potential to recur,[79] including viral hepatitis, malignant tumours, alcoholic and non-alcoholic steatohepatitis,[80-82] Budd–Chiari syndrome and variants of veno-occlusive disease,[83] autoimmune hepatitis, primary biliary cirrhosis and primary sclerosing cholangitis.[83a] The diagnosis of recurrent disease on liver biopsy can be controversial because some of these pre-transplant disorders have histopathological features which overlap with those seen in rejection or post-transplantation biliary obstruction.

Although the incidence of **recurrent viral hepatitis** in patients transplanted for severe liver disease due to hepatitis B, C and D varies at different transplantation centres, without prophylactic therapy it is an expected outcome in most cases. There are varied histopathological expressions of **recurrent hepatitis B**, including acute hepatitis, chronic hepatitis, cirrhosis, a carrier state with minimal histological disease, and fibrosing cholestatic hepatitis[84,85] (see below). Recurrent hepatitis B may evolve from chronic hepatitis to cirrhosis within a year after transplantation.[86] Hepatitis B and D (delta) antigens can be demonstrated by immunohistochemistry in allografts as early as 1–3 weeks after transplantation.[86] For patients with **co-infection by hepatitis B and hepatitis D** in the native liver, recurrence may follow a variable course. In some patients, delta virus recurs without demonstrable hepatitis B virus (HBV) replication (absence of HBV core antigen on immunohistochemistry) or histological evidence of hepatitis.[87] Once HBV replication recurs and core antigen is present in the allograft, chronic hepatitis may then be seen on biopsy.[88] A minority of patients with recurrent hepatitis B infection may show a **fibrosing cholestatic hepatitis** with large numbers of ground-glass inclusions, 'cytopathic' liver-cell ballooning, cholestasis and a network of periportal fibrosis[85,89–93] (**Figs 16.13, 16.14**). This pattern of disease recurrence is associated with a high rate of graft failure.

Recurrent hepatitis C after transplantation results in a characteristic sequence of pathological changes.[94] Within the first several months, increased numbers of apoptotic bodies appear, an important histological marker of recurrence[95] (**Fig. 16.15**). Their number and close proximity within the lobule far exceed that seen in acute rejection alone. Steatosis is often present and variable in degree, sometimes severe when genotype 3 infection recurs.[96] Increased lobular necroinflammation and liver-cell ballooning[97] follow and by 6 months to 1 year the portal lesion of recurrent chronic hepatitis becomes established. This is manifested by the presence of lymphoid aggregates or follicles (sometimes an isolated

Figure 16.13 Fibrosing cholestatic hepatitis.
Hepatocytes are swollen and many contain ground-glass inclusions. A bile thrombus is seen to the right of centre. (Explanted donor liver, H&E.) (Case kindly provided by Dr Bernard Portmann, London, UK.)

Figure 16.14 Fibrosing cholestatic hepatitis. Trichrome stain from the case depicted in **Fig. 17.12** shows an intricate network of fibrosis emanating from the portal tract (centre). (Explanted donor liver, trichrome.) (Case kindly provided by Dr Bernard Portmann, London, UK.)

Figure 16.15 Early recurrent hepatitis C after transplantation. The numerous acidophilic (apoptotic) bodies shown here were the earliest histopathological evidence of recurrent hepatitis C in this case. (Needle biopsy, H&E.)

finding in the first few months after transplant), lymphocytic or lymphoplasmacytic inflammation and variable degrees of interface hepatitis. The disease is frequently mild.[98,99] The inflammatory cell infiltrates are often polarised towards the edges of the portal tracts and periportal regions, in contrast to acute rejection where the infiltrates are more centrally localised around the bile ducts and portal-vein branches. A ductular reaction is sometimes

**Figure 16.16
Cholestatic
recurrent chronic
hepatitis C.**
The portal tract
shows mild chronic
inflammation and
fibrosis, with a
prominent periportal
ductular reaction
(arrowheads). *Inset*:
Hepatocytes show
considerable
ballooning,
cytopathic damage
and cholestasis.
(Needle biopsy, H&E.)

present in combination with the features of chronic hepatitis (**Fig. 16.16**) or may be the predominant portal lesion in the more serious **cholestatic recurrent hepatitis C** which resembles fibrosing cholestatic hepatitis B.[100] These cases often show pronounced cholestasis and liver-cell ballooning (**Fig. 16.16**, Inset), features attributed to direct cytopathic effects of the virus. Serum bilirubin and HCV titres are usually high.[101,102] The degree of fibrosis is more variable than in fibrosing cholestatic hepatitis B. Other forms of severe recurrent hepatitis C show confluent necrosis, liver-cell ballooning, bridging fibrosis and cirrhosis.[101,102] Occasional cases of recurrent chronic hepatitis C show numerous **portal and periportal plasma cells** resembling autoimmune hepatitis, often with accompanying lymphoplasmacytic central perivenulitis[103] (**Fig. 16.17**). This picture sometimes follows a reduction in immunosuppression or introduction of interferon therapy[104] and may be a variant form of *alloimmune* rejection[105] with a worse outcome.[105a] Such complex cases warrant discussion with the clinical team. Distinction of recurrent chronic hepatitis C from acute rejection is often a considerable diagnostic problem,[94,106] especially compounded when evidence of both processes is present in a given biopsy. Many histological parameters must therefore be evaluated (**Table 16.4**). The major pathological process should be emphasised in the pathology report whenever possible.

Following transplantation for **primary biliary cirrhosis** (PBC), serum anti-mitochondrial antibodies may persist or recur, liver function tests (particularly serum alkaline phosphatase activity) may worsen, and liver biopsy may demonstrate recurrent damage to bile ducts.[107] Florid bile-duct lesions and adjacent epithelioid granulomas are the most useful histological signs of recurrent disease. Ductular reaction and progressive copper deposition are other helpful features. There may also be portal lymphoid aggregates and mononuclear inflammation as well as ductopenia, but these can also be seen in HCV infection and rejection. If there is uncertainty, HCV infection should be serologically excluded. Recurrent PBC can progress to cirrhosis within several years.[108] **Autoimmune hepatitis** (AIH) with high levels of serum globulins and typical liver biopsy features has also been reported in patients transplanted for PBC.[109] AIH with high biochemical and histological activity pre-transplantation may presage recurrence in the allograft.[109a]

Figure 16.17 Recurrent chronic hepatitis C with plasma-cell-rich inflammation.
A: The portal tract shows an expansive chronic inflammatory infiltrate rich in plasma cells with considerable interface hepatitis (long arrows). The bile duct (BD) and portal-vein branch (V) show no significant changes of rejection. This patient's immunosuppression had recently been reduced. The field at upper right (short arrow) is shown at higher magnification in Panel B. **B:** The interface hepatitis features clusters of plasma cells and eosinophils. Such changes may represent a form of alloimmune rejection.

Table 16.4 Comparative features of acute rejection versus recurrent chronic hepatitis C

Feature	Acute rejection	Recurrent hepatitis C
Lobular necroinflammation	No	Yes
Apoptotic bodies	Few	Many
Cholestasis	Mild	May be marked
Interface hepatitis	No (unless severe)	Often
Lymphoid aggregates/follicles	No	Yes
Portal inflammation	Heterogeneous	Lymphocytes, plasma cells
Fat	No (except with corticosteroid therapy)	Yes (genotype 3 especially)
Ductular reaction	No	Variable (common in cholestatic type)
Central venulitis	Often, diffuse	Uncommon, focal
Bile-duct damage	Yes, diffuse	Focal or none
Portal/periportal fibrosis	No	Often

Recurrence of **primary sclerosing cholangitis** (PSC) after transplantation is reported[110] but has been controversial, because the radiological and histopathological features of PSC resemble those seen in biliary complications of the transplant procedure, such as biliary stricture due to hepatic artery thrombosis and bile-duct or choledochojejunostomy-anastomotic obstruction.[79] Biopsy features of cholestasis and portal obstructive changes therefore require cautious interpretation in the context of radiological and other data. Fibro-obliterative lesions (**see Ch. 5**) are more specific for recurrence.[110] Perihilar xantho-granulomatous cholangitis in the explanted PSC liver (**see Ch. 5**) has been associated with increased post-transplantation morbidity and mortality.

Studies of patients transplanted for AIH are at variance with regard to the incidence of recurrence.[79] An abrupt rise in serum aminotransferases, detectable autoantibodies, hyper-gammaglobulinaemia and portal inflammation with interface hepatitis on biopsy are consistent with recurrent disease. Lobular hepatitis may be the first sign of recurrence.[66] In children, recurrent AIH may be an aggressive disease resulting in cirrhosis and re-transplantation.[111]

Recurrence of **alcoholic** or **non-alcoholic fatty liver disease** may be manifested by steatosis and steatohepatitis after transplantation.[112] Corticosteroid immunosuppression or weight gain with recurrent or new metabolic syndrome are additional causes of post-transplant fatty liver and steatohepatitis.[113] Steatosis, steatohepatitis and cirrhosis also are seen after transplantation for progressive familial intrahepatic cholestasis type 1.[114]

De novo autoimmune hepatitis

Children and adults who have undergone liver transplantation for conditions other than AIH infrequently develop *de novo* AIH, with elevated serum immunoglobulin levels and a variety of autoantibodies.[115] Lymphoplasmacytic interface hepatitis is the major histo-logical criterion for this condition. The centrilobular necroinflammatory lesion of AIH (**see Fig. 9.16**) may also be present. A related, severe form of post-transplant liver disease, **graft dysfunction mimicking autoimmune hepatitis,**[116] can result in graft loss.

**Figure 16.18
Post-transplant
lymphoprolifera-
tive disease.**
The portal tract is
infiltrated and
overrun by a B-cell
proliferation. *Inset*:
The cytological
features are
consistent with an
immunoblastic
lymphoma but
immunotyping
and other studies
are necessary
for definitive
characterisation.
(Needle biopsy, H&E.)

Neoplastic disease

Post-transplant lymphoproliferative disease (PTLD), chiefly B-cell lymphoma in lymph nodes and extranodal sites, is a complication of immunosuppression in patients with organ transplants. Special studies are important in determining whether the PTLD is polymorphic or monomorphic according to the current World Health Organization classification.[117] B-cell lymphoma in the liver has been reported as early as 2 months after liver transplantation[118] but usually occurs 1 year or more after adult liver transplantation and within a year in children.[117] Lymphoma usually originates in recipient lymphoid tissue, but rarely it may be derived from donor lymphoid tissue present in the allograft.[119] Hepatic involvement consists of diffuse lymphoma nodules or portal tract infiltration by lymphoma cells (**Fig. 16.18**). Biopsy demonstration of Epstein–Barr virus, which is involved in the pathogenesis of most cases of PTLD,[117] is helpful in distinguishing this from rejection.[120] *De novo*[121,122] or recurrent[123] **hepatocellular carcinoma** has also developed in patients transplanted for chronic hepatitis B and C, even after viral clearance.[123a]

Late liver allograft dysfunction

Most transplant recipients with abnormal liver function tests or symptoms at 1 year or later after transplantation show biopsy changes related to recurrent disease or biliary stricture.[124] However, as with earlier biopsies, several pathological processes may be evident, and helpful histological guidelines for sorting these out have been provided by the Banff Working Group.[124] Examination for changes of acute or chronic rejection is always important. Particular attention should be paid to perivenular regions since certain cases of ongoing or late acute rejection may be confined to these areas as **isolated central perivenulitis** (ICP)[42,125,126] (**Fig. 16.19**). The changes are similar to those of central perivenulitis earlier after transplantation, but there may also be perivenular fibrosis and possible evolution to ductopenic rejection. The degree of terminal venule involvement and associated perivenular hepatocyte dropout and necrosis in ICP should be specifically described in the diagnosis.[124]

Figure 16.19 Isolated central perivenulitis.
The rejection lesion in this 1-year post-transplant biopsy chiefly involves terminal venules (V) where lymphocytic infiltrates, congestion and perivenular fibrosis are seen. The portal tract at upper right is relatively spared, with only sparse lymphocytes and no bile-duct or portal-vein damage. (Needle biopsy, H&E.) *Inset*: Connective tissue stain highlights the collagenous scar surrounding the venule. (Trichrome stain.)

Late biopsies sometimes show non-specific portal or lobular lymphocytic infiltrates of uncertain aetiology in the absence of more diagnostic changes of rejection. Unexplained periportal fibrosis in paediatric allograft biopsies several years after transplant has also been reported.[3] A small number of late paediatric and adult allograft biopsies show histological changes of chronic hepatitis or cirrhosis that are unexplained by chronic hepatitis B or C or AIH. These instances of **'idiopathic chronic hepatitis'** may represent a variant form of chronic rejection.[127] Reports suggesting hepatitis E virus as an aetiological factor[128,129] require further validation.

Differential diagnosis in transplant biopsies

Most problems in biopsy interpretation after liver transplantation arise in distinguishing rejection from other conditions (**Table 16.5**). It should be kept in mind that rejection and other allograft disorders can coexist. Difficult pathological problems are usually resolved by discussion with clinicians, assessment of viral serologies and microbial culture results, and review of drug therapy. When necessary, patency of vascular or biliary anastomoses may need to be radiologically demonstrated.

While **endotheliitis** may be seen in several forms of liver disease,[130] when it is found in combination with bile-duct damage and a mixed portal inflammatory infiltrate the diagnosis of acute rejection is usually clear. Endotheliitis involving central veins (**central venulitis**) sometimes presents diagnostic difficulties.[41] Regular involvement of most central

Table 16.5 Differential diagnostic features in transplant biopsies

Histological feature	Rejection	Condition		Biliary obstruction	Ischaemia
		Recurrent HBC	Recurrent HCV		
Cholestasis	+/−	Unusual (except in fibrosing cholestatic hepatitis)	Unusual	Yes	No
Portal inflammation					
Mixed (L,P,N,E)*	Yes	+/−	+/−	No	No
Lymphocytes, plasma cells	+/−	Yes	Yes	No	No
Neutrophils	+/−	No	No	Yes	No
Bile-duct damage	Yes	Unusual	Yes	No	No
Endotheliitis	Yes	Unusual	Unusual	No	Occasional
Zone 3 necrosis	Yes, if chronic	No	No	No	Yes
Sinusoidal inflammation	No	+/−	++	No	No
Apoptotic bodies	+/−	+	+++	No	No

+/− indicates a feature which is not characteristic, but which may sometimes be present.
*Mixed portal inflammation includes lymphocytes (L), plasma cells (P), neutrophils (N) and eosinophils (E).

veins in a biopsy specimen favours rejection or the less common development of *de novo* AIH. Central venulitis due to viral and drug hepatitis is more irregular in distribution. **Bile-duct damage** represents a more difficult histological problem, because it is a feature seen in rejection, chronic hepatitis C and PBC. Portal tract lymphoid aggregates, numerous apoptotic bodies, interface hepatitis and prominent sinusoidal inflammation support the diagnosis of chronic hepatitis C. As noted earlier, the presence of a granulomatous, destructive cholangitis in a hepatitis C-seronegative patient transplanted for PBC is important evidence of recurrent PBC.

Neutrophils may be seen in the vicinity of damaged bile ducts in rejection (**Fig. 16.5**) and should not be mistaken for evidence of biliary obstruction. Obstruction can usually be excluded if portal tract oedema and ductular reaction are absent. **Eosinophils** are often prominent in rejection but can be seen in fewer numbers in recurrent viral or autoimmune hepatitis. Subendothelial eosinophils in portal-vein branches favours rejection. Drug hepatitis as a cause of eosinophil infiltrates may need consideration when there is antibiotic prophylaxis with sulfa agents such as trimethoprim–sulphamethoxazole, but the parenchymal changes of acute hepatitis usually help to distinguish this from rejection. **Plasma cells** in small numbers are often present in acute rejection infiltrates, but are also seen admixed with lymphocytes as periportal interface hepatitis in recurrent diseases such as chronic hepatitis B or C or AIH. Interface hepatitis with large numbers of plasma cells in clusters in biopsies from transplant recipients without such antecedent native liver diseases suggests possible *de novo* AIH which should be further substantiated by the presence of serum autoantibodies and elevated γ-globulin level. Post-transplant recurrent chronic hepatitis C with plasma-cell infiltrates was discussed earlier.

Cholestasis may pose significant diagnostic problems because of several potential causes,[19] including biliary obstruction, rejection and sepsis. In biopsies obtained early (1–2 weeks) after transplantation, cholestasis is usually functional in nature. Small-for-size living donor grafts may also develop cholestasis. Cholestasis accompanied by portal oedema and a ductular reaction should prompt an assessment of the biliary anastomosis. The distinctive pattern of 'bile ductular cholestasis' is usually associated with sepsis.

Steatosis of large-droplet type in post-transplant biopsies may be due to several factors, including corticosteroid immunosuppression and recurrent hepatitis C virus infection. Genotype 3 re-infection particularly may result in severe fatty change.[96] Considerable fat also develops in allografts of children transplanted for progressive familial intrahepatic cholestasis type 1.[131]

Hepatitis B virus-negative recipients of liver and other transplants occasionally develop **ground-glass-like hepatocellular inclusions** that are periodic acid–Schiff-positive and represent an abnormal form of glycogen.[132–134] These should be distinguished from other types of ground-glass inclusions.[135]

Renal transplantation

Patients who have undergone renal transplantation are exposed to many viruses capable of causing acute or chronic hepatitis, particularly hepatitis B[136] and hepatitis C.[137] Steatosis, chronic hepatitis and cirrhosis are often found on biopsy.[138] Fibrosing cholestatic hepatitis is infrequently seen in recipients with chronic hepatitis C.[139] There may be lesions related to administration of potentially hepatotoxic drugs such as azathioprine, which may cause cholestasis, veno-occlusive disease, nodular regenerative hyperplasia and other lesions.[72,140–142] Cirrhosis develops in a small proportion of patients. Incrimination of a single aetiological agent is often difficult. Transfusions may cause substantial siderosis involving both hepatocytes and macrophages.[143,144] Vascular lesions following renal transplantation include narrowing or occlusion of efferent veins,[145] peliosis hepatis[146] and non-cirrhotic portal hypertension.[147] Portal hypertension associated with dilatation of sinusoids in acinar zones 2 and 3, with eventual development of fibrosis or cirrhosis, has also been reported.[148]

Patients who have been treated by **haemodialysis** may have birefringent material, probably derived from silicone tubing, in portal tracts. In some instances this material gives rise to a giant-cell or granulomatous reaction.[149–151] Haemodialysis patients often have Kupffer-cell siderosis.

Bone marrow transplantation

Graft recipients are liable to liver damage from graft-versus-host disease, chemotherapy-related sinusoidal obstruction syndrome/veno-occlusive disease, infection and idiosyncratic drug jaundice. Siderosis is often present because of prior transfusions. **Graft-versus-host disease** (GVHD) involving the liver has varying histological features depending on the stage of evolution.[152–154] The most characteristic features of acute (less than 90 days after transplant) GVHD are **bile-duct damage** and **cholestasis**.[152,153] The ducts often appear attenuated, tapering and stretched lengthwise. The duct epithelium is irregular, with vacuolated or acidophilic cytoplasm, nuclear pleomorphism and multilayering, and increased nucleus–cytoplasm ratio[152,155] (**Fig. 16.20**). Lymphocytes infiltrate the portal tracts and duct epithelium, but are sparse. In early GVHD (less than 35 days), duct changes are less apparent and numerous parenchymal acidophilic bodies may be present.[152] Endotheliitis is uncommon in comparison with acute liver allograft rejection. In **chronic GVHD** (after 90 days) there is progressive bile-duct dystrophy and senescence, ductopenia and portal fibrosis.[156] The clinical and radiological picture may mimic intrahepatic primary sclerosing cholangitis.[157] Rarely, there are parenchymal changes of an acute hepatitis.[158] Cirrhosis of biliary type may finally develop.[159] Chemotherapy for leukaemia/lymphoma may damage sinusoidal endothelium leading to **sinusoidal obstruction syndrome/veno-occlusive**

Figure 16.20 Graft-versus-host disease.
The bile-duct epithelium shows dyspolarity and attenuation. A small apoptotic nuclear fragment is seen at top (arrowhead) near an intracellular degenerative vacuole. The surrounding lymphocytic infiltrate is relatively mild. (Needle biopsy, H&E.)

Figure 16.21 Sinusoidal obstruction syndrome.
A: There is marked congestion and several venules and nearby sinusoids contain plugs of young fibrous tissue (arrows). The terminal venule at centre is injured. The injury was attributed to recent busulphan conditioning chemotherapy prior to hematopoietic stem cell transplantation for leukaemia.

disease[160] (also discussed in **Ch. 12**). Such cases show variable perivenular or more diffuse sinusoidal congestion with disruption and effacement of endothelium, intravasation of erythrocytes into the space of Disse and patchy fibrosis of sinusoids and terminal venules[161] (**Fig. 16.21**). Eosinophilic cytoplasmic inclusions in hepatocytes of patients dying after bone marrow transplantation have been described.[162]

Figure 16.21, cont'd

B: The endothelium of this terminal venule is partially denuded and detached (long arrow) with extrusion of hepatocytes into the vessel lumen (short arrows). (Needle biopsy, H&E.)

References

1 Henley KS, Lucey MR, Appelman HD, et al. Biochemical and histopathological correlation in liver transplant: the first 180 days. *Hepatology* 1992; **16**: 688–693.

2 Abraham SC, Poterucha JJ, Rosen CB, et al. Histologic abnormalities are common in protocol liver allograft biopsies from patients with normal liver function tests. *Am J Surg Pathol* 2008; **32**: 965–973.

3 Ekong UD, Melin-ALdana H, Seshadri R, et al. Graft histology characteristics in long-term survivors of pediatric liver transplantation. *Liver Transplant* 2008; **14**: 1582–1587.

4 Minervini MI, Ruppert K, Fontes P, et al. Liver biopsy findings from healthy potential living liver donors: reasons for disqualification, silent diseases and correlation with liver injury tests. *J Hepatol* 2009; **50**: 501–510.

5 Demetris AJ, Kelly DM, Eghtesad B, et al. Pathophysiologic observations and histopathologic recognition of the portal hyperperfusion or small-for-size syndrome. *Am J Surg Pathol* 2006; **30**: 986–993.

6 Kasahara M, Takada Y, Fujimoto Y, et al. Impact of right lobe with middle hepatic vein graft in living-donor liver transplantation. *Am J Transplant* 2005; **5**: 1339–1346.

7 Ayata G, Pomfret E, Pomposelli JJ, et al. Adult-to-adult live donor liver transplantation: a short-term clinicopathologic study. *Hum Pathol* 2001; **32**: 814–822.

8 Gaffey MJ, Boyd JC, Traweek ST, et al. Predictive value of intraoperative biopsies and liver function tests for preservation injury in orthotopic liver transplantation. *Hepatology* 1997; **25**: 184–189.

9 de Vera ME, Lopez-Solis R, Dvorchik I, et al. Liver transplantation using donation after cardiac death donors: long-term follow-up from a single center. *Am J Transplant* 2009; **9**: 773–781.

10 Pungpapong S, Krishna M, Abraham SC, et al. Clinicopathologic findings and outcomes of liver transplantation using grafts from donors with unrecognized and unusual diseases. *Liver Transplant* 2006; **12**: 310–315.

11 Verran D, Kusyk T, Painter D, et al. Clinical experience gained from the use of 120 steatotic donor livers for orthotopic liver transplantation. *Liver Transplant* 2003; **9**: 500–505.

12 Bzeizi KI, Jalan R, Plevris JN, et al. Primary graft dysfunction after liver transplantation: from pathogenesis to prevention. *Liver Transplant Surg* 1997; **3**: 137–148.

13 Trevisani F, Colantoni A, Caraceni P, et al. The use of donor fatty liver for liver transplantation: a challenge or a quagmire? *J Hepatol* 1996; **24**: 114–121.

14 Fishbein TM, Fiel MI, Emre S, et al. Use of livers with microvesicular fat safely expands the donor pool. *Transplantation* 1997; **64**: 248–251.

15 Eggink HF, Hofstee N, Gips CH, et al. Histopathology of serial graft biopsies from liver transplant recipients. *Am J Pathol* 1984; **114**: 18–31.

16. Ludwig J, Lefkowitch JH. Histopathology of the liver following transplantation. In: Maddrey WC, Schiff ER, Sorrel MF, eds. Transplantation of the Liver, 3rd edn. Philadelphia: Lippincott Williams & Wilkins, 2001; Ch. 15: 229–250.

17 Williams JW, Vera S, Peters TG, et al. Cholestatic jaundice after hepatic transplantation. A nonimmunologically mediated event. *Am J Surg* 1986; **151**: 65–70.

18 Jaeschke H, LeMasters JJ. Apoptosis versus oncotic necrosis in hepatic ischemia/reperfusion injury. *Gastroenterology* 2003; **125**: 1246–1257.

19 Ben-Ari Z, Pappo O, Mor E. Intrahepatic cholestasis after liver transplantation. *Liver Transplant* 2003; **9**: 1005–1018.

20 Ng IOL, Burroughs AK, Rolles K, et al. Hepatocellular ballooning after liver transplantation: a light and electronmicroscopic study with clinicopathological correlation. *Histopathology* 1991; **18**: 323–330.

21 Goldstein NS, Hart J, Lewin KJ. Diffuse hepatocyte ballooning in liver biopsies from orthotopic liver transplant patients. *Histopathology* 1991; **18**: 331–338.

22 Russo PA, Yunis EJ. Subcapsular hepatic necrosis in orthotopic liver allografts. *Hepatology* 1986; **6**: 708–713.

23 Cha I, Bass N, Ferrell LD. Lipopeliosis. An immunohistochemical and clinicopathologic study of five cases. *Am J Surg Pathol* 1994; **18**: 789–795.

24 International Working Party. Terminology for hepatic allograft rejection. *Hepatology* 1995; **22**: 648–654.

25 Snover DC, Sibley RK, Freese DK, et al. Orthotopic liver transplantation: a pathological study of 63 serial liver biopsies from 17 patients with special reference to the diagnostic features and natural history of rejection. *Hepatology* 1984; **4**: 1212–1222.

26 Demetris AJ, Lasky S, Van Thiel DH, et al. Pathology of hepatic transplantation: a review of 62 adult allograft recipients immunosuppressed with a cyclosporine/steroid regimen. *Am J Pathol* 1985; **118**: 151–161.

27 Hubscher SG. Histological findings in liver allograft rejection – new insights into the pathogenesis of hepatocellular damage in liver allografts. *Histopathology* 1991; **18**: 377–383.

28 Freese DK, Snover DC, Sharp HL, et al. Chronic rejection after liver transplantation: a study of clinical, histopathological and immunological features. *Hepatology* 1991; **13**: 882–891.

29 Wiesner RH, Ludwig J, Krom RAF, et al. Hepatic allograft rejection: new developments in terminology, diagnosis, prevention, and treatment. *Mayo Clin Proc* 1993; **68**: 69–79.

30 Haga H, Egawa H, Shirase T, et al. Periportal edema and necrosis as diagnostic histological features of early humoral rejection in ABO-incompatible liver transplantation. *Liver Transplant* 2004; **10**: 16–27.

31 Demetris AJ, Jaffe R, Tzakis A, et al. Antibody-mediated rejection of human orthotopic liver allografts. A study of liver transplantation across ABO blood group barriers. *Am J Pathol* 1988; **132**: 489–502.

32 Wardle EN. Kupffer cells and their function. *Liver* 1987; **7**: 63–75.

33 Clavien P-A, Camargo CA, Cameron R, et al. Kupffer cell erythrophagocytosis and graft-versus-host hemolysis in liver transplantation. *Gastroenterology* 1996; **110**: 1891–1896.

34 Wiesner RH, Demetris AJ, Belle SH, et al. Acute hepatic allograft rejection: incidence, risk factors and impact on outcome. *Hepatology* 1998; **28**: 638–645.

35 DeGroen PC, Kephart GM, Gleich GJ, et al. The eosinophil as an effector cell of the immune response during hepatic allograft rejection. *Hepatology* 1994; **20**: 654–662.

36 Nagral A, Ben-Ari Z, Dhillon AP, et al. Eosinophils in acute cellular rejection in liver allografts. *Liver Transplant Surg* 1998; **4**: 355–362.

37 International Panel. Banff schema for grading liver allograft rejection: an international consensus document. *Hepatology* 1997; **25**: 658–663.

38 Khettry U, Backer A, Ayata G, et al. Centrilobular histopathologic changes in liver transplant biopsies. *Hum Pathol* 2002; **33**: 270–276.

39 Lovell MO, Speeg KV, Halff GA, et al. Acute hepatic allograft rejection: a comparison of patients with and without centrilobular alterations during first rejection episode. *Liver Transplant* 2004; **10**: 369–373.

40 Sundaram SS, Melin-ALdana H, Neighbors K, et al. Histologic characteristics of late cellular rejection, significance of centrilobular injury, and long-term outcome in pediatric liver transplant patients. *Liver Transplant* 2006; **12**: 58–64.

41 Demetris AJ. Central venulitis in liver allografts: considerations of differential diagnosis. *Hepatology* 2001; **33**: 1329–1330.

42 Hübscher SG. Central perivenulitis: a common and potentially important finding in late posttransplant liver biopsies. *Liver Transplant* 2008; **14**: 596–600.

43 International Panel. Update of the international Banff schema for liver allograft rejection: working recommendations for the histopathologic staging and reporting of chronic rejection. *Hepatology* 2000; **31**: 792–799.

44 Weisner RH, Batts KP, Krom RAF. Evolving concepts in the diagnosis, pathogenesis and treatment of chronic hepatic allograft rejection. *Liver Transplant Surg* 1999; **5**: 388–400.

45 Wiesner RH, Demetris AJ, Seaberg EC. Chronic hepatic allograft rejection: defining clinical risk factors and assessing impact on graft outcome. *Hepatology* 1998; **28**: 314A.

46 Ludwig J, Hashimoto E, Porayko MK, et al. Failed allografts and causes of death after orthotopic liver transplantation from 1985 to 1995: decreasing prevalence of irreversible hepatic allograft rejection. *Liver Transplant Surg* 1996; **2**: 185–191.

47 McCaughan GW, Bishop GA. Atherosclerosis of the liver allograft. *J Hepatol* 1997; **27**: 592–598.

48 Demetris AJ, Belle SH, Hart J, et al. Intraobserver and interobserver variation in the histopathological assessment of liver allograft rejection. *Hepatology* 1991; **14**: 751–755.

49 Thung SN, Gerber MA. Histological features of liver allograft rejection: do you see what I see? *Hepatology* 1991; **14**: 949–951.

50 Sebagh M, Blakolmer K, Falissard B, et al. Accuracy of bile duct changes for the diagnosis of chronic liver allograft rejection: reliability of the 1999 Banff schema. *Hepatology* 2002; **35**: 117–125.

51 Liu G, Butany J, Wanless IR, et al. The vascular pathology of human hepatic allografts. *Hum Pathol* 1993; **24**: 182–188.

52 Ludwig J, Gross JB, Perkins JD, et al. Persistent centrilobular necroses in hepatic allografts. *Hum Pathol* 1990; **21**: 656–661.

53 Arnold JC, Portmann BC, O'Grady JG, et al. Cytomegalovirus infection persists in the liver graft in the vanishing bile duct syndrome. *Hepatology* 1992; **16**: 285–292.

54 Donaldson PT, Alexander GJM, O'Grady J, et al. Evidence for an immune response to HLA Class I antigens in the vanishing-bile duct syndrome after liver transplantation. *Lancet* 1987; **1**: 945–948.

55 O'Grady JG, Alexander GJM, Sutherland S, et al. Cytomegalovirus infection and donor/recipient HLA antigens: interdependent co-factors in pathogenesis of vanishing bileduct syndrome after liver transplantation. *Lancet* 1988; **2**: 302–305.

56 Lautenschlager I, Höckerstedt K, Jalanko H, et al. Persistent cytomegalovirus in liver allografts with chronic rejection. *Hepatology* 1997; **25**: 190–194.

57 Conti F, Grude P, Calmus Y, et al. Expression of the membrane attack complex of complement and its inhibitors during human liver allograft transplantation. *J Hepatol* 1997; **27**: 881–889.

58 Hubscher SG, Buckels JAC, Elias E, et al. Vanishing bile-duct syndrome following liver transplantation – is it reversible? *Transplantation* 1991; **51**: 1004–1010.

59 Tabatabai L, Lewis WD, Gordon F, et al. Fibrosis/cirrhosis after orthotopic liver transplantation. *Hum Pathol* 1999; **30**: 39–47.

60 Seehofer D, Rayes N, Tullius SG, et al. CMV hepatitis after liver transplantation: incidence, clinical course, and long-term follow-up. *Liver Transplant* 2002; **8**: 1138–1146.

61 MacDonald GA, Greenson JK, DelBuono EA, et al. Mini-microabscess syndrome in liver transplant patients. *Hepatology* 1997; **26**: 192–197.

62 Theise ND, Conn M, Thung SN. Localization of cytomegalovirus antigens in liver allografts over time. *Hum Pathol* 1993; **24**: 103–108.

63 Alshak NS, Jimenez AM, Gedebou M, et al. Epstein–Barr virus infection in liver transplantation patients: correlation of histopathology and semiquantitative Epstein–Barr virus-DNA recovery using polymerase chain reaction. *Hum Pathol* 1993; **24**: 1306–1312.

64 Markin RS. Manifestations of Epstein–Barr virus-associated disorders in liver. *Liver* 1994; **14**: 1–13.

65 Hubscher SG, Williams A, Davison SM, et al. Epstein–Barr virus in inflammatory diseases of the liver and liver allografts: an in situ hybridization study. *Hepatology* 1994; **20**: 899–907.

66 Pessoa MG, Terrault NA, Ferrell LD, et al. Hepatitis after liver transplantation: the role of the known and unknown viruses. *Liver Transplant Surg* 1998; **4**: 461–468.

67 Blair JE, Kusne S. Bacterial, mycobacterial, and protozoal infections after liver transplantation – Part I. *Liver Transplant* 2005; **11**: 1452–1459.

68 Hertzler GL, Millikan WJ. The surgical pathologist's role in liver transplantation. *Arch Pathol Lab Med* 1991; **115**: 273–282.

69 Oh C-K, Pelletier SJ, Sawyer RG, et al. Uni- and multivariate analysis of risk factors for early and late hepatic artery thrombosis after liver transplantation. *Transplantation* 2001; **71**: 767–772.

70 Harper PL, Edgar PR, Luddington RJ, et al. Protein C deficiency and portal thrombosis in liver transplantation in children. *Lancet* 1988; **2**: 924–927.

71 Ludwig J, Batts KP, MacCarty RL. Ischemic cholangitis in hepatic allografts. *Mayo Clin Proc* 1992; **67**: 519–526.

72 Sterneck M, Wiesner R, Ascher N, et al. Azathioprine hepatotoxicity after liver transplantation. *Hepatology* 1991; **14**: 806–810.

73 Dhillon AP, Burroughs AK, Hudson M, et al. Hepatic venular stenosis after orthotopic liver transplantation. *Hepatology* 1994; **19**: 106–111.

74 Gulbis B, Adler M, Ooms HA, et al. Liver-function studies in heart-transplant recipients treated with cyclosporin A. *Clin Chem* 1988; **34**: 1772–1774.

75 Kadmon M, Klünemann C, Böhme M, et al. Inhibition by cyclosporin A of adenosine triphosphate-dependent transport from the hepatocyte into bile. *Gastroenterology* 1993; **104**: 1507–1514.

76 Arias IM. Cyclosporin, the biology of the bile canaliculus, and cholestasis. *Gastroenterology* 1993; **104**: 1558–1560.

77 Thomson AW. FK-506 enters the clinic. *Immunol Today* 1990; **11**: 35–36.

78 Fung JJ, Todo S, Tzakis A, et al. Current status of FK 506 in liver transplantation. *Transplant Proc* 1991; **23**: 1902–1905.

79 Davern TJ, Lake JR. Recurrent disease after liver transplantation. *Semin Gastrointest Dis* 1998; **9**: 86–109.

80 Kim WR, Poterucha JJ, Porayko MK, et al. Recurrence of nonalcoholic steatohepatitis following liver transplantation. *Transplantation* 1996; **62**: 1802–1805.

81 Molloy RM, Komorowski R, Varma RR. Recurrent nonalcoholic steatohepatitis and cirrhosis after liver transplantation. *Liver Transplant Surg* 1997; **3**: 177–178.

82 Carson K, Washington MK, Treem WR, et al. Recurrence of nonalcoholic steatohepatitis in a liver transplant recipient. *Liver Transplant Surg* 1997; **3**: 174–176.

83 Fiel MI, Schiano TD, Klion FM, et al. Recurring fibroobliterative venopathy in liver allografts. *Am J Surg Pathol* 1999; **23**: 734–737.

83a Duclos-Vallee J-C, Sebagh M. Recurrence of autoimmune disease, primary sclerosing cholangitis, primary biliary cirrhosis, and autoimmune hepatitis after liver transplantation. *Liver Transplant* 2009; **15**: S25–S34.

84 Walker N, Apel R, Kerlin P, et al. Hepatitis B virus infection in liver allografts. *Am J Surg Pathol* 1993; **17**: 666–677.

85 Lucey MR, Graham DM, Martin P, et al. Recurrence of hepatitis B and delta hepatitis after orthotopic liver transplantation. *Gut* 1992; **33**: 1390–1396.

86 ten Kate FJW, Schalm SW, Willemse PJA, et al. Course of hepatitis B and D virus infection in auxiliary liver grafts in hepatitis B-positive patients. A light-microscopic and immunohistochemical study. *J Hepatol* 1992; **14**: 168–175.

87 Ottobrelli A, Marzano A, Smedile A, et al. Patterns of hepatitis delta virus reinfection and disease in liver transplantation. *Gastroenterology* 1991; **101**: 1649–1655.

88 David E, Rahier J, Pucci A, et al. Recurrence of hepatitis D (delta) in liver transplants: histopathological aspects. *Gastroenterology* 1993; **104**: 1122–1128.

89 Davies SE, Portmann BC, O'Grady JG, et al. Hepatic histological findings after transplantation for chronic hepatitis B virus infection, including a unique pattern of fibrosing cholestatic hepatitis. *Hepatology* 1991; **13**: 150–157.

90 O'Grady JG, Smith HM, Davies SE, et al. Hepatitis B virus reinfection after orthotopic liver transplantation. Serological and clinical implications. *J Hepatol* 1992; **14**: 104–111.

91 Benner KG, Lee RG, Keeffe EB, et al. Fibrosing cytolytic liver failure secondary to recurrent hepatitis B after liver transplantation. *Gastroenterology* 1992; **103**: 1307–1312.

92 Lau JYN, Bain VG, Davies SE, et al. High-level expression of hepatitis B viral antigens in fibrosing cholestatic hepatitis. *Gastroenterology* 1992; **102**: 956–962.

93 Phillips MJ, Cameron R, Flowers MA, et al. Post-transplant recurrent hepatitis B viral liver disease. Viral-burden, steatoviral, and fibroviral hepatitis B. *Am J Pathol* 1992; **140**: 1295–1308.

94 Demetris AJ, Eghtesad B, Marcos A, et al. Recurrent hepatitis C in liver allografts. Prospective assessment of diagnostic accuracy, identification of pitfalls, and observations about pathogenesis. *Am J Surg Pathol* 2004; **28**: 658–669.

95 Saxena R, Crawford JM, Navarro VJ, et al. Utilization of acidophil bodies in the diagnosis of recurrent hepatitis C infection after orthotopic liver transplantation. *Mod Pathol* 2002; **15**: 897–903.

96 Gordon FD, Pomfret EA, Pomposelli JJ, et al. Severe steatosis as the initial histologic manifestation of recurrent hepatitis C genotype 3. *Hum Pathol* 2004; **35**: 636–638.

97 Guerrero RB, Batts KP, Burgart LJ, et al. Early detection of hepatitis C allograft reinfection after orthotopic liver transplantation: a molecular and histologic study. *Mod Pathol* 2000; **13**: 229–237.

98 Ferrell LD, Wright TL, Roberts J, et al. Hepatitis C viral infection in liver transplant recipients. *Hepatology* 1992; **16**: 865–876.

99 Böker KHW, Dalley G, Bahr MJ, et al. Long-term outcome of hepatitis C virus infection after liver transplantation. *Hepatology* 1997; **25**: 203–210.

100 Dickson RC, Caldwell SH, Ishitani MB, et al. Clinical and histologic patterns of early graft failure due to recurrent hepatitis C in four patients after liver translantation. *Transplantation* 1996; **61**: 701–705.

101 Taga SA, Washington MK, Terrault N, et al. Cholestatic hepatitis C in liver allografts. *Liver Transplant Surg* 1998; **4**: 304–310.

102 Schluger LK, Sheiner PA, Thung SN, et al. Severe recurrent cholestatic hepatitis C following orthotopic liver transplantation. *Hepatology* 1996; **23**: 971–976.

103 Khettry U, Huang W-Y, Simpson MA, et al. Patterns of recurrent hepatitis C after liver transplantation in a recent cohort of patients. *Hum Pathol* 2007; **38**: 443–452.

104 Berardi S, Lodato F, Gramenzi A, et al. High incidence of allograft dysfunction in liver transplanted patients treated with pegylated-interferon alpha-2b and ribavirin for hepatitis C recurrence: possible de novo autoimmune hepatitis? *Gut* 2007; **56**: 237–242.

105 Demetris AJ, Sebagh M. Plasma cell hepatitis in liver allografts: variant of rejection or autoimmune hepatitis? *Liver Transplant* 2008; **14**: 750–755.

105a Ward SC, Schiano TD, Thung SN, Fiel MI. Plasma cell hepatitis in hepatitis C virus patients post-liver transplantation: case control study showing poor outcome and predictive features in the liver explant. *Liver Transplant* 2009; **15**: 1826–1833.

106 Souza P, Prihoda TJ, Hoyumpa AM, et al. Morphologic features resembling transplant rejection in core biopsies of native livers from patients with hepatitis C. *Hum Pathol* 2009; **40**: 92–97.

107 Sylvestre PB, Batts KP, Burgart LJ, et al. Recurrence of primary biliary cirrhosis after liver transplantation: histologic estimate of incidence and natural history. *Liver Transplant* 2003; **9**: 1086–1093.

108 Hubscher SG, Elias E, Buckels JAC, et al. Primary biliary cirrhosis. Histological evidence of disease recurrence after liver transplantation. *J Hepatol* 1993; **18**: 173–184.

109 Khettry U, Anand N, Faul PN, et al. Liver transplantation for primary biliary cirrhosis: a long-term pathologic study. *Liver Transplant* 2003; **9**: 87–96.

109a Montano-Loza AJ, Mason AL, Ma M, Bastiampillai RJ, Bain VG, Tandon P. Risk factors for recurrence of autoimmune hepatitis after liver transplantation. *Liver Transplant* 2009; **15**: 1254–1261.

110 Graziadei IW, Wiesner RH, Batts KP, et al. Recurrence of primary sclerosing cholangitis following liver transplantation. *Hepatology* 1999; **29**: 1050–1056.

111 Birnbaum AH, Benkov KJ, Pittman NS, et al. Recurrence of autoimmune hepatitis in children after liver transplantation. *J Pediatr Gastroenterol Nutr* 1997; **25**: 20–25.

112. Malik SM, deVera ME, Fontes P, Shaikh O, Sasatomi E, Ahmed J. Recurrent disease following liver transplantation for nonalcoholic steatohepatitis cirrhosis. *Liver Transplant* 2009; **15**: 1843–1851.

113 Bianchi G, Marchesini G, Marzocchi R, et al. Metabolic syndrome in liver transplantation: relation to etiology and immunosuppression. *Liver Transplant* 2008; **14**: 1648–1654.

114 Miyagawa-Hayashino A, Egaqa H, Yorifuji T, et al. Allograft steatohepatitis in progressive familial intrahepatic cholestasis type 1 after living donor liver transplantation. *Liver Transplant* 2009; **15**: 610–618.

115 Mieli-Vergani G, Vergani D. De novo autoimmune hepatitis after liver transplantation. *J Hepatol* 2004; **40**: 3–7.

116 Heneghan MA, Portmann BC, Norris SM, et al. Graft dysfunction mimicking autoimmune hepatitis following liver transplantation in adults. *Hepatology* 2001; **34**: 464–470.

117 Leblond V, Choquet S. Lymphoproliferative disorders after liver transplantation. *J Hepatol* 2004; **40**: 728–735.

118 Palazzo JP, Lundquist K, Mitchell D, et al. Rapid development of lymphoma following liver transplantation in a recipient with hepatitis B and primary hemochromatosis. *Am J Gastroenterol* 1991; **88**: 102–104.

119 Spiro IJ, Yandell DW, Li C, et al. Brief report: lymphoma of donor origin occurring in the porta hepatis of a transplanted liver. *N Engl J Med* 1993; **329**: 27–29.

120 Lones MA, Shintaku IP, Weiss LM, et al. Posttransplant lymphoproliferative disorder in liver allograft biopsies: a comparison of three methods for the demonstration of Epstein–Barr virus. *Hum Pathol* 1997; **28**: 533–539.

121 Luketic VA, Shiffman ML, McCall JB, et al. Primary hepatocellular carcinoma after orthotopic liver transplantation for chronic hepatitis B infection. *Ann Intern Med* 1991; **114**: 212–213.

122 Saxena R, Ye MQ, Emre S, et al. De novo hepatocellular carcinoma in a hepatic allograft with recurrent hepatitis C cirrhosis. *Liver Transplant Surg* 1999; **5**: 81–82.

123 McPeake JR, O'Grady JG, Zaman S, et al. Liver transplantation for primary hepatocellular carcinoma: tumor size and number determine outcome. *J Hepatol* 1993; **18**: 226–234.

123a Morita K, Taketoni A, Soejima Y, et al. De novo hepatocellular carcinoma in a liver graft with sustained hepatitis C virus clearance after living donor liver transplantation. *Liver Transplant* 2009; **15**: 1412–1416.

124 Banff Working Group. Liver biopsy interpretation for causes of late liver allograft dysfunction. *Hepatology* 2006; **44**: 489–501.

125 Krasinskas AM, Demetris AJ, Poterucha JJ, et al. The prevalence and natural history of untreated isolated central perivenulitis in adult allograft livers. *Liver Transplant* 2008; **14**: 625–632.

126 Abraham SC, Freese DK, Ishitani MB, et al. Significance of central perivenulitis in pediatric liver transplantation. *Am J Surg Pathol* 2008; **32**: 1479–1488.

127 Shaikh OS, Demetris AJ. Idiopathic posttransplantation hepatitis? *Liver Transplant* 2007; **13**: 943–946.

128 Kamar N, Selves J, Mansuy J-M, et al. Hepatitis E virus and chronic hepatitis in organ–transplant recipients. *N Engl J Med* 2008; **358**: 811–817.

129. Pischke S, Suneetha PV, Baechlein C, et al. Hepatitis E virus infection as a cause of graft hepatitis in liver transplant recipients. *Liver Transplant* 2010; **16**: 74–82.

130 Nonomura A, Mizukami Y, Matsubara F, et al. Clinicopathological study of lymphocyte attachment to endothelial cells (endothelialitis) in various liver diseases. *Liver* 1991; **11**: 78–88.

131 Lykavieris P, van Mil S, Cresteil D, et al. Progressive familial intrahepatic cholestasis type 1 and extrahepatic features: no catch-up of stature growth, exacerbation of diarrhea, and appearance of liver steatosis after liver transplantation. *J Hepatol* 2003; **39**: 447–452.

132 Lefkowitch JH, Lobritto SJ, Brown RS Jr, et al. Ground-glass, polyglucosan-like hepatocellular inclusions: a 'new' diagnostic entity. *Gastroenterology* 2006; **131**: 713–718.

133 Bejarano PA, Garcia MT, Rodriguez MM, et al. Liver glycogen bodies: ground-glass hepatocytes in transplanted patients. *Virchows Arch* 2006; **449**: 539–545.

134 Wisell J, Boitnott J, Haas M, et al. Glycogen pseudoground glass change in hepatocytes. *Am J Surg Pathol* 2006; **30**: 1085–1090.

135 Vázquez JJ. Ground glass hepatocytes: light and electron microscopy. Characterization of the different types. *Histol Histopathol* 1990; **5**: 379–386.

136 Degos F, Degott C. Hepatitis in renal transplant recipients. *J Hepatol* 1989; **9**: 114–123.

137 Chan T-M, Lok ASF, Cheng IKP, et al. A prospective study of hepatitis C virus infection among renal transplant recipients. *Gastroenterology* 1993; **104**: 862–868.

138 Rao KV, Anderson WR, Kasiske BL, et al. Value of liver biopsy in the evaluation and management of chronic liver disease in renal transplant recipients. *Am J Med* 1993; **94**: 241–250.

139 Delladetsima JK, Boletis JN, Makris F, et al. Fibrosing cholestatic hepatitis in renal transplant recipients with hepatitis C virus infection. *Liver Transplant Surg* 1999; **5**: 294–300.

140 Sopko J, Anuras S. Liver disease in renal transplant recipients. [Review.] *Am J Med* 1978; **64**: 139–146.

141 Ware AJ, Luby JP, Hollinger B, et al. Etiology of liver disease in renal-transplant patients. *Ann Intern Med* 1979; **91**: 364–371.

142 Weir MR, Kirkman RL, Strom TB, et al. Liver disease in recipients of long-functioning renal allografts. *Kidney Int* 1985; **28**: 839–844.

143 Rao KV, Anderson WR. Hemosiderosis: an unrecognized complication in renal allograft recipients. *Transplantation* 1982; **33**: 115–117.

144 Rao KV, Anderson WR. Hemosiderosis and hemochromatosis in renal transplant recipients. Clinical and pathological features, diagnostic correlations, predisposing factors, and treatment. *Am J Nephrol* 1985; **5**: 419–430.

145 Marubbio AT, Danielson B. Hepatic veno-occlusive disease in a renal transplant patient receiving azathioprine. *Gastroenterology* 1975; **69**: 739–743.

146 Degott C, Rueff B, Kreis H, et al. Peliosis hepatis in recipients of renal transplants. *Gut* 1978; **19**: 748–753.

147 Nataf C, Feldmann G, Lebrec D, et al. Idiopathic portal hypertension (perisinusoidal fibrosis) after renal transplantation. *Gut* 1979; **20**: 531–537.

148 Gerlag PG, Lobatto S, Driessen WM, et al. Hepatic sinusoidal dilatation with portal hypertension during azathioprine treatment after kidney transplantation. *J Hepatol* 1985; **1**: 339–348.

149 Krempien B, Bommer J, Ritz E. Foreign body giant cell reaction in lungs, liver and spleen. A complication of long term haemodialysis. *Virchows Arch [A]* 1981; **392**: 73–80.

150 Leong AS, Disney AP, Gove DW. Refractile particles in liver of haemodialysis patients [letter]. *Lancet* 1981; **1**: 889–890.

151 Parfrey PS, O'Driscoll JB, Paradinas FJ. Refractile material in the liver of haemodialysis patients [letter]. *Lancet* 1981; **1**: 1101–1102.

152 Shulman HM, Sharma P, Amos D, et al. A coded histologic study of hepatic graft-versus-host disease after human bone marrow transplantation. *Hepatology* 1988; **8**: 463–470.

153 McDonald GB, Shulman HM, Sullivan KM, et al. Intestinal and hepatic complications of human bone marrow transplantation. Part I. *Gastroenterology* 1986; **90**: 460–477.

154 McDonald GB, Shulman HM, Sullivan KM, et al. Intestinal and hepatic complications of human bone marrow transplantation. Part II. *Gastroenterology* 1986; **90**: 770–784.

155 Snover DC, Weisdorf SA, Ramsay NK, et al. Hepatic graft versus host disease: a study of the predictive value of liver biopsy in diagnosis. *Hepatology* 1984; **4**: 123–130.

156 Shulman HM, Kleiner D, Lee SJ, et al. Histopathologic diagnosis of chronic graft-versus-host disease: National Institutes of Health consensus development project on criteria for clinical trials in chronic graft-versus-host disease. II. Pathology Working Group report. *Biol Blood Marrow Transplant* 2006; **12**: 31–47.

157 Geubel AP, Cnudde A, Ferrant A, et al. Diffuse biliary tract involvement mimicking primary sclerosing cholangitis after bone marrow transplantation. *J Hepatol* 1990; **10**: 23–28.

158 Strasser SI, Shulman HM, Flowers ME, et al. Chronic graft-versus-host disease of the liver: presentation as an acute hepatitis. *Hepatology* 2000; **32**: 1265–1271.

159 Knapp AB, Crawford JM, Rappeport JM, et al. Cirrhosis as a consequence of graft–versus-host disease. *Gastroenterology* 1987; **92**: 513–519.

160 DeLeve LD, Shulman HM, McDonald GB. Toxic injury to hepatic sinusoids: sinusoidal obstruction syndrome (veno-occlusive disease). *Semin Liver Dis* 2002; **22**: 27–42.

161 Shulman HM, Fisher LB, Schoch HG, et al. Venoocclusive disease of the liver after marrow transplantation: histological correlates of clinical signs and symptoms. *Hepatology* 1994; **19**: 1171–1180.

162 Zubair I, Herrera GA, Pretlow TG, et al. Cytoplasmic inclusions in hepatocytes of bone marrow transplant patients: light and electron microscopic characterization. *Am J Clin Pathol* 1985; **83**: 65–68.

General reading

Banff Working Group. Liver biopsy interpretation for causes of late liver allograft dysfunction. *Hepatology* 2006; **44**: 489–501.

Demetris AJ, Crawford JM, Minervini MI, et al. Transplantation pathology of the liver. In: Odze RD, Goldblum JR, eds. Surgical Pathology of the GI Tract, Liver, Biliary Tract, and Pancreas, 2nd edn. Philadelphia, PA: Saunders/Elsevier, 2009: 1169–1230.

Hübscher S, Portmann BC. Transplantation pathology. In: Burt AD, Portmann BC, Ferrell LD, eds. MacSween's Pathology of the Liver, 5th edn. Edinburgh: Churchill Livingstone/Elsevier, 2007: 815–880.

International Panel. Banff schema for grading liver allograft rejection: an international consensus document. *Hepatology* 1997; **25**: 658–663.

International Panel. Update of the international Banff schema for liver allograft rejection: working recommendations for the histopathologic staging and reporting of chronic rejection. *Hepatology* 2000; **31**: 792–799.

Lefkowitch JH. Diagnostic issues in liver transplantation pathology. *Clin Liver Dis* 2002; **6**: 555–570.

Ludwig J, Lefkowitch JH. Histopathology of the liver following transplantation. In: Maddrey WC, Schiff ER, Sorrell MF, eds. Transplantation of the Liver, 3rd edn. Philadelphia, PA: Lippincott Williams & Wilkins, 2001: 229–250.

Electron Microscopy and Other Techniques

Introduction

This chapter will focus primarily on the role of transmission electron microscopy in the assessment of liver ultrastructure and disease. It also describes, in brief, the principles and uses of other methodologies. The special conditions required for tissue processing in each of these techniques (**Table 17.1**) should be carefully planned for in advance of obtaining specimens. While some of these methods are not universally available in pathology departments, other departments at one's institution or at other centres of investigation may be consulted in cases of particular diagnostic or research interest. Procedures for fixation and processing for transmission electron microscopy are available in several of the General reading references at the end of the chapter.

Electron microscopy of liver biopsies

Transmission electron microscopy (TEM) continues to provide important information about the normal cellular and extracellular constituents of the liver and their alterations in disease. Recent interest in the relationships between the various sinusoidal cells of the liver has benefited from TEM studies[1,2] as has investigations of hepatic progenitor cells.[3] Data from standard TEM studies can be enhanced by the application of immunohisto-chemical stains (see Immunoelectron microscopy), digitised three-dimensional computer reconstructions[4–6] and morphometry. TEM is sometimes limited by the lack of specificity of certain ultrastructural changes and the problem of sampling error in lesions that may not be uniformly distributed. The first of these limitations is well illustrated in cholestasis; various features of cholestasis such as loss of canalicular microvilli are easily recognised under the electron microscope, but many causes produce these changes. Sampling error can sometimes be reduced by the combination of light and electron microscopy in a single instrument.[7]

In diagnostic work TEM should be seriously considered under five circumstances:

1 *To establish the nature of an inborn error of metabolism.* In a number of storage diseases the ultrastructural changes are diagnostic or give an indication of the type of disease to be considered.[8,9] Specific features are seen, for example, in type II glycogenosis, in Gaucher's disease and in Niemann–Pick disease (**Fig. 17.1**). Storage diseases can and should often be diagnosed by other, usually biochemical, methods, but even then electron microscopy can reduce the period of investigation by drawing attention to a

©2010 Elsevier Ltd
DOI: 10.1016/B978-0-7020-3410-7.00023-X

Figure 17.1 Liver tissue from a patient with Niemann–Pick disease.
Macrophages (M) and hepatocytes (H) contain abundant vacuoles in which there are lamellar lipid inclusions. (Needle biopsy, lead citrate; ×4600.)

Table 17.1 Liver tissue processing for various techniques

Technique	Tissue preparation
Transmission electron microscopy	Glutaraldehyde fixation
Scanning electron microscopy	Perfusion-fixation; critical point drying; coating with gold or platinum
Immunoelectron microscopy	Glutaraldehyde/paraformaldehyde fixation
Immunoperoxidase of tissue sections	Fixation in 10% neutral formalin or alternative fixative
Immunoperoxidase and immunofluorescence of frozen sections	Snap freeze after embedding in OCT compound
In situ hybridisation	Snap freeze after embedding in OCT compound
Flow cytometry	Fresh tissue
Confocal laser scanning microscopy	Snap freeze after embedding in OCT compound
Laser capture microdissection	Conventional tissue sections for light microscopy
Gene array analysis	Snap freeze in liquid nitrogen; store at −80°C

OCT, optimal cutting temperature.

likely diagnosis. Electron microscopy may show whether a liver-cell pigment is lipofuscin or the pigment of the Dubin–Johnson syndrome (**Fig. 17.2**), and can therefore be helpful when this syndrome is suspected but not fully proved by light microscopy.[10] In some patients with Wilson's disease characteristic changes may be seen in liver-cell mitochondria (see below).

Figure 17.2
Dubin–Johnson syndrome.
Large, characteristically complex dense bodies are seen near a bile canaliculus (BC). (Needle biopsy, lead citrate; ×18 900.)

2 *To establish the presence of viral infection.* Electron microscopy of liver biopsies may prove to be important when serological test results or cultures for suspected viral infection are unavailable or incomplete. Both intranuclear and intracytoplasmic virions may be identified by the appearances of their spherical or hexagonal capsids, dense core material, surface envelopes and paracrystalline and lattice-like arrays. These features can be compared with published micrographs for identification of the candidate virion.[11,12] For example, some adult patients with the unusual finding of giant-cell hepatitis on routine light microscopy have been shown to have paramyxovirus-like particles in the liver as a result of electron microscopic studies of biopsy material.[13,14] Electron microscopy can also be applied to cell cultures, as shown in a recent study demonstrating 50–90 nm hepatitis C virions.[15] Glutaraldehyde fixation of biopsy specimens is preferred, but viral particles can also be identified in formalin-fixed tissues which are washed and then processed for electron microscopy.

3 *To establish the nature of a tumour of doubtful histogenesis.* The ultrastructural features of many tumours, including neuroendocrine tumours and malignant melanomas, help in making a firm diagnosis.[16] The more obvious features such as neurosecretory granules in neuroendocrine tumours survive paraffin embedding; re-embedding of paraffin material for electron microscopy should therefore be considered.

4 *To establish the presence of specific drug-related changes.* In liver damage due to a small number of drugs, including perhexiline maleate[17] and amiodarone,[18-21] hepatocytes contain lysosomes filled with lamellar phospholipid material (**Fig. 17.3**).

5 *To provide material for research.* Electron microscopy offers wide potential for research into human liver disease, and it may be that future research will increase the diagnostic value of electron microscopy in this field. If liver biopsy is performed in a patient having a disease with potentially helpful or interesting ultrastructural features, small pieces of the specimen can be embedded for electron microscopy and

Figure 17.3 Amiodarone-induced phospholipidosis.
An enlarged lysosome (asterisk), resembling a myelin figure, contains densely packed, concentrically arranged osmiophilic lipids, thought to represent drug–lipid complexes. A smaller membranous whorl (arrowhead) is seen in the cytoplasm. L, lipid. (Ferrocyanide, ×38,000). (Illustration kindly provided by Dr S. Poucell and Professor M. J. Phillips, Toronto, Canada.)

stored indefinitely in block form. The extent to which this is done clearly depends on the resources of the particular laboratory.

Whenever electron microscopy of a liver biopsy specimen is considered, the laboratory should be contacted beforehand and arrangements made for collection and fixation of the specimen at the bedside. Proper processing of the tissue, including optimal fixation, provides the basis for accurate analysis of ultrastructural changes.

The normal liver and examples of ultrastructural changes in disease

The following description of the liver under the transmission electron microscope is a general one. It should be noted that the quality of fixation will influence the appearance of cells and organelles. The labels in the description of normal liver refer to **Figs 17.4 and 17.5**.

Several cell types are found in the hepatic lobules. The hepatocytes or parenchymal cells (PC) are separated from the sinusoidal endothelial cells (EC) by the space of Disse (SD), in which there are collagen fibres and stellate cells (SC), formerly known as perisinusoidal cells, Ito cells or fat-storing cells. Within the sinusoidal lumen are Kupffer cells (KC), the hepatic macrophages and large granular lymphocytes (also called pit cells) with natural killer activity.

Figure 17.4
Normal human liver.
At the edge of a liver-cell plate the parenchymal cell (PC) is separated from the sinusoidal lumen (S) by an endothelial cell (EC) and Kupffer cell (KC). SC, stellate cell; SD, space of Disse. (Needle biopsy, lead citrate, ×10,000.)

Hepatocyte (liver cell, parenchymal cell)

Hepatocytes have similar features in different lobular regions but vary in detailed structure. For example, there are more lysosomes and mitochondria in periportal than in perivenular hepatocytes, while the converse is true for the smooth-surfaced endoplasmic reticulum. The hepatocyte is a highly polarised cell with surfaces facing the space of Disse, other hepatocytes and the bile canaliculus. The plasma membrane is specialised in these three areas. Many microvilli project into the space of Disse and into the bile canaliculus. This

Figure 17.5
Normal human
liver.
Two parenchymal cells have formed a bile canaliculus (BC) delimited by junctional complexes (JC). Lysosomes (Ly) have varying density, the darker ones corresponding to lipofuscin as seen under the light microscope. N, nucleus; M, mitochondria; Gly, glycogen; RER, rough-surfaced endoplasmic reticulum; G, Golgi apparatus. (Needle biopsy, lead citrate, ×24,000.)

is a potential space formed by two or three hepatocytes in normal liver, and sometimes more in disease. The intercellular membrane of the hepatocyte is relatively smooth and forms several types of intercellular junctions.

The nucleus

The nucleus (N) is normally limited by a double membrane, the nuclear envelope, which is continuous with the rough-surfaced endoplasmic reticulum. The nuclear envelope has

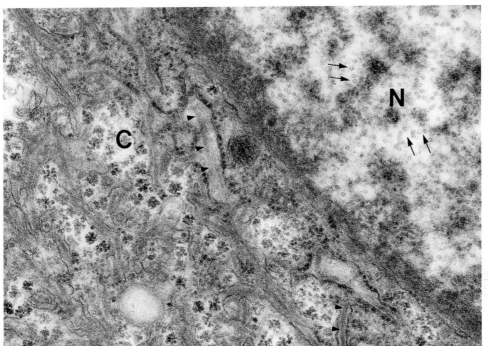

Figure 17.6
Hepatocyte in hepatitis B surface material (HBsAg)-positive chronic hepatitis.
In the nucleus (N) there are numerous core particles (arrows). The cytoplasm (C) contains irregularly shaped cisternae of the endoplasmic reticulum in which there are tubules (arrowheads), the morphological *in situ* counterpart of surface antigen. (Needle biopsy, lead citrate, ×45,000.)

small pores which are thought to serve as a route of communication between the nucleo-plasm and the cytoplasm. Within the nucleus there is irregularly distributed chromatin, and a nucleolus is often visible.

Structural changes

Large amounts of monoparticulate glycogen are seen in some adult hepatocyte nuclei in diabetes mellitus and in insulin resistance, and also in children. In type B hepatitis, core virus particles are seen (**Fig. 17.6**). Intranuclear virions are also seen in infections due to cytomegalovirus, herpesvirus, echovirus and adenovirus.

Mitochondria

Mitochondria (M) are the sites of oxidative enzyme activity, and are involved in the metabolism of amino acids, lipids and carbohydrates. There are an average of 2200 mito-chondria within the hepatocyte.[22] A smooth outer limiting membrane and an inner mem-brane with deep infoldings, the cristae, give the mitochondria a characteristic appearance. The inner membrane surrounds the mitochondrial matrix which contains many dense granules.

Structural changes

Cristae of atypical shape, crystalline inclusions and enlarged or unusually scanty granules are found in a wide variety of conditions, and sometimes also in normal liver. Giant mitochondria are seen most often in alcoholic liver disease[23] but are also found in non-alcoholic fatty liver disease[24] and other conditions.[25] Immunohistochemistry and immuno-electron microscopy can assist in their detection.[26] They are frequently found in patients with systemic sclerosis.[27] In the early stages of Wilson's disease mitochondria show varia-tion in shape, increased electron density, widening of the spaces between membranes, vacuolation, enlargement of matrix granules and deposition of crystalline material[28,29]

367

**Figure 17.7
Wilson's disease.**
Hepatocyte
cytoplasm with
mitochondria
showing dilatation
of intracristal spaces
(arrowheads). Some
are microcystic and
their contents finely
granular (asterisk).
Dense granules
are prominent.
(Ferrocyanide,
×11 400.) (Illustration
kindly supplied by
Professor M. J.
Phillips and Ms J. S.
Patterson, Toronto,
Canada.)

(**Fig. 17.7**). Three types of Wilsonian mitochondria are described which show intrafamilial concordance.[30] Abnormal, swollen and irregular mitochondria are found in hepatocytes in Reye's syndrome[31] and other microvesicular fat syndromes.[32]

Endoplasmic reticulum

This is an important site of protein synthesis and transport. It also contains enzymes involved in drug and steroid metabolism. Morphologically, the endoplasmic reticulum is a cisternal membrane-bound system continuous with the nuclear envelope. It is the morphological counterpart of the microsomes. Two main types of endoplasmic reticulum can be recognised. The **rough-surfaced endoplasmic reticulum** (RER) is studded with ribosomes and is often arranged in a lamellar pattern. The **smooth-surfaced endoplasmic reticulum** (SER) lacks ribosomes and has a tubular or vesicular appearance.

Structural changes

Dilatation, degranulation, vesiculation and proliferation of the endoplasmic reticulum can be seen in many conditions. Some of these 'changes' are also influenced by the fixation procedure, making them difficult to evaluate. Their accurate quantification requires carefully controlled processing conditions and morphometric analysis. However, in α_1-antitrypsin deficiency the dilatation of endoplasmic reticulum is striking, and finely granular material accumulates in the cisternae (**Fig. 17.8**). In chronic type B hepatitis the cisternae are also dilated and contain tubular structures representing the surface material of the hepatitis B virus (**Fig. 17.6**), and sometimes complete Dane particles.

Lysosomes

Lysosomes (Ly) are organelles that carry many different lytic enzymes and are involved in the breakdown of proteins, carbohydrates and lipids. **Primary lysosomes** are small vesicles containing enzymes, but not yet involved in catabolic processes. **Secondary lysosomes**

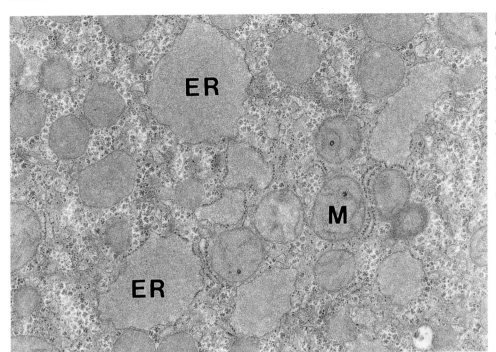

Figure 17.8
α₁-Antitrypsin deficiency.
In this parenchymal cell the cisternae of the endoplasmic reticulum (ER) are dilated and filled with finely granular material. M, mitochondrion. (Needle biopsy, lead citrate; ×16,000.)

are membrane-bound, often irregularly shaped electron-dense bodies in which the breakdown processes take place. When undigested residues accumulate and enzyme activity is diminished, the secondary lysosomes are called residual bodies. These are the lipofuscin granules. All types of secondary lysosomes tend to be concentrated around the bile canaliculi.

Structural changes

Lysosomes accumulate iron pigment in various forms of iron overload, including hereditary haemochromatosis.[33] They can be strikingly enlarged in inborn errors of metabolism, such as Niemann–Pick disease (**Fig. 17.1**) and type II glycogenosis, or show characteristic changes, such as in the Dubin–Johnson syndrome (**Fig. 17.2**). Lamellar and reticular inclusions are seen within them in acquired, drug-related phospholipidosis.[16–20]

Peroxisomes

These are round or oval bodies with an even, granular matrix bounded by a single membrane. Human peroxisomes infrequently have a nucleoid, whereas this is often seen in other species. They are most numerous in perivenular hepatocytes. They contain numerous oxidative enzymes and are involved in β-oxidation of long-chain fatty acids and synthesis of bile acids and prostaglandins. Their catalase enzyme mediates conversion of peroxide to water.

Structural changes

Peroxisomes are absent in Zellweger's syndrome (cerebro-hepato-renal syndrome).[34] In alcoholic and drug hepatitis, catalase content of peroxisomes is decreased[33] and they show irregular shapes.[34–36] Increased numbers of peroxisomes are seen in alcoholic and drug hepatitis[35] as well as in cirrhosis.[37]

Golgi apparatus

The Golgi apparatus (G) is a membranous system involved in excretory functions of the cell. It contains enzymes such as glycosyl transferases and is involved in glycoprotein metabolism. Morphologically it is composed of small groups of flattened sacs with associated vesicles.

Structural changes

The appearance of the Golgi apparatus is influenced by fixation, and changes are therefore difficult to quantify, but dilatation is evident in regenerating liver and in hepatocellular carcinoma. Electron-dense liposomes accumulate in the system during the development of fatty liver.

Cell sap (cytosol)

The soluble portion of the cytoplasm (cell sap) contains variable amounts of glycogen, free ribosomes, microtubules, intermediate filaments and microfilaments. A few lipid droplets and scanty iron-containing granules are also seen.

Structural changes

Ferritin particles accumulate in iron storage disorders.[33] Fat droplets are numerous in fatty liver, but the amount of fat varies greatly with the patient's state of nutrition. Core particles of hepatitis B virus can be identified in the cytoplasm in many cases of chronic type B hepatitis. Cytoplasmic crystalline inclusions are seen both in normal and in diseased livers. In alcoholic hepatitis, the Mallory bodies found in ballooned hepatocytes are composed of accumulations of cytokeratin and other proteins in the form of filaments (**Fig. 17.9**).

**Figure 17.9
Mallory bodies.**
Irregular electron-dense material (arrow) is seen in the cytoplasm of a hepatocyte. The fibrillar nature of the material is evident at the higher magnification shown in the inset. (Needle biopsy, uranyl acetate and lead citrate; ×8600; *inset*: ×27,000.)

Bile canaliculus

The bile canaliculus (BC) measures approximately 0.75 μm and is formed by membranes of several contiguous hepatocytes which are joined by tight junctions.[38] Surface microvilli covered with a thin glycoprotein coat project into the canalicular lumen. Actin filaments are present within the microvilli and extend downward into a pericanalicular web also composed of actin, functioning in canalicular contraction.

Structural changes

Alterations in the bile canaliculus are similar in many forms of cholestasis. Loss of microvilli, formation of surface membrane blebs and disorganisation of the pericanalicular actin filament web are common features. In the cholestasis related to preservation injury after liver transplantation, for example, ischaemia and reperfusion injury result in canalicular dilatation, loss of microvilli and compaction of actin filaments.[39] Intracanalicular bile appears as electron-dense filamentous material. Coarsely granular canalicular bile ('Byler bile') is a characteristic of progressive familial intrahepatic cholestasis type 1 (Byler disease) seen in Amish children[40] (**Fig. 17.10**).

Kupffer cell

The Kupffer cell (KC) has an irregular outline, with many finger-like protrusions of the cell surface by which it anchors to endothelial cells. It is rich in phagocytic vacuoles (phagosomes), lysosomes and mitochondria, while the endoplasmic reticulum is only

**Figure 17.10
Progressive familial intrahepatic cholestasis, type 1 (PFIC-1).**
The dilated bile canaliculus (BC) contains coarsely granular bile ('Byler bile'), a feature associated with cholestasis in Amish children. The canaliculus is delimited by several junctional complexes (arrows) and has a reduced number of microvilli. (Needle biopsy, lead citrate; ×24475.) (Illustration kindly provided by Dr A. S. Knisely, Galveston, TX, USA.)

moderately well developed. The nucleus is irregular in shape, with a tendency for the chromatin to be concentrated at the nuclear periphery.

Structural changes

Hypertrophied Kupffer cells can be seen in all conditions of parenchymal cell destruction (e.g. hepatitis) and in pigment overload (e.g. cholestasis, siderosis). Many storage disorders affect the Kupffer cells; in Niemann–Pick disease, for example, both Kupffer cells and hepatocytes are enlarged and filled with vacuoles containing accumulated sphingomyelin (**see Fig. 17.1**).

Endothelial cell

The endothelial cell (EC) is a flattened cell with a smooth surface, showing small fenestrae organised into sieve plates which provide direct communication between the sinusoidal lumen and the space of Disse.[41] Fenestrae show open and multifolded labyrinth-like configurations.[42] The cytoplasmic volume is relatively small. Many micropinocytotic vesicles can be seen beneath the plasma membrane.

Structural changes

In hepatitis and other conditions, endothelial cells undergo several changes, including the accumulation of iron-rich siderosomes and the formation of basement membrane material on the aspect of the cells facing the space of Disse.[43] In patients with chronic viral hepatitis and AIDS, **tubuloreticular structures** and **cylindrical confronting cisternae** develop within the rough endoplasmic reticulum of endothelial cells and sometimes within Kupffer cells, stellate cells (see below) and lymphocytes.[44,45] Tubuloreticular structures are reticular aggregates of branching tubules within the cisternae of the endoplasmic reticulum and sometimes the perinuclear envelope. Cylindrical confronting cisternae are cylinders of fused membranous lamellae derived from two or more cisternae of endoplasmic reticulum, one inside the other. They appear to be a result of increased endogenous levels of α- and β-interferon. Membrane-bound dense bodies, seen on light microscopy as diastase–periodic acid–Schiff (PAS)-positive cytoplasmic granules, are sometimes present in chronic hepatitis B and C and autoimmune hepatitis[46] (**see Fig. 9.12**).

Stellate cell

The stellate cell (SC), previously known as the Ito cell, fat-storing cell, perisinusoidal cell or lipocyte, is a major storage site for vitamin A. In liver injury, it becomes a transitional cell or myofibroblast-like cell capable of synthesising collagen types I, III and IV as well as laminin.[47] Stellate cells are located within the space of Disse (**see Fig. 7.6**) and have conspicuous rough endoplasmic reticulum, a large Golgi apparatus and large lipid droplets containing vitamin A. In alcoholic liver disease, hypervitaminosis A and methotrexate toxicity stellate cells undergo hyperplasia and are associated with increased collagen fibres within the space of Disse. Multivesicular stellate cells with numerous lipid droplets have been reported in primary biliary cirrhosis.[48]

Pit cell (large granular lymphocyte)

This cell is located within the sinusoidal lumen, preferentially in the periportal region compared to acinar zone 3.[49] Its surface uropodia and pseudopodia are often in close contact with endothelial cells or Kupffer cells. The nucleus is dense, eccentrically located in the cell and indented. The cell's name derives from its characteristic electron-dense, membrane-bound granules of cytotoxic enzymes which resemble 'pits' or pips in fruit. The cytoplasm contains profiles of rough endoplasmic reticulum, a well-developed Golgi apparatus, centrioles and occasional rod-cored vesicles. Pit cells function as natural killer cells and have been identified in autoimmune hepatitis and in increased numbers in livers with malignant tumours.[50]

Immunoelectron microscopy

The principles employed in immunohistochemical staining of liver biopsy sections for light microscopy (see Immunohistochemistry, below) can be adapted for use in electron microscopy.[51] Following fixation of the specimen in a mixture of glutaraldehyde and paraformaldehyde, the tissue is treated with borohydride, cryoprotected and frozen for storage. Thick sections of 20–40 μm are later cut from the thawed samples and stained by either a direct or indirect immunoperoxidase method.[52] The stained sections are then post-fixed in osmium tetroxide, dehydrated and embedded in Epon. Under the electron microscope, electron-dense immunoreactive material is seen at the site of the target antigen.

Availability of a wide variety of monoclonal and polyclonal antibodies to tissue antigens and receptors has greatly expanded investigations of interactions of hepatocytes with immune cells and with the extracellular matrix. Intercellular adhesion molecules, histocompatibility antigens and interferon receptors are among the potential list of antigens that can be studied by immunoelectron microscopy.[53-55] An example of this technique is shown in **Fig. 17.11**, which demonstrates the up-regulation of the type A receptor for tumour necrosis factor on hepatocyte membranes in a patient with chronic hepatitis B.[56]

Scanning electron microscopy

The three-dimensional structure of the liver can be assessed by scanning electron microscopy of specially prepared tissues,[57] or even of sections from paraffin blocks[58] (**Fig. 17.12**). X-ray microanalysis may be combined with the scanning technique and is useful in elemental analysis. Laboratories with scanning electron microscopes are best equipped to provide details on appropriate tissue fixation, critical point drying and coating of specimens with gold or platinum. Scanning electron microscopy is useful in examining bile ducts[59] and resin casts of hepatic vasculature.[60-63]

Immunohistochemistry

Immunohistochemical techniques are now widely available in pathology laboratories and the methods for both immunoperoxidase stains and immunofluorescence microscopy are covered in standard textbooks.[64] Both direct and indirect labelling methods are used to detect antigens in liver biopsy tissue; the indirect method is the more popular and more sensitive. Important variables that may affect results include the type and duration of fixation, the vendor or other source used to obtain the antibodies, and the type of label attached to the antibody for detection of the antigen. Microwave treatment of tissue sections in certain cases may improve antigen exposure for staining. While fixation in 10% neutral formalin is acceptable for many immunohistochemical stains, some will require alternative fixatives or cryostat sections, and these factors should be considered when the biopsy specimen is initially processed.

In routine diagnostic work immunohistochemistry is helpful in four major areas:

1 *To ascertain the histogenesis of malignant tumours in the liver.* In distinguishing metastatic carcinoma from primary hepatocellular carcinoma, the former usually stain positively for epithelial membrane antigen and with the pooled monoclonal anti-keratin antibody AE1/AE3. Hepatocellular carcinomas show negative staining

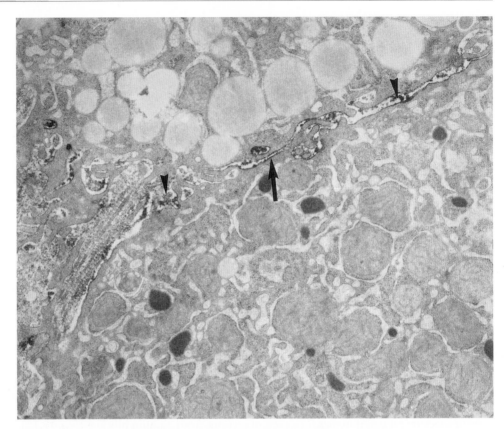

Figure 17.11 Type A receptor for tumour necrosis factor (TNF).
A case of hepatitis B virus-positive chronic hepatitis stained with monoclonal antibody Utr-1 (directed against type A receptor of TNF) shows positive staining on the membranes of two adjacent hepatocytes in a discontinuous pattern (arrow) and in the intercellular space (arrowheads). (Immunoelectron microscopy, ×18 400.) (Illustration kindly provided by Drs V. J. Desmet, R. Volpes, J. Van den Oord and R. De Vos, Leuven, The Netherlands.)

for cytokeratin 7 and 20.[65] α-Fetoprotein staining gives disappointing results in many hepatocellular carcinomas but is usually positive in hepatoblastomas. This is discussed further in **Chapter 11**.

2 *Staining for α_1-antitrypsin* (**see Fig. 13.14**) is important in confirming the identity of diastase-resistant, PAS-positive periportal granules in chronic hepatitis, cirrhosis and in neonatal hepatitis.

3 *Identification of bile-duct epithelium.* Biopsy specimens which show an apparent paucity of interlobular bile ducts may benefit from specific staining for biliary cytokeratins 7 and 19 of the catalogue of Moll.[66] Biliary epithelium that may be obscured by inflammatory cell infiltrates in chronic biliary disease, drug-related hepatitis or liver transplant rejection can thereby be identified (**see Figs. 5.24, 5.25**). Residual duct epithelium in segments of atretic ducts resected at the time of Kasai surgery for extrahepatic biliary atresia can also be demonstrated. Unusual patterns of the ductular reaction or remnants of the bile-duct plate (**see Fig. 13.5**) can be studied with cytokeratin stains. AE1/AE3 pooled antibody generally gives good staining results.

4 *Localisation of viral antigens.* For patients with hepatitis B virus infection, immunohistochemical demonstration of surface antigen is more sensitive than

Figure 17.12 Colourised scanning electron micrograph of liver.
Sinusoids (S) (light pink) course between the hepatic cords (green). The network of bile canaliculi (BC) is well demonstrated. Note the narrow space of Disse (spD) between the sinusoidal endothelial lining cells and the surfaces of hepatocytes. (Micrograph kindly provided by Jackie Lewin, UCL Medical School, London, UK.)

non-immunohistochemical methods such as orcein or Victoria blue. In addition, assessment of the distribution of core and surface antigens when correlated with serum markers of viral replication and biopsy features on light microscopy usually provides a more comprehensive perspective regarding viral liver disease in any given patient. In some patients, demonstration of hepatitis D antigen by immunohistochemistry is the first evidence of delta virus infection or recurrence. Attempts at immunohistochemical staining of hepatitis C virus antigens using commercially available reagents have met with mixed results, and other techniques such as *in situ* hybridisation[67] or polymerase chain reaction[68,69] may be more sensitive. This topic is also discussed in **Chapter 9**. Immunohistochemical staining for cytomegalovirus in post-transplantation liver biopsies is frequently required.[70]

Scientific questions of a more basic nature concerning the interaction of the immune system with the liver in various forms of injury, the composition of the extracellular matrix and factors involved in hepatocellular proliferation can be addressed with immunohisto-chemistry. For example, expression of intercellular adhesion molecules on the surfaces of hepatocytes for binding lymphocytes is of fundamental importance in interface hepatitis associated with chronic viral hepatitis[53] (**Fig. 17.13**). A histological index of liver-cell proliferation in acute and chronic liver disease can be obtained by staining for proliferat-ing cell nuclear antigen, an intranuclear auxiliary protein of DNA polymerase-α,[71-74] and other markers.

In situ hybridisation

In this technique, radioactively labelled probes for specific RNA or DNA sequences are applied to cryostat tissue sections. Biotinylated probes can also be used on formalin-fixed,

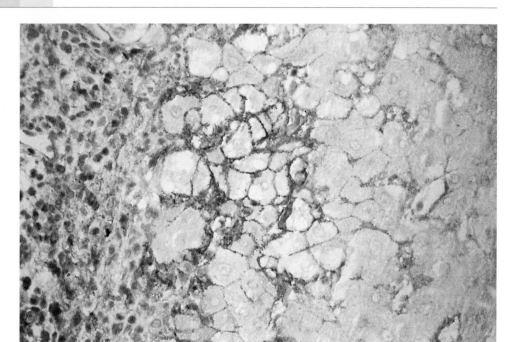

Figure 17.13 Intercellular adhesion molecule-1 (ICAM-1) expression on hepatocytes.
Brown immunoreaction product to ICAM-1 is seen on periportal hepatocyte membranes in a case of chronic hepatitis. An inflamed portal tract is seen at left. The section was stained with monoclonal antibody 84H10 directed against ICAM-1. (Illustration kindly provided by Drs V. J. Desmet, R. Volpes, J. Van den Oord and R. De Vos, Leuven, The Netherlands.)

paraffin-embedded sections.[75] Probes are prepared by cloning of genetic material and subcloning into plasmids. After preparation of the tissue sections, the probe is applied directly and hybridised. Slides treated with radiolabelled probes are then exposed to photographic emulsion for 1–2 weeks, resulting in a distribution of silver grains over cells containing the target RNA or DNA sequences. *In situ* hybridisation is widely used in research laboratories to localise gene sequences encoding hepatic secretory proteins such as albumin and extracellular matrix proteins. One of its major applications is in the identification of viral sequences, including cytomegalovirus,[75] hepatitis B virus and hepatitis C virus.[67] The sensitivity of *in situ* hybridisation can be improved by combination with **polymerase chain reaction**[76,77] (see below).

Flow cytometry of lymphocytes from liver biopsies

In order to immunotype lymphocytes present in liver biopsy specimens, fresh samples of liver tissue are treated with enzymatic digestion and gradient centrifugation.[78] This technique has been used to analyse lymphocyte subpopulations in various forms of liver disease, including chronic hepatitis, primary biliary cirrhosis and alcoholic liver disease.[79,80]

Confocal laser scanning microscopy

The confocal laser scanning microscope has been referred to as an 'opto-digital microtome'[81] because of its capacity to obtain two-dimensional images from very thin optical sections of tissues or cells and to process them into three-dimensional data with digitised computer software. The primary advantages of this form of microscopy are its high resolution and enhanced contrast. These two advantages are obtained by using a very thin plane of focus provided by a laser light source (usually argon ion) filtered through several dichroic mirrors. The light emanating from a focal point in the specimen is imaged by back projection onto a detector pinhole aperture; the emanating light and the imaged light are in common focus, hence the name 'confocal'.

Following specimen fixation (usually by an aldehyde agent), one or more fluorescent reagents are used to label the specific antigen(s) under investigation. A series of two-dimensional images in a thin focal plane of approximately 0.6–1.5 μm are obtained through the confocal laser scanning microscope. These images are then aligned pixel-by-pixel using specific software image processing in order to generate three-dimensional data. Elements to be considered in planning confocal microscopy include the wavelength of light which the laser source can provide for excitation of the fluorochrome, appropriate stability of the antigen in tissue after fixation, mounting medium used, and type(s) of fluorochrome to be utilised.[81] Dyes with widely separated excitation and emission wavelengths are optimal, such as fluorescein or acridine orange for simultaneous DNA and RNA staining.

This technique is versatile; one can examine protein traffic in cells, localisation of matrix proteins,[82] metabolites produced in chemical hepatotoxicity,[83] DNA of individual chromosomes and ploidy status of tumours. *In situ* hybridisation can also be performed.

Polymerase chain reaction

Polymerase chain reaction (PCR) is an *in vitro* method of nucleic acid synthesis by which small targeted segments of DNA (or RNA) can be amplified from biological samples. The ingredients for this method include two oligonucleotide primers that complement opposite ends of each strand in the target sequence, thermostable *Taq* DNA polymerase (or reverse transcriptase, in detecting RNA) and four deoxynucleotide triphosphates (dNTPs) in a buffered solution. The DNA strands are first separated by boiling. The oligonucleotide primers are then annealed to the target DNA, after which the primers are extended by *Taq* DNA polymerase. These extension products or daughter strands are complementary to and can bind the two primers, thereby allowing repeated cycles of denaturation and amplification and an exponential (2n) production of the target segment.[84–87]

Liver samples for PCR must be frozen in most instances.[88] However, extraction of nucleic acids from formalin-fixed, paraffin-embedded sections is also feasible, and can be used in the diagnosis of genetic mutations, for example in the *HFE* gene in hereditary haemochromatosis.[89]

Laser capture microdissection

This technique obtains well-defined target cell populations (including immunostained cells) from formalin-fixed, paraffin-embedded tissue sections for molecular analysis using PCR. A thermoplastic polymer coating attached to a rigid support is placed in contact with a tissue section and is bonded to microscopically selected cell clusters by a near-infrared laser pulse.[90] The selected cells are then subjected to PCR. Laser capture microdissection improves the sensitivity of detecting genetic alterations in archival tissue samples[91] and can be applied to diagnostic and research problems in hepatic pathology, such as detection of hepatitis C virus RNA sequences in liver biopsies.[92]

Gene array analysis

The recent elucidation of the human genome has resulted in a number of functional genomics techniques by which gene profiling in normal and disease states can be undertaken. The liver transcriptosome expresses some 25–40% of the 39,000 genes in the human genome.[93] Snap frozen liver tissue can be used for comparative studies utilising oligonucleotide gene chip arrays and other methods. The relevance of this technique to liver disease has been reviewed.[93] Appropriate control tissue is important.[94] Data are now available for a wide range of liver diseases, including gene signatures associated with fibrosis in recurrent chronic hepatitis C after transplantation,[95] chronic hepatitis C with dysplasia[96] and hepatocellular carcinoma.[97]

References

1 Burt AD, Le Bail B, Balabaud C, et al. Morphologic investigation of sinusoidal cells. *Semin Liver Dis* 1993; **13:** 21–38.

2 Rieder H, Meyer zum Büschenfelde K-H, Ramadori G. Functional spectrum of sinusoidal endothelial liver cells. Filtration, endocytosis, synthetic capacities and intercellular communication. *J Hepatol* 1992; **15:** 237–250.

3 Xiao J-C, Ruck P, Adam A, et al. Small epithelial cells in human liver cirrhosis exhibit features of hepatic stem-like cells: immunohistochemical, electron microscopic and immunoelectron microscopic findings. *Histopathology* 2003; **42:** 141–149.

4 Nagore N, Howe S, Boxer L, et al. Liver cell rosettes: structural differences in cholestasis and hepatitis. *Liver* 1989; **9:** 43–51.

5 Nagore N, Howe S, Scheuer PJ. The three-dimensional liver. In: Popper H, Schaffner F, eds. Progress in Liver Diseases, Vol. IX. Philadelphia, PA: WB Saunders, 1989: 1–10.

6 Ludwig J, Ritman EL, LaRusso NF, et al. Anatomy of the human biliary system studied by quantitative computer-aided three-dimensional imaging techniques. *Hepatology* 1998; **27:** 893–899.

7 Jones S, Chapman SK, Crocker PR, et al. Combined light and electron microscope in routine histopathology. *J Clin Pathol* 1982; **35:** 425–429.

8 Spycher MA. Electron microscopy: a method for the diagnosis of inherited metabolic storage diseases. Electron microscopy in diagnosis. *Pathol Res Pract* 1980; **167:** 118–135.

9 Ishak KG, Sharp HL. Metabolic errors and liver disease. In: MacSween RNM, Anthony PP, Scheuer PJ, et al., eds. Pathology of the Liver, 3rd edn. Edinburgh: Churchill Livingstone, 1994; Ch. 4: 123–218 .

10 Toker C, Trevino N. Hepatic ultrastructure in chronic idiopathic jaundice. *Arch Pathol* 1965; **80:** 453–460.

11 Miller SE. Detection and identification of viruses by electron microscopy. *J Electron Microsc Tech* 1986; **4:** 265–301.

12 Phillips MJ, Poucell S, Patterson J, et al. The Liver. An Atlas and Text of Ultrastructural Pathology. New York: Raven Press, 1987.

13 Phillips MJ, Glendis LM, Paucell S, et al. Syncytial giant-cell hepatitis. Sporadic hepatitis with distinctive pathologic features, a severe clinical course, and paramyxoviral features. *N Engl J Med* 1991; **324:** 455–460.

14 Fimmel CJ, Guo L, Compans RW, et al. A case of syncytial giant cell hepatitis with features of a paramyxoviral infection. *Am J Gastroenterol* 1998; **93:** 1931–1937.

15 Lazaro CA, Chang M, Tang W, et al. Hepatitis C virus replication in transfected and serum-infected cultured human fetal hepatocytes. *Am J Pathol* 2007; **170:** 478–489.

16 Lloreta-Trull J, Serrano S. The current role of electron microscopy in the diagnosis of epithelial and epithelioid tumors. *Semin Diagn Pathol* 2003; **20:** 46–59.

17 Pessayre D, Bichara M, Degott C, et al. Perhexiline maleate-induced cirrhosis. *Gastroenterology* 1979; **76:** 170–177.

18 Poucell S, Ireton J, Valencia-Mayoral P, et al. Amiodarone-associated phospholipidosis and fibrosis of the liver. Light, immunohistochemical, and electron microscopic studies. *Gastroenterology* 1984; **86:** 926–936.

19 Simon JB, Manley PN, Brien JF, et al. Amiodarone hepatotoxicity simulating alcoholic liver disease. *N Engl J Med* 1984; **311:** 167–172.

20 Pirovino M, Müller O, Zysset T, et al. Amiodarone-induced hepatic phospholipidosis: correlation of morphological and biochemical findings in an animal model. *Hepatology* 1988; **8:** 591–598.

21 Lewis JH, Ranard RC, Caruso A, et al. Amiodarone hepatotoxicity: prevalence and clinicopathologic correlations among 104 patients. *Hepatology* 1989; **9:** 679–685.

22 Rohr HP, Lüthy J, Gudat F, et al. Stereology: a new supplement to the study of human liver biopsy specimens. In: Popper H, Schaffner F, eds. Progress in Liver Diseases, Vol. V. New York: Grune & Stratton, 1976: 24–34.

23 Uchida T, Kronborg I, Peters RL. Alcoholic hyalin-containing hepatocytes – a characteristic morphologic appearance. *Liver* 1984; **4:** 233–243.

24 Caldwell SH, de Freitas AR, Park SH, et al. Intramitochondrial crystalline inclusions in nonalcoholic steatohepatitis. *Hepatology* 2009; **49:** 1888–1895.

25 Chedid A, Jao W, Port J. Megamitochondria in hepatic and renal disease. *Am J Gastroenterol* 1980; **73**: 319–324.

26 Foschini MP, Macchia S, Losi L, et al. Identification of mitochondria in liver biopsies. A study by immunohistochemistry, immunogold and Western blot analysis. *Virchows Arch* 1998; **433**: 267–273.

27 Feldmann G, Maurice M, Husson JM, et al. Hepatocyte giant mitochondria: an almost constant lesion in systemic scleroderma. *Virchows Arch [A]* 1977; **374**: 215–227.

28 Sternlieb I. Evolution of the hepatic lesion in Wilson's disease (hepatolenticular degeneration). In: Popper H, Schaffner F, eds. Progress in Liver Diseases, Vol. IV. New York: Grune & Stratton, 1972; Ch. 29: 511–525.

29 Scheinberg IH, Sternlieb I. Wilson's disease. Major Problems in Internal Medicine XXIII. Philadelphia, PA: WB Saunders, 1984.

30 Sternlieb I. Fraternal concordance of types of abnormal hepatocellular mitochondria in Wilson's disease. *Hepatology* 1992; **16**: 728–732.

31 Tonsgard JH. Effect of Reye's syndrome serum on the ultrastructure of isolated liver mitochondria. *Lab Invest* 1989; **60**: 568–573.

32 Lichtenstein GR, Kaiser LR, Tuchman M, et al. Fatal hyperammonemia following orthotopic lung transplantation. *Gastroenterology* 1997; **112**: 236–240.

33 Iancu TC, Deugnier Y, Halliday JW, et al. Ultrastructural sequences during liver iron overload in genetic hemochromatosis. *J Hepatol* 1997; **27**: 628–638.

34 Mooi WJ, Dingemans KP, Van Den Bergh Weerman MA, et al. Ultrastructure of the liver in cerebrohepatorenal syndrome of Zellweger. *Ultrastruct Pathol* 1983; **5**: 135–144.

35 De Craemer D, Kerckaert I, Roels F. Hepatocellular peroxisomes in human alcoholic and drug-induced hepatitis: a quantitative study. *Hepatology* 1991; **14**: 811–817.

36 Sternlieb I, Quintana N. The peroxisomes of human hepatocytes. *Lab Invest* 1977; **36**: 140–149.

37 De Craemer D, Pauwels M, Roels F. Peroxisomes in cirrhosis of the human liver: a cytochemical, ultrastructural and quantitative study. *Hepatology* 1993; **17**: 404–410.

38 Arias IM, Che M, Gatmaitan Z, et al. The biology of the bile canaliculus, 1993. *Hepatology* 1993; **17**: 318–329.

39 Cutrin JC, Cantino D, Biasi F, et al. Reperfusion damage to the bile canaliculi in transplanted human liver. *Hepatology* 1996; **24**: 1053–1057.

40 Bull LN, Carolton VEH, Stricker NL, et al. Genetic and morphological findings in progressive familial intrahepatic cholestasis (Byler disease [PFIC-1] and Byler syndrome): evidence for heterogeneity. *Hepatology* 1997; **26**: 155–164.

41 Horn T, Lyon H, Christoffersen P. The blood hepatocytic barrier: a light microscopical, transmission and scanning electron microscopic study. *Liver* 1986; **6**: 233–245.

42 Braet F, Riches J, Geerts W, et al. Three-dimensional organization of fenestrae labyrinths in liver sinusoidal endothelial cells. *Liver Int* 2009; **29**: 603–613.

43 Bardadin KA, Scheuer PJ. Endothelial cell changes in acute hepatitis. A light and electron microscopic study. *J Pathol* 1984; **144**: 213–220.

44 Schaff Z, Hoofnagle JH, Grimley PM. Hepatic inclusions during interferon therapy in chronic viral hepatitis. *Hepatology* 1986; **6**: 966–970.

45 Luu J, Bockus D, Remington F, et al. Tubuloreticular structures and cylindrical confronting cisternae: a review. *Hum Pathol* 1989; **20**: 617–627.

46 Iwamura S, Enzan H, Saibara T, et al. Appearance of sinusoidal inclusion-containing endothelial cells in liver disease. *Hepatology* 1994; **20**: 604–610.

47 Friedman SL. The cellular basis of hepatic fibrosis. *N Engl J Med* 1993; **328**: 1828–1835.

48 Cameron RG, Neuman MG, Shear N, et al. Multivesicular stellate cells in primary biliary cirrhosis. *Hepatology* 1997; **26**: 819–822.

49 Luo D, Vanderkerken K, Bouwens L, et al. The number and distribution of hepatic natural killer cells (pit cells) in normal rat liver: an immunohistochemical study. *Hepatology* 1995; **21**: 1690–1694.

50 Bouwens L, Wisse E. Pit cells in the liver. *Liver* 1992; **12**: 3–9.

51 De Vos R, De Wolf-Peeters C, van den Oord JJ, et al. A recommended procedure for ultrastructural immunohistochemistry on small human tissue samples. *J Histochem Cytochem* 1985; **33**: 959–964.

52 Elia JM. Immunohistopathology. A Practical Approach to Diagnosis. Chicago, IL: ASCP Press, 1990.

53 Volpes R, van den Oord JJ, Desmet VJ. Can hepatocytes serve as 'activated' immunomodulating cells in the immune response? *J Hepatol* 1992; **16**: 228–240.

54 Horiike N, Onji M, Kumon I, et al. Intercellular adhesion molecule-1 expression on the hepatocyte membrane of patients with chronic hepatitis B and C. *Liver* 1993; **13**: 10–14.

55 Volpes R, van den Oord JJ, De Vos R, et al. Expression of interferon-gamma receptor in normal and pathological human liver tissue. *J Hepatol* 1991; **12**: 195–202.

56 Volpes R, van den Oord JJ, De Vos R, et al. Hepatic expression of type A and type B receptors for tumor necrosis factor. *J Hepatol* 1992; **14**: 361–369.

57 Vonnahme F-J. The Human Liver. A Scanning Electron Microscopic Atlas. Basel and Freiburg: Karger, 1993.

58 Ishak KG. Applications of scanning electron microscopy to the study of liver disease. In: Popper H, Schaffner F, eds. Progress in Liver Diseases, Vol. VIII. Orlando, FL: Grune & Stratton, 1986: 1–32.

59 Petersen C, Grasshoff S, Luciano L. Diverse morphology of biliary atresia in an animal model. *J Hepatol* 1998; **28**: 603–607.

60 Haratake J, Hisaoka M, Furuta A, et al. A scanning electron microscopic study of postnatal development of rat peribiliary plexus. *Hepatology* 1991; **14**: 1196–1200.

61 Haratake J, Hisaoka M, Yamamoto O, et al. Morphological changes of hepatic microcirculation in experimental rat cirrhosis: a scanning electron microscopic study. *Hepatology* 1991; **13**: 952–956.

62 Gaudio E, Pannarale L, Onori P, et al. A scanning electron microscopic study of liver microcirculation disarrangement in experimental rat cirrhosis. *Hepatology* 1993; **17**: 477–485.

63 Terada T, Ishida F, Nakanuma Y. Vascular plexus around intrahepatic bile ducts in normal livers and portal hypertension. *J Hepatol* 1989; **8**: 139–149.

64 Taylor CR, Cote RJ. Immunomicroscopy: a Diagnostic Tool for the Surgical Pathologist (Major Problems in Pathology, Vol. 19). Philadelphia, PA: WB Saunders, 1994.

65 Wang NP, Zee S, Zarbo RJ, et al. Coordinate expression of cytokeratins 7 and 20 defines unique subsets of carcinomas. *Appl Immunohistochem* 1995; **3**: 99–107.

66 Moll R, Franke WW, Schiller D, et al. The catalog of human cytokeratins: pattern of expression in normal epithelia, tumors and cultured cells. *Cell* 1982; **31**: 11–24.

67 Felger RE, Montone KT, Furth EE. A rapid method for the detection of hepatitis C virus RNA by *in situ* hybridization. *Mod Pathol* 1996; **9**: 696–702.

68 Park YN, Abe K, Li H, et al. Detection of hepatitis C virus RNA using ligation-dependent polymerase chain reaction in formalin-fixed, paraffin-embedded liver tissues. *Am J Pathol* 1996; **149**: 1485–1491.

69 Lau GKK, Davis GL, Wu SPC, et al. Hepatic expression of hepatitis C virus RNA in chronic hepatitis C: a study by *in situ* reverse-transcription polymerase chain reaction. *Hepatology* 1996; **23**: 1318–1323.

70 Theise ND, Conn M, Thung SN. Localization of cytomegalovirus antigens in liver allografts over time. *Hum Pathol* 1993; **24**: 103–108.

71 Wolf HK, Michalopoulos GK. Hepatocyte regeneration in acute fulminant and nonfulminant hepatitis: a study of proliferating cell nuclear antigen expression. *Hepatology* 1992; **15**: 707–713.

72 Kayano K, Yasunaga M, Kubota M, et al. Detection of proliferating hepatocytes by immunohistochemical staining for proliferating cell nuclear antigen (PCNA) in patients with acute hepatic failure. *Liver* 1992; **12**: 132–136.

73 Kawakita N, Seki S, Sakaguchi H, et al. Analysis of proliferating hepatocytes using a monoclonal antibody against proliferating cell nuclear antigen/cyclin in embedded tissues from various liver diseases fixed in formaldehyde. *Am J Pathol* 1992; **140**: 513–520.

74 Siitonen SM, Kallioniemi O-P, Isola JJ. Proliferating cell nuclear antigen immunohistochemistry using monoclonal antibody 19A2 and a new antigen retrieval technique has prognostic impact in archival paraffin-embedded node-negative breast cancer. *Am J Pathol* 1993; **142**: 1081–1089.

75 Naoumov NV, Alexander GJM, O'Grady JG, et al. Rapid diagnosis of cytomegalovirus infection by in-situ hybridisation in liver grafts. *Lancet* 1988; **1**: 1361–1364.

76 Nuovo GJ, Lidonnici K, MacConnell P, et al. Intracellular localization of polymerase chain reaction (PCR)-amplified hepatitis C cDNA. *Am J Surg Pathol* 1993; **17**: 683–690.

77 Komminoth P, Long AA, Ray R, et al. *In situ* polymerase chain reaction detection of viral DNA, single-copy genes, and gene rearrangements in cell suspensions and cytospins. *Diagn Mol Pathol* 1992; **1**: 85–97.

78 Hata K, Zhang XR, Iwatsuki S, et al. Isolation, phenotyping and functional analysis of lymphocytes from human liver. *Clin Immunol Immunopathol* 1990; **56**: 401–419.

79 Hata K, Van Thiel DH, Herberman RB, et al. Phenotypic and functional characteristics of lymphocytes isolated from liver biopsy specimens from patients with active liver disease. *Hepatology* 1992; **15**: 816–823.

80 Li X, Jeffers LJ, Reddy KR, et al. Immunophenotyping of lymphocytes in liver tissue of patients with chronic liver diseases by flow cytometry. *Hepatology* 1991; **14**: 121–127.

81 Neri LM, Martelli AM, Previati M, et al. From two dimensional (2D) to three dimensional (3D) analysis by confocal microscopy. *Liver* 1992; **12**: 268–279.

82 Vassy J, Rigaut JP, Briane D, et al. Confocal microscopy immunofluorescence localization of desmin and other intermediate filament proteins in fetal rat livers. *Hepatology* 1993; **17**: 293–300.

83 Pompella A, Comporti M. Imaging of oxidative stress at subcellular level by confocal laser scanning microscopy after fluorescent derivatization of cellular carbonyls. *Am J Pathol* 1993; **142**: 1353–1357.

84 Berk PD, Worman HJ. An introduction to molecular biology and recombinant DNA technology for the hepatologist. *Semin Liver Dis* 1992; **12**: 227–245.

85 Rose EA. Applications of the polymerase chain reaction to genome analysis. *FASEB J* 1991; **5**: 46–54.

86 Mullis KB. The unusual origin of the polymerase chain reaction. *Sci Am* 1990; **262**: 56–65.

87 Eisenstein BI. The polymerase chain reaction. A new method of using molecular genetics for medical diagnosis. *N Engl J Med* 1990; **322**: 178–183.

88 Shieh YSC, Shim K-S, Lampertico P, et al. Detection of hepatitis C virus sequences in liver tissue by the polymerase chain reaction. *Lab Invest* 1991; **65**: 408–411.

89 Press RD, Flora K, Gross C, et al. Hepatic iron overload. Direct HFE (HLA-H) mutation analysis vs. quantitative iron assays for the diagnosis of hereditary hemochromatosis. *Am J Clin Pathol* 1998; **109**: 577–584.

90 Suarez-Quian CA, Goldstein SR, Pohida T, et al. Laser capture microdissection of single cells from complex tissues. *Biotechniques* 1999; **26**: 328–335.

91 Giercksky HE, Thorstensen L, Qvist H, et al. Comparison of genetic changes in frozen biopsies and microdissected archival material from the same colorectal liver metastases. *Diagn Mol Pathol* 1997; **6**: 318–325.

92 Saito K, Sullivan D, Haruna Y, et al. Detection of hepatitis C virus RNA sequences in hepatocellular carcinoma and its precursors by microdissection polymerase chain reaction. *Arch Pathol Lab Med* 1997; **121**: 400–403.

93 Shackel NA, Gorrell MD, McCaughan GW. Gene array analysis and the liver. *Hepatology* 2002; **36**: 1313–1325.

94 Asselah T, Bieche I, Laurendeau I, et al. Significant gene expression differences in histologically 'normal' liver biopsies: implications for control tissue. *Hepatology* 2008; **48**: 953–962.

95 Smith MW, Walters K-A, Korth MJ, et al. Gene expression patterns that correlate with hepatitis C and early progression to fibrosis in liver transplant patients. *Gastroenterology* 2006; **130**: 179–187.

96 Wurmbach E, Chen Y, Khitrov G, et al. Genome-wide molecular profiles of HCV-induced dysplasia and hepatocellular carcinoma. *Hepatology* 2007; **45**: 938–947.

97 Hoshida Y, Villanueva A, Kobayashi M, et al. Gene expression in fixed tissues and outcome in hepatocellular carcinoma. *N Engl J Med* 2008; **359**: 1995–2004.

General reading

Berk PD, Worman HJ. An introduction to molecular biology and recombinant DNA technology for the hepatologist. *Semin Liv Dis* 1992; **12:** 227–245.

Ghadially FN. Ultrastructural Pathology of the Cell and Matrix. 3rd edn. London: Butterworths, 1988.

Phillips MJ, Poucell S, Patterson J, Valencia P. The Liver. An Atlas and Text of Ultrastructural Pathology. New York: Raven Press, 1987.

Shackel NA, Gorrell MD, McCaughan GW. Gene array analysis and the liver. *Hepatology* 2002; **36:** 1313–1325.

Smedsrod B, Le Couteur D, Ikejima K, et al. Hepatic sinusoidal cells in health and disease: update from the 14th International Symposium. *Liver Int* 2009; **29:** 490–499.

Taylor CR, Cote RJ. Immunomicroscopy: a Diagnostic Tool for the Surgical Pathologist (Major Problems in Pathology, Vol. 19), 2nd edn. Philadelphia, PA: WB Saunders, 1994.

Vonnahme F-J. The Human Liver. A Scanning Electron Microscopic Atlas. Basel and Freiburg: Karger, 1993.

Watson JD, Gilman M, Witkowski J, Zoller M. Recombinant DNA, 2nd edn. New York: Scientific American Books, 1992.

Glossary

Note: Words in *italics* are defined elsewhere in the glossary.

Acidophil body (Figs 6.2 and 16.15) A *hepatocyte* which has undergone apoptosis; now often referred to as an apoptotic body. See also *Councilman bodies*.

Acinus (Fig. 3.1) An anatomical unit based on blood supply, its three parenchymal zones containing successively less oxygenated blood. Zone 1 is nearest to the terminal portal vessels in a small portal tract.

Activity (Figs 9.7, 9.8) In histological terms, an expression of the degree of hepatocellular damage and associated inflammation. Especially used in chronic hepatitis and cirrhosis, in which it forms the basis of *grading*.

Apoptosis (Figs 6.2 and 16.15) Shrinkage and fragmentation of cells, seen in the liver mainly in the form of densely-stained rounded structures derived from hepatocytes but lying free outside the liver-cell plates.

Autoimmune hepatitis A form of hepatitis associated with high titres of autoantibodies in serum. Usually responds to immunosuppressive therapy.

Ballooning degeneration Swelling and rounding of hepatocytes, with loss of their normal polygonal shape. Different forms of ballooning are seen in viral hepatitis (Fig. 6.2) and steatohepatitis (Fig. 7.8C).

Bile canaliculus (Figs 1.8D and 5.2) The tubular space formed between the biliary poles of two or three *hepatocytes*, or more in diseased liver. The canaliculus has no separate epithelial lining of its own.

Bile duct (Fig. 3.2) The smallest ducts, the interlobular bile ducts, are centrally located in small portal tracts and are usually accompanied by blood vessels. In practice they are sometimes difficult to distinguish from *bile ductules*, the transition being gradual.

Bile ductule and canal of Hering (Fig. 3.3) At the portal–parenchymal interface the canalicular system drains into the *canals of Hering* which are partly lined by hepatocytes and partly by biliary epithelial cells (*cholangiocytes*). These in turn connect with bile ductules, fully lined by biliary epithelium.

Bile extravasate (Fig. 5.9) Leakage of bile from a duct into the connective tissue of the portal tract, occasionally seen in large bile-duct obstruction.

Bile infarct (Fig. 5.4) An area of liver-cell death in a cholestatic liver; often periportal whereas canalicular cholestasis is mainly perivenular. Bile staining is variable and may be absent. Bile infarcts are easily mistaken for accumulations of foamy macrophages.

Bile lake An accumulation of bile outside a liver-cell plate.

Bile thrombus (Fig. 5.2) Synonymous with bile plug: the accumulation of visible bile in a *bile canaliculus*.

Bilirubinostasis A term sometimes used for histological cholestasis.

Bridging fibrosis (Fig. 7.17) Linking of portal tracts and/or efferent venules by fibrous tissue.

Bridging necrosis (Fig. 6.8) Confluent hepatocellular necrosis and *collapse* linking vascular structures; usually and preferably confined to linking of portal tracts to efferent venules.

Canals of Hering (Fig. 3.3) Structures lined partly by *hepatocytes* and partly by bile ductular epithelium. They are a probable site of progenitor cells.

Central perivenulitis (Fig. 16.19) A feature of liver transplant rejection in which efferent venules are targeted by lymphocytes and other effector immune cells. Dropout and *apoptosis* of perivenular *hepatocytes* and focal congestion are also frequently present. This common manifestation of pediatric allograft rejection is sometimes present in combination with classical portal tract rejection changes and occasionally is seen late (>1 yr after transplantation) as the isolated expression of rejection.

DOI: 10.1016/B978-0-7020-3410-7.00024-1

Ceroid pigment (Fig. 6.4) Brown pigment in macrophages, found after hepatocellular injury; rich in oxidised lipids and PAS-positive after diastase digestion. Distinct from *lipofuscin*.

Cholangiocyte Epithelial cell of the biliary tract.

Cholate stasis (Fig. 5.10) A term sometimes used for chronic cholestasis, on the assumption that the hepatocellular changes result from the accumulation of toxic bile salts. Also known as *precholestasis* or *pseudoxanthomatous change*.

Cholestasis (Fig. 5.2) In morphological terms, *bilirubinostasis* or visible bile in a section of liver. Also defined as failure of bile to reach the duodenum and biochemically as a type of jaundice with dark urine, pale stools, conjugated hyperbilirubinaemia and raised serum alkaline phosphatase level.

Cirrhosis The transformation of the normal hepatic architecture into nodules separated by *fibrosis*.

Collapse (Fig. 4.2) Condensation of pre-existing reticulin framework as a result of necrosis. May be followed by *fibrosis*.

Confluent necrosis (Fig. 8.4) Death of groups of adjacent *hepatocytes*.

Councilman bodies *Hepatocytes* which have undergone *apoptosis*. The term is best restricted to yellow fever, the disease in which they were described by Dr Councilman.

Disse space (Fig. 17.4) The space between the sinusoidal endothelium and *hepatocytes*; contents include extracellular matrix and *hepatic stellate cells*.

Ductopenia (Figs 13.6 and 16.9) Loss of significant numbers of interlobular *bile ducts*. Causes include rejection of liver grafts, graft-versus-host disease, primary biliary cirrhosis, primary sclerosing cholangitis and drug injury. Diseases characterised by ductopenia are known as *vanishing bile duct syndromes*.

Ductular proliferation Use of this term is discouraged for the reason given in the next definition.

Ductular reaction (Figs 1.8B and 4.6) A reaction of ductular phenotype, seen as an increase in ductular structures. This may be the result of proliferation of pre-existing ductules, but the new structures could also arise from biliary metaplasia of *hepatocytes* or from transformation of *progenitor cells*.

Dysmetabolic hepatic iron overload (DHIO) (Fig. 7.7) *Siderosis* of *Kupffer cells* and/or *hepatocytes* due to insulin resistance and its effects on iron homeostasis. Most often evident histologically as iron overload in the setting of macrovesicular *steatosis* in non-alcoholic fatty liver disease.

Dysplasia (Figs 10.8, 10.9) A change in the size, nucleus : cytoplasm ratio and/or nuclear appearances of *hepatocytes*, usually in chronic hepatitis and *cirrhosis*. Large-cell and small-cell types are described. Also known as large- and small-cell change.

Fat-storing cells *Hepatic stellate cells*.

Fatty liver disease Includes both *steatosis* and *steatohepatitis*, as in alcoholic fatty liver disease (AFLD) and non-alcoholic fatty liver disease (NAFLD).

Feathery degeneration (Fig. 5.3) A type of liver-cell injury in *cholestasis*, attributed to toxic effects of bile salts. Affected *hepatocytes*, often single cells lying within normal *parenchyma*, are swollen and have pale-staining feathery cytoplasm.

Fibrosis Formation of new collagen fibres. It may follow *collapse* of pre-existing connective tissue framework or arise *de novo*.

Focal necrosis (Fig. 9.8) Death of *hepatocytes*, singly or in small groups. Because of the rapid disappearance of the dead cells, focal necrosis is usually recognised by the presence of inflammatory cells and by a break in continuity of a *liver-cell plate* rather than by the presence of necrotic tissue.

Follicle See *lymphoid follicle*.

Glycogen vacuolation See *nuclear vacuolation*.

Grading Semi-quantitative scoring of the various processes comprising hepatocellular damage and inflammation, usually in chronic hepatitis. Numerical assessment of histological activity.

Granuloma (Fig. 15.1) A focal accumulation of epithelioid cells, which are modified macrophages with abundant cytoplasm and often curved, elongated nuclei. To be distinguished from simple accumulations of macrophages.

Ground-glass hepatocytes (Fig. 9.13) *Hepatocytes* with a well-defined, lightly eosinophilic homogeneous area occupying much of the cytoplasm. The commonest form is seen in the livers of patients infected with the hepatitis B virus.

Haemochromatosis (See also *siderosis*) A condition in which hepatic *fibrosis* and *cirrhosis* ultimately develop as a result of iron overload. The common form, hereditary haemochromatosis, is usually the result of mutations of the *HFE* gene on chromosome 6.

Hepatic stellate cells (Figs 7.6 and 17.4) Cells containing vacuoles rich in vitamin A, lying within the *Disse space*. In pathological conditions, they are able to transform into myofibroblasts and produce extracellular matrix components. Previously used synonyms include *fat-storing cells*, *Ito cells*, *lipocytes*, *parasinusoidal cells* and *perisinusoidal cells*.

Hepatocytes Liver cells.

Interface hepatitis (Figs 9.3, 9.4) Death of *hepatocytes* at the interface of connective tissue and *parenchyma* in chronic liver disease, accompanied by inflammatory-cell infiltration. Characteristic of chronic hepatitis and synonymous with the older term *piecemeal necrosis*.

Ito cells *Hepatic stellate cells*.

Kupffer cells The resident macrophages of the liver, straddling the sinusoidal lumens.

Limiting plate The layer of *hepatocytes* next to a portal tract.

Lipocytes *Hepatic stellate cells*.

Lipofuscin (Fig. 3.6) Pigmented granular material in *hepatocytes*, of lysosomal origin and most abundant at the biliary poles of the cells. Found in normal liver in greatly varying amounts.

Liver-cell plates (Fig. 3.5) Interconnecting walls of *hepatocytes*, one-cell thick in adults. Thicker plates are found in children and in regenerating liver.

Lobular activity (Fig. 9.8) Inflammation and hepatocellular damage deep within the lobules, in contrast to *interface hepatitis*.

Lobule (Fig. 3.1) An anatomical unit with an efferent (centrilobular) vein at its centre and portal tracts peripherally.

Lupoid hepatitis An old term for *autoimmune hepatitis*, no longer in use.

Lymphoid follicle (Figs 9.16 and 9.17) A structured accumulation of lymphocytes resembling the follicles of normal lymph nodes.

Mallory bodies (Figs 7.15 and 17.9) Irregular, dense cytoplasmic inclusions with a cytokeratin component, often in the form of strands or garlands. Electron microscopy reveals a filamentous structure.

Massive necrosis (Figs 4.6D and 6.11) *Multilobular necrosis* involving a substantial part of the whole liver. This usually leads to severe liver insufficiency.

Metabolic syndrome The association of insulin resistance with central (truncal) obesity, diabetes mellitus, hyperlipidaemia and systemic arterial hypertension. Non-alcoholic fatty liver disease (NAFLD) is considered the hepatic expression of the metabolic syndrome.

Multilobular necrosis (Figs 4.6D and 6.11) Confluent necrosis involving the whole of several adjacent lobules. The clinical effects are variable, depending on the extent of the lesion.

Non-alcoholic steatohepatitis (NASH) (Fig. 7.18) A form of hepatitis resembling alcoholic *steatohepatitis* but associated with other causes such as obesity, diabetes or drugs.

Nuclear vacuolation (Fig. 7.10) Empty *hepatocyte* nuclei in paraffin sections. May be due to glycogen accumulation, lipid, or invagination of cytoplasm. Glycogen nuclei, common in the young, the obese and the diabetic, are typically enlarged and have prominent nuclear membranes. The glycogen may be demonstrable histochemically but is often lost during processing.

Panacinar necrosis (Fig. 6.11) *Necrosis of an entire acinus*.

Panlobular necrosis (Fig. 6.11) *Necrosis of an entire lobule*.

Parasinusoidal cells *Hepatic stellate cells*.

Parenchyma The specialised tissue of the liver, as opposed to the connective tissue. Often used loosely to describe the contents of the *lobules* as opposed to the portal tracts.

Periportal The part of the hepatic *lobule* or *acinus* next to a small portal tract.

Perisinusoidal cells *Hepatic stellate cells*.

Piecemeal necrosis *Interface hepatitis* is now often used for this process, because it almost certainly involves *apoptosis* rather than, or as well as, *necrosis*.

Polyploidy (Fig. 3.9) The coexistence of different classes of nuclei containing multiple sets of chromosomes (e.g. quadriploid, octaploid); a normal state in adult human liver.

Portal triad (Fig. 3.2) The triad of artery, vein and *bile duct* present in most portal tracts.

Precholestasis (Fig. 5.10) See *cholate stasis*.

Progenitor cell A partly committed cell capable of producing a range of specialised cell types. In the liver, progenitor cells are probably located in *bile ductules* or *canals of Hering*. See also *stem cell*.

Pseudoacini *Rosettes*.

Pseudoxanthomatous change (Fig. 5.10) See *cholate stasis*.

Regeneration (Fig. 10.6) Loosely used to describe hepatocellular hyperplasia following injury or loss. Not easily recognised in conventional sections because of low mitotic rate; characterised by increase in the thickness of the cell plates.

Rosettes (Figs 4.4, 9.9 and 9.18) In liver pathology this term refers to a change of the normal plate pattern of *hepatocytes* to glandular structures formed by several *hepatocytes*. Different types of rosette formation are seen in *cholestasis* and in chronic hepatitis.

Septa (Figs 10.15 and 10.16) Walls of fibrous tissue, seen in two-dimensional sections as lines or bands. Septa may be formed by *collapse* ('passive septa'), by new fibre formation ('active septa') or by both.

Siderosis The presence of stainable iron in any component of liver tissue. The many causes of siderosis include several diseases under the heading of *haemochromatosis*, in which progressive iron accumulation leads to *fibrosis* and *cirrhosis*. However, at an early stage of hereditary *haemochromatosis* there is iron deposition without *fibrosis*.

Sinusoidal obstruction syndrome (Fig. 16.21) Circulatory obstruction within hepatic sinusoids and efferent venules following endothelial damage due to myeloablative chemotherapy or exposure to toxins such as pyrrolizine alkaloids.

The term is often used as an alternative to veno-occlusive disease.

Spotty necrosis Widespread, but patchy hepatocellular *necrosis*, typical of acute hepatitis.

Staging The semi-quantitative assessment of structural changes including *fibrosis* and *cirrhosis*.

Steatohepatitis (Fig. 7.12) A form of hepatitis characterised by *steatosis*, hepatocellular *ballooning, Mallory bodies* and pericellular *fibrosis*.

Steatosis (Figs 7.1, 7.2) The accumulation of excess lipid in *hepatocytes*

Stellate cells See *hepatic stellate cells*.

Stem cell A self-renewing cell with the potential to give rise to a variety of cells including *progenitor cells*.

Vanishing bile duct syndromes Disorders characterised by loss of *bile ducts* leading to *ductopenia* (paucity of ducts) with consequent *cholestasis*.

Index

Bold numbers denote **main entries**

Abscess 55
Aceruloplasminaemia 282, 287
Acetaminophen (paracetamol) 370
Acidophil body *see* Apoptotic body
Acidophilic change of hepatocytes 76
Acinus 9, **17–18**
  definition 384
Acquired immune deficiency syndrome
      (AIDS) 301
  cholangiopathy 302, **303**
  hepatobiliary lesions 301–302
  opportunistic infections and
      infestations **302–303**
Activity 183, 192, 196, 205, 208, 260,
      266, 307–308, 337, 340, 347,
      364, 367, 369
  definition 384
Acute fatty liver of pregnancy 97
Adaptive changes, drug-induced 117
Adenofibroma biliary 187
Adenoma
  bile-duct 181–184, **186–187**, 194,
      197–200, 206, 210–212, 214,
      249–254, 256–257, 259, 266,
      268
  liver-cell **181–183**, 185–186,
      189–191, 195, 202–203, 206,
      211, 214, 241, 250–251, 260,
      263, 265–266
    cytopathology 231
Adenomatosis 181, 183
Adenovirus 75
Adhesion molecules 19, 22
Ageing **14–25**
AIDS (acquired immune deficiency
      syndrome) 57, 118
  cholangiopathy 57
  hepatobiliary lesions 301–302
  opportunistic infections and
      infestations **302–303**
Ajmaline 127
Alagille's syndrome 8–9, 40
Alcohol aversion therapy 237–238,
      244, 351
Alcoholic cardiomyopathy 244, 282
Alcoholic fatty liver disease (AFLD)
      367, 384
Alcohol-related liver disease 9, **98–106**
  cardiomyopathy 111
  chronic hepatitis and 317, 320, 353
  cirrhosis 111
  fatty liver 93, 98
  fetal alcohol syndrome 111
  fibrosis 110
  foamy degeneration 97, 110
  hepatocellular carcinoma 111
  pancreatitis and 110
  perivenular fibrosis 105
  portal fibrosis 110
  siderosis 98
  steatohepatitis **99–106**
  venous occlusion 111
Algorithmic approach to cholestasis 37
Allopurinol 116, 127
Alper's disease 269
Alphafetoprotein 195, 197, 203, 208, 374
Alphamethyldopa 223
Aluminium 45
Amiodarone 107, 116, 118, 123
Ammonia metabolism 9
Amoebiasis 310
Amoxycillin 64, 116, 127
Amyloid amyloidosis 205, 233, 302,
      304, 315, 317–319, 334
Amylopectinosis 260
Anabolic steroids 185
Angiomyelolipoma 188
Angiomyolipoma 188–189, 197
Angiosarcoma 116
  cytopathology 231
Antibody-mediated graft rejection 335
α_1-Antichymotrypsin 195, 263
Anti-convulsant drugs 185, 206
Antimitochondrial antibodies (AMA)
      61, 70, 98, 147
α_1-Antitrypsin 9, 13
  deficiency 12, 40, 150
Apoptosis 31, 44, 48
  definition 384
  in normal liver 22, 44

Apoptotic body **75–78**, 98
Arsenic 118, 123
Artefacts 5–6
Arteries 181, 183, 191, 233, 237, 254,
      307, 317, 341, 343–344
  relation to bile duct numbers 341
Arteriohepatic dysplasia 254
Arteriopathy in liver transplantation
      360
Arteritis
  giant-cell 233, 249, 251, 268, 287,
      298–299, 304, 317
  necrotising 295–296, 305, 307, 315,
      317
Arthropods 314
Ascariasis 314
Atresia, biliary 249–254, 374
Augmentin 127
Autoantibodies 349, 352
  in autoimmune hepatitis 147, 150
  in non-alcoholic fatty liver disease 98
Autoimmune cholangitis **70**
Autoimmune hepatitis **147–150**
  acute onset 88, 148–149
  definition 384
  drug-related 120, 122
  histological features **147–149**
  after liver transplantation 70
  perivenular necrosis 149
  plasma cells 147, 149
  primary sclerosing cholangitis and
      59, 69–70, 147
  overlap syndromes 69–70
Autoimmune pancreatitis 61
Azathioprine 344, 353

Bacillary peliosis 238, 302–304
Bacterial diseases 238
Ballooning degeneration 76, 104
  definition 76
Banff scoring system for acute
      rejection 340
Barbiturates 43
Bartonella henselae 302–303, 305
BCG 305
Behçet's disease 185, 241

©2010 Elsevier Ltd
DOI: 10.1016/B978-0-7020-3410-7.00025-3